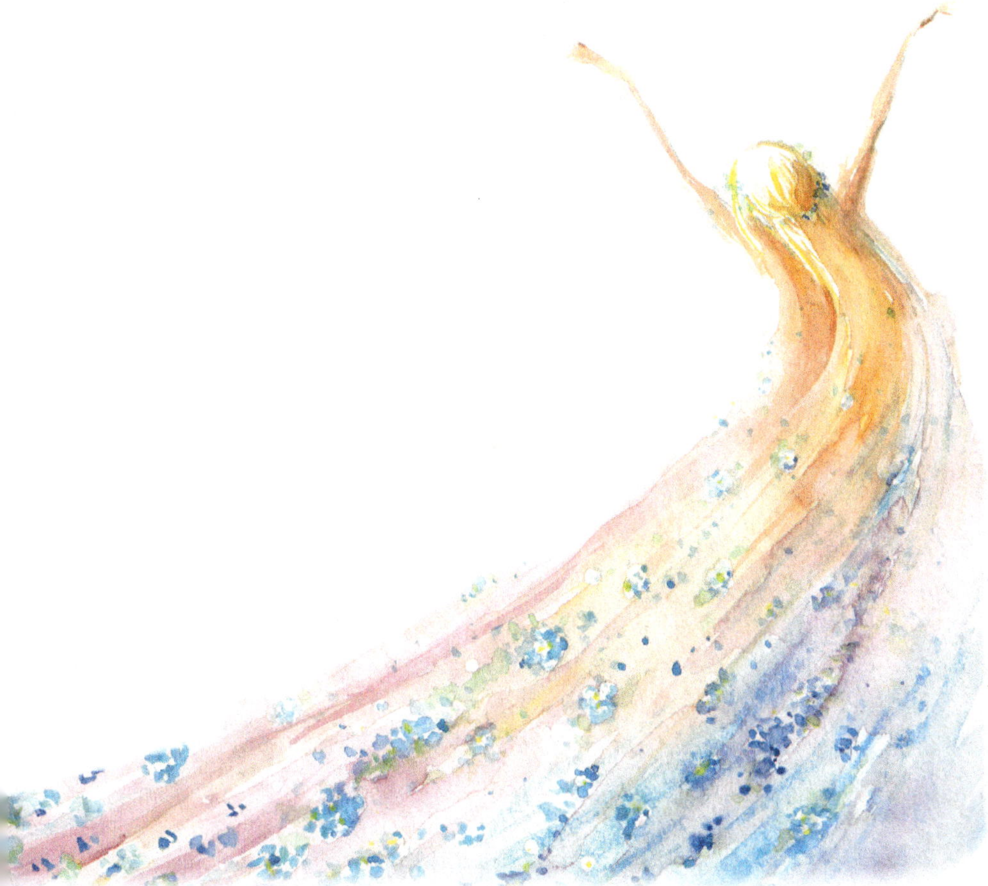

Health-a-Pedia™ *presents*

The Essence of a Woman

Unleash the Feminine Soul

Featuring:

Tiffany Haddish

Dr. Khalilah Camacho-Ali
HRH Princess Dr. Moradeun Ogunlana

Dr. Jo Dee Baer, PhD   Dr. James Marinakis,
                                ND, HmD, Acu.Phys.

Foreword by:
Dr. Glen Depke, ND

STORIES BY THE FOLLOWING HEALING WORLD CHANGERS

TIFFANY HADDISH

DR. KHALILAH CAMACHO-ALI

HRH PRINCESS DR. MORADEUN OGUNLANA

DR. JAMES MARINAKIS, ND, HMD, ACU.PHYS.

DR. JO DEE BAER, PHD * DR. GLEN DEPKE, ND

SHANNON L. ROPER, FNP-BC * DR. NEPHETINA L. SERRANO

DEBBIE MORALES * DESIREE PEACOCK

DR. NITIKUL SOLOMON, MD, MSHM, ABIHM

JENNIFER LOUISE KERR * KATHY STRAUSS, CCFC

LORINA K. SANCHEZ, MSN, RN * BETTY NORLIN

ANNE BOROW-LAWRENCE, MED * RENÉE BROWN

SONJA RECHNITZER * KAREN RUDOLF

CYNTHIA HAMMEL-KNIPE, CPE * MARBETH DUNN

BARBIE LAYTON * LEILANI ALESH, ESQ * ANNA M. MCKEE

CATHY VERGARA, APRN * DR. JACQUELINE MOHAIR, PHD

DR. TYRA GOOD * DR. ANNETTE WATSON-JOHNSON

DR. SHIRLEY LUU * DR. HEPSHARAT AMADI, MD, LAC

DR. GOLDA JOSEPH, PHD * DONNA DAWSON, FCCA

DOMINIQUE BRUN * LAURA IBARRA, ABD

GLORIA KURZ, JD, SRS * KIM JACOBS, MBA, BD

DEBORAH DENNIS * CRISTINA CANDULLO-DODY

Copyright © 2024 by Dr. Jo Dee Baer, PhD All rights reserved.

The Essence of a Woman is a collaborative work featuring contributions from multiple authors. Health-a-Pedia Publishing serves as the publisher.

No part of this book may be utilized or reproduced in any manner without the express written consent of the principal author, Dr. Jo Dee Baer, PhD, and/or Health-a-Pedia Publishing. This restriction applies to all forms of reproduction and usage, including but not limited to photocopying, electronic distribution, or any other means of dissemination.

Exceptions are granted solely for brief quotations incorporated within critical articles and reviews, provided that appropriate attribution is made to the source. Because of the dynamic nature of the Internet, any web addresses or links contained in this book may have changed since publication and may no longer be valid.

For more information, visit: www.DrJoDee.com and www.healthapedia365.com

ISBN: 979-8-990062-46-7 (Hardback)

ISBN: 979-8-990062-45-0 (Paperback)

ISBN: 979-8-990062-44-3 (E-book)

First published in 2024.

Disclaimer

The information provided in this book is for informational purposes only and is not intended to be a source of advice with respect to the material presented. The information contained in this book does not constitute legal, financial, medical, or health advice. The publisher does not make any guarantee or other promise as to any results that may be obtained from using the content of this book. To the maximum extent permitted by law, the publisher disclaims any and all liability in the event any information, commentary, analysis, opinions, advice, and/or recommendations contained in this book prove to be inaccurate, incomplete, or unreliable or result in any investment, medical, or health-related losses. Content contained or made available through this book is not intended to and does not constitute legal advice, financial advice, medical advice, or health advice, and no attorney-client or doctor-patient relationship is formed. The contents of this book, including any health-related information, should not be considered a substitute for professional medical advice, diagnosis, or treatment. Always consult with a qualified health professional.

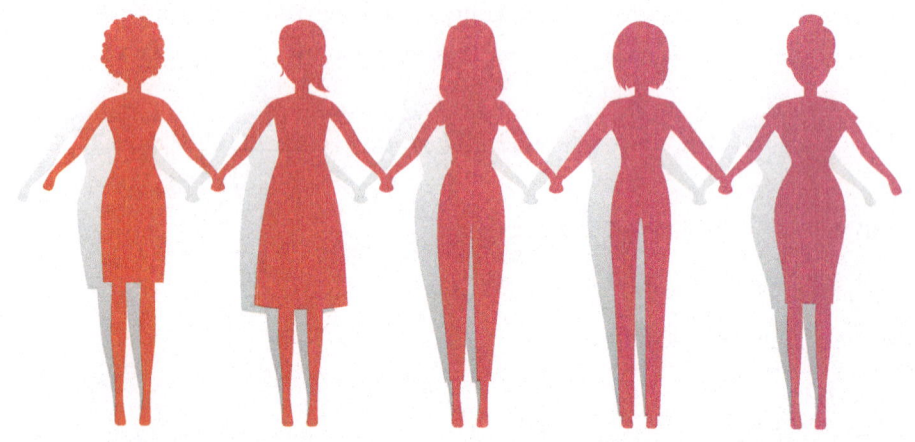

Contents

Acknowledgements vii
Foreword xi
Dedication xiii
Endorsements xvii
Preface xxix
Introduction xxxiii
Disclaimers xxxv

CHAPTER ONE: SPIRITUAL PILLAR 1

Dr Khalilah Camacho-Ali	The Essence of Faith and Forgiveness 3
Dr. James Marinakis, ND, HmD, Acu.Phys.	Humanity's Core 19
Shannon L. Roper, FNP-BC	The Virtuous Path of a Family Nurse Practitioner 29
Dr. Nephetina L. Serrano	My Dream Personified— A Woman's Spiritual Mandate 39
Debbie Morales	Love's Formula: Forgiveness and Healing 49
Desiree Peacock	Finding My Identity 59
Dr. Nitikul Solomon, MD, MSHM, ABIHM	The Divine Feminine Essence 69

CHAPTER TWO: MENTAL PILLAR 79

Jennifer Louise Kerr	You Versus Your Armour 81
Kathy Strauss, CCFC	The Transformative Power of Creativity 91
Lorina K. Sanchez, MSN, RN	From Fear to Faith: Becoming a Forensic Nurse 101
Anne Borow-Lawrence	Discover Your Fountain of Youth: Myth to Mindset 111
Betty (Elizabeth) A. Norlin	Our Bodies: The Optimal Design 121
Renée Brown	Unbreakable: From Trenches to Triumph! 131

CHAPTER THREE: EMOTIONAL PILLAR 141

Dr. Jacqueline Mohair, PhD	The Journey of Healing, Trust, and Transformation	143
Sonja Rechnitzer	The Full Power of Intuition and Purposeful Living	155
Karen Rudolf	Dancing with The Divine: A Graceful Journey Within	165
Cynthia Hammel-Knipe, CPE	Self-Esteem: The Road to Self-Empowerment	175
MarBeth Dunn	Your Body Loves You	185
Barbie Layton	A Woman's Weight is Not Her Worth	195
Leilani Alesh, Esq.	Indomitable Joy: Ours for the Taking	205
Anna M. McKee	Harmonic Conversions	215

CHAPTER FOUR: PHYSICAL PILLAR: 225

Dr. Glen Depke, ND	Healthy Hormones are Your Superpower	227
Cathy Vergara, APRN	The Prescription Glass: an Unlimited Life	237
Dr. Annette Watson-Johnson	Just Get Well, The Sea Moss Way	247
Dr. Hepsharat Amadi, MD, LAc	Natural Hormone Balance at Any Age	257
Dr. Tyra Good	My #GOOD and Lasting Healing	267
Dr. Golda Joseph, PhD	She-oric Journey Through the Circle of Time©	277

CHAPTER FIVE: FINANCIAL PILLAR 287

Dr. Shirley Luu	How to Win the Financial Health Game of Life	289
Donna Dawson, FCCA	Proverbs for the Soul: My Legacy	299
Dominique Brun	The Turning Point: Embracing the Domino Effect	309
Laura Ibarra, AbD	Healthy Mindset: Game, Set, and Match!	319
Gloria Kurz, JD, SRS	Pursuing My American Dream	329

CHAPTER SIX: SOCIAL PILLAR		339
Tiffany Haddish	Woman Up!	341
Dr. Jo Dee Baer, PhD	The Woman in a White Robe	353
Kim Jacobs, MBA, BD	Who Knew? God Knew!	363
Deborah Dennis	Parenting Xtra-Growth Families	373
Cristina Candullo-Dody	The Loyalty of Love	383
HRH Princess Dr. Moradeun Ogunlana	The All-Empowered Woman	393

Author Testimonials 405
High Heel Moment 415
Legacy Lady 435
Author Resources 453
Author Acknowledgements 469

CONCLUSION 481
  Love Freely 483
  We Women of Essence Write 489
  Universal QR Code 490

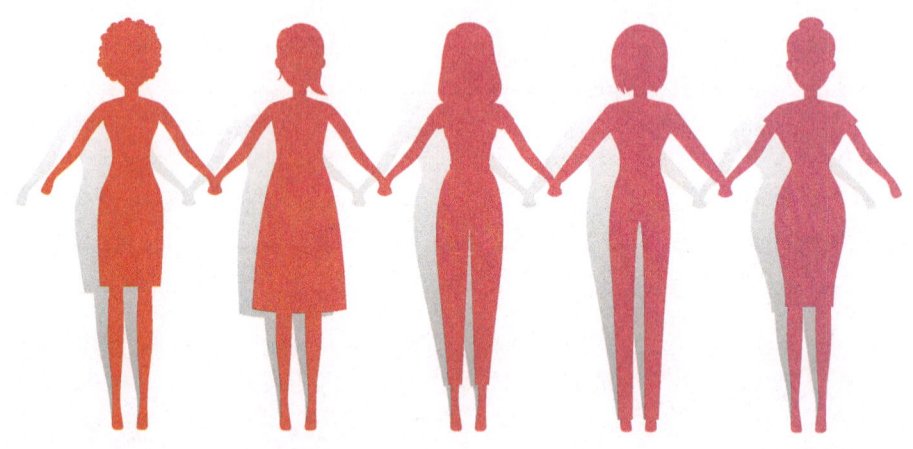

Acknowledgements

I have spent four decades as a Health Coach, sixty percent of my time with women, grew up in a household full of women, 24 years as a part of a Women's Retreat and Movement on relationships, and my entire life as a woman having focused much of my life and practice ascribing to master the **tree of life**, a fundamental archetype in many of the world's **mythological**, **religious**, and philosophical traditions. The above nuggets of the 'Tree of Life,' emanate as an example of the wisdom, knowledge, and understanding from my years of mentorship by the World Renowned Physician and Co-Founder of *Health-a-Pedia*: Dr. James Marinakis, ND, HmD, Acu.Phys.—I honor you! The following people and businesses have all added a branch of this sacred tree in our *Essence of a Woman* project. Wisdom, knowledge, and love have overflowed together in part to create our creative flow.

Graphic Designer:

Kathy Strauss: Multi-faceted magician of graphics, book 'be-in-charge' project manager, photographer, artist, and author, typifying one word: BRAVO! www.imagewerks.net.

Media Marvels:

Robert Towns: Videographer with a personal and profound vision behind the camera: www.trycityworks.com.

Tom Chesser: who has an amazing talent for your story and initiative to get out to the world—one of the reasons that *Health-a-Pedia* has become a household word. www.riseupmarketingandmedia.com.

Allison Martin: my 'mind' reader and creator with artistic flair. www.virtualidealsolutions.com.

Denise Burkhardt: CEO and Co-Founder Trey Duplain of Traverse TV who generously provided their platform and advertising. www.traversetv.com.

Tony and Cristina Dody: Phenomenal film producers, connectors, and visionaries. www.dreammakeragency.com.

Dr. (hon) Lawrence Martin Pratt of Unidial Media who integrated essential components from website development to organic social media content. www.askdrpratt.com.

Vice and Parsa: Two of the most marketing marvel GenZ'ers I've ever met. www.purgion.com.

Health-a-Pedia Sponsors, who initially shared our vision, knowing that *Health-a-Pedia* was more than a book, events, eventually movies, it's a movement!

- Gravity Ball: www.gravityball.com
- Tranquil SOULutions: www.tranquilsoulutions.com
- Medical Mindshare: www.medicalmindshare.org
- Personal Performance Institute www.personal-performance-institute.com
- Be Great: www.thedreampromoter.com
- Money and You: www.moneyandyoudistinctions.com
- Rise Up Marketing and Media: https://riseupmedia-marketing.vcardinfo.com/
- Roper's Health Oasis: www.ropershealthoasis.com
- Mansions and Manors: www.mansionsandmanors.com
- Vital Essence: www.vitalessence.com
- Author Launchpad: www.christrammellcoaching.com
- 3-G Effect: www.noahcrane.com
- Lumi-Consciousness: www.modernconsciousness.com

Essence Ambassadors:

Kathy Strauss, Renée Brown, Shannon Roper, Anna McKee, Cynthia Hammel-Knipe, Karen Rudolf, and Betty Norlin—who collectively volunteered their gifts, vision, and love as liaisons. Gratitude unbounded from me! Proverbs 3:18 says that wisdom is *"A tree of life to those who grasp her, and whoever holds on to her is happy."*

Editors:

Anna McKee of AM Developments: graphic artist, editor, proofreader, and amazingly intuitively author.

Betty Norlin, owner of What Is Holistic Health and podcast host of Be Healthy in a Hurry: whose editing skills transmuted to 'editing' in a hurry.

Authors:

Lorina Sanchez, NP for her heartfelt care with our Six Pillar Quotes I entitled: "Women's Wisdom." And to all 40 *The Essence of a Woman* authors who poured into their life stories with wisdom, love, and vulnerability—each a she-roes journey to "Unleash the Feminine Soul."

In memoriam:

Carrie Fisher, LMT-CRT, who graced her life's story in *Health-a-Pedia: Putting Together the Pieces in Foundational Health*. Her chapter was profoundly titled: "Healing the Wounded Healer." As she has transitioned to her eternal healing, her life, words, and story will live on the legacy of healing and hope.

Family:

To Yahuah and my sons, Carl and Evan, who've taught me and illustrated the innate qualities of 'mercy and severity' of the *Essence of a Woman*. I continually learn from both of you to this day.

To my Yahuah (commonly known as God), lastly and most importantly, who instilled this desire in me at inception, whose pages live in this book as a testimony and legacy of health for humanity.

And finally and most appropriately, to the dearest man I've ever met, known, and loved, my husband, Bob Baer, who supported, advised, and eternally steadfast with my mission—unexpectedly passed away before this book was published. When he saw the proof print copy, he fluttered through the pages like any successful author would. His resounding words will always resonate in my heart and soul, "I always just wanted to give you a platform for you and your gifts." That you did, my Big Baer. In every way, you made me realize my own 'essence of a woman.'

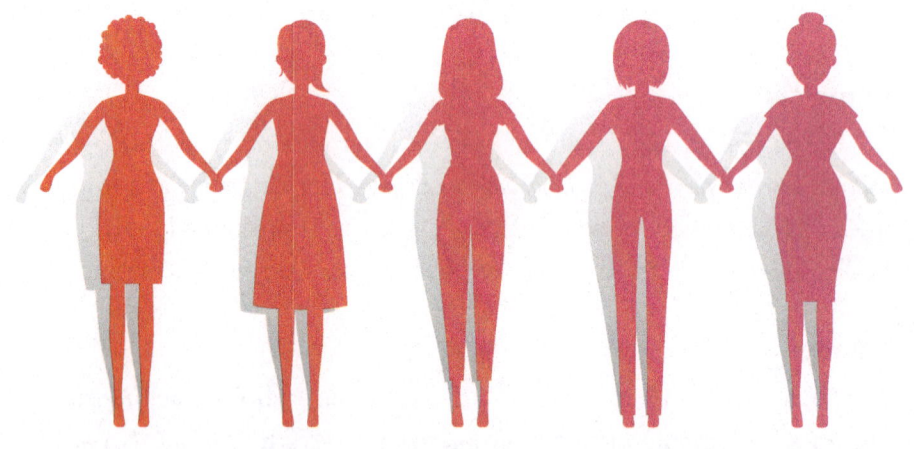

Foreword

By Dr. Glen Depke, ND, Traditional Naturopath

You have to love the passion and compassion in *The Essence of a Woman* by Dr. Jo Dee Baer and the host of equally amazing co-authors who have chosen to share their expertise and knowledge with you.

And all of your gifted authors are always keeping in mind your intention to reach the full potential of the essence of who you are as a woman.

I understand this because as a Traditional Naturopath, I have been assisting women in balancing hormones during the menopause season of their life for over 20 years.

I see firsthand how often women are lied to, put down, and even ridiculed at times.

Well, that's about to change…

The time for change is NOW!

Women have been lied to for far too long, and even worse, the essence of women is being lost.

Perhaps you are thinking to yourself right now, "This is me!"

As a woman, you may feel some type of pain in the moment, without truly being able to identify the source of this pain, whether this is physical, mental, emotional, vibrational, or spiritual.

And you may feel as if you've lost the "flow" of who you are, and maybe even worse, you no longer have your finger on who you're becoming?

The journey you are about to embark on by reading and living *The Essence of a Woman*, is a dream come true of Dr. Jo Dee Baer, PhD.

Dr. Jo Dee is the founder of Health-a-Pedia and has been helping women find their essence for over 45 years. She's done this with her emphasis on what is referred to as the six pillars of health: Spiritual, Mental, Emotional, Physical, Financial, and Social.

And every author you will adore in *The Essence of a Woman* as they focus their healing on these six pillars of health.

So, as you move excitedly from chapter to chapter, you will notice real women, with real life experiences.

Together, this will provide you with three significant life-altering benefits, including answers, actions, and opportunities.

Just imagine living into the action steps of your newfound golden nuggets within these six pillars of health, to become the woman that you desire to become, and more importantly, deserve to become.

And the beauty of this book, *The Essence of a Woman*, provides something you have always had, and always will have—which is choice.

So, it is up to you.

You can read this book, learn all the golden nuggets provided, and most importantly, you can take action on these steps provided, to reach your true essence.

Or you can read this book, put it on the shelf and allow it to be another piece of "shelf help" in which you will never take the action steps needed to reach the true potential of your essence.

While that choice is yours, and yours only, I trust you will take that action that is most important to you!

Remember, the time for change is now, and it is your time to reach for your true Essence of a Woman!

And to leave you with powerful words direct from the most beautiful and inspiring poem written by Dr. Jo Dee Baer, *"Others will always be drawn to the woman who is certain of who she is, And She? Who is unafraid to freely express her true Creator-inspired Nature."*

Dedication

"I am She, and She is Me." We women are the connectivity, the glue, sometimes Velcro and duct tape, but always mirrors of each other. Gazing into another woman's eyes, without a sound or gesture, only women feel another woman's essence—looking into but beyond and behind another woman's eyes. We collectively feel pain, joy, love, sadness, depression, grief, delight, passion, confidence, and gratitude, to name a few.

Those sets of eyes are currently represented by the global population of all women which is approximately 3.9 billion. Globally, we string our Global Oneness together each with their "Essence of a Woman" like a string of paper dolls collectively locked—'arm in arm'—as a display of tenacity, resilience, peace, in love and unity for all Humanity to witness.

We dedicate *The Essence of a Woman* to those who have *'unleashed'* their *'feminine souls'* like the assortment of passionate, renowned, and acclaimed women who blazed the trail and forever changed the landscape of Planet Earth:

Imelda Marcos—First Lady of the Philippines, stood tall in the gap for her husband; the ultimate supportive partner in trial and triumph.

Margaret Thatcher—Prime Minister from the United Kingdom. Britain's first female Prime Minister, earned the legacy and moniker of "Iron Lady."

Sandra Day O'Connor—First U.S. Supreme Court Justice to don a lace collar, rather than a man's nehru collar with her black robe, enumerated brilliance with compassion.

Mother Teresa—Spiritual symbol and servant dedicated her life to caring for "the poorest of the poor."

Malala Yousafzai—Pakistani activist shot in the head by the Taliban, miraculously recovered now stands in the gap as a Global Activist for female education and equality.

Jennifer Lopez—Hollywood SuperStar, one of the highest-paid actresses and best-selling music artists of all time.

Mary Golda Ross—First African American Engineer at NASA, broke through two barriers, commanding the entire Apollo Program.

Rosa Parks—Alabama seamstress courageous enough to just "sit" for her rights on a bus, became the emblematic face of the entire Civil Rights Movement.

Wilma Rudoph—American Olympian American Sprinter who overcame significant health challenges, including polio to win three Gold Medals.

Leontyne Price—Metropolitan Opera Soprano, known for her bravura, paved the way for future generations of African-American opera singers and musicians.

Wilma Mankiller—First female Principal Chief of the Cherokee Nation revitalized her Native American Heritage and People.

Each of these world renowned woman of the Universe—representing politics, entertainment, science and technology, philanthropy, activism, music, law, and religion acculturate Traditional Chinese Medicine's concepts of *Yin and Yang*—balance, life force, and interconnectedness within the Natural and Spiritual Worlds. This interwoven tapestry of the golden thread within the cultural, religious, and scientific fabric of Planet Earth is intertwined for each woman together—in birth, life, health, and death. Whether as a famous, notable, or every day woman, these stories of healing and hope are for you. We feel each of you in the pages of our book. You all embody the true "Essence of a Woman," Unleash *your* feminine soul and join us to empower the Universe!

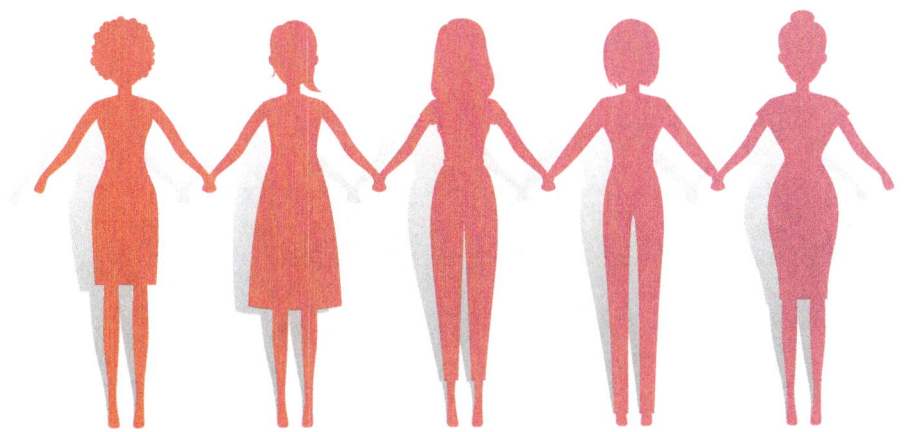

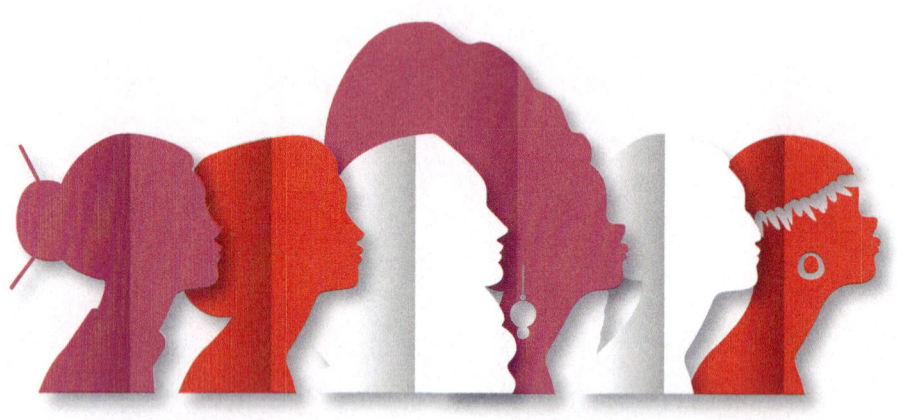

Endorsements

Few collections in literature manage to capture the multifaceted essence of womanhood as poignantly as *The Essence of a Woman: Unleash the Feminine Soul*. This anthology is a powerful testament to the strength, resilience, grace, and beauty that define the feminine experience. Each story, poem, and narrative thread weaves together to create a rich tapestry that celebrates the diversity and depth of women's lives.

From the ancient myths that first tried to capture women's enigma to the contemporary voices that continue to redefine and reclaim their narratives, this book is filled with a symphony of voices. These voices, each unique yet universally relatable, offer glimpses into the joys, struggles, triumphs, and reflections that shape every woman's journey.

The contributors to this anthology come from varied backgrounds and walks of life, bringing with them a wealth of perspectives and experiences. Their stories are not just tales to be read but experiences to be felt, offering readers a profound connection to the shared human experience. Whether it's a poem that stirs the soul, a story that brings tears, or an essay that challenges perceptions, *The Essence of a Woman* stands as a testament to the enduring spirit and indomitable will of women everywhere.

As you turn these pages, allow yourself to be immersed in the voices and stories that await you. Let them inspire, challenge, and move you. For in understanding the essence of a woman, we come to appreciate the boundless potential and unyielding strength that lies within us all.

It is with great honor and deep respect that I invite you to explore *The Essence of a Woman*. May it enrich your understanding, touch your heart, and celebrate the extraordinary journey of womanhood.

—*Dr. Jacqueline Mohair, PhD*
President Trinity Business School
Teenage Girls Empowerment

This powerful and transformative work speaks directly to the heart of what it means to embrace our full selves. This book is not just a guide; it's an invitation to reconnect with the deep, intrinsic power within each of us. It beautifully captures the complexities of our experiences, the strength in our vulnerability, and the boundless potential that we hold.

It's an empowering read for anyone looking to deepen their understanding of their inner strength, embrace her authenticity, and unleash her full potential. It's a must-read for anyone committed to living with purpose, passion, and power.

—Tricia Benn
Partner & Chief Executive Officer
C-Suite Network™
Podcast & TV Host, Business Disruptor

Stories empower and encourage us. Dr. Jo Dee Baer's new book: *The Essence of a Woman* gifts us with incredible stories of women who transformed their lives, and who can transform ours. Each story gives us a glimpse of women who have pursued their dreams and their passions allowing each one to become the fullest version of herself. A community of women is revealed. Women who are bold, passionate, leaning into their giftedness despite obstacles, defying all expectations, and inspirational in their aspirations and dreams. A must-read to learn how to navigate life's challenges in every arena. Accessing and recognizing "giftedness," fueling your dreams with hard work and determination, incorporating flexibility and willingness to learn from mistakes, staying healthy with good "self-care," and celebrating small victories along the way. These stories illuminate the way for all of us.

—Judith Scott Mayer, PhD
Chemistry, MA in Theology

Dr. Jo Dee Baer's love and commitment to bringing the best tools and information, especially to women, is extraordinary. Never miss the opportunity to 'devour' her wisdom and of those whom she brings to you—this time with 39 other healers and world changers for the betterment of humanity—which is my Global Vision as well. Read, absorb these golden nuggets by each author, and share it with another female friend for collective empowerment.:

—Dame Doria (DC) Cordova
CEO/Owner, Excellerated Business Schools® / Money & You®
www.MoneyandYou.com

What an immensely healing book! We as women all have something we are dealing with in our lives, and if you just need to feel a little bit better or a little bit more supported or even to find something to bring a soft smile to your face, this is the book to read. Dr. Jo Dee Baer and Dr. Jim Marinakis have created beautiful healing words from beautiful, strong, yet sensitive women.

—Dame Didi Wong
Angel Investor, Speaker
Movie Producer, Philanthropist

As an author in the Financial Pillar in Health-a-Pedia's premier anthology: *Health-a-Pedia: Putting the Pieces Together in Foundational Health*. Our book had key experts in every pillar where I was honored to be featured in the financial pillar. With Deborah Dennis being selected in the Social Pillar of Health, the reader will be in for a treat! Deborah is an amazing mother. I have been so honored to see her with her incredible kids and I know when I step into fatherhood I will be going to her for advice. Her story will do just that for anyone who reads and applies her wisdom.

—Jason Estes
www.jasonesstes.org
www.mtvo.org
www.alignedearth.org
www.voidspacetech.org

At the very core of every human being lies a well of untapped potential. Often, our life's journey takes us through rough waters of uncertainty blanketed with worry, fear, anxiety, resentment, and bewilderment, leaving us confused and unsure of what to do.

These brave women embarked *'the dark night of the soul'* and took an inward journey giving new empowering meaning to the events and circumstances of their lives—providing powerful stories—to help anyone struggling in similar situations to overcome and become victorious.

Life is truly happening for us, from us, and when we change the lens through which we view the world, the world changes right before our eyes.

Embracing and activating our divine feminine and finding balance through the Six Pillars is a sure way to solve any of life's challenges. It is my honor and privilege to personally know, Dr. Khalilah Camacho-Ali, and Dr. Jo Dee Baer—and now feel as though I know the rest of these dynamic and courageous women—their lives and inner souls, as well. It is a must-read for men and women alike.

—Eric Claussen, EC, Actor, Motivational Speaker;
Recovered Alcoholic/Addict and Fitness Enthusiast
IG: @eric_claussen

The world needs more women leaders. We need leaders with a heart who are compassionate and helpful. I was honored to be a part of the original book: *Health-a-Pedia: Putting the Pieces Together in Foundational Health.* Now, this anthology is a book filled with women leaders sharing their insights, which is what everyone needs. Both women and men need to read this book. I am excited that young girls and boys have an opportunity to see what is possible when we have great role models. Thanks for writing and publishing *The Essence of a Woman: Unleash the Feminine Soul.*

—Rex Sikes
Speaker, Actor, Trainer, Best Selling Author:
Life on Your Terms

This is one of the most well-thought-out and written books on the divine energy and true *Essence of a Woman.* I am humbled to learn from mama nature, the essence of a woman, her rhythms, and working with mainly women for most of my wellness/holistic career.

I can say that the 40 women who have collaborated to create this masterpiece, "Unleash The Feminine Soul" work of art, really take women and humanity to the next level of awareness. Through the depth of each woman's journey, you read and see the integrity within their words and feel the emotional and mental depth of each one's story and the practices that transformed their lives, which made them who and what they truly are today.

Each one is a Wonder Woman within their own universe, and each one is an extraordinary guide to change, all in one book.

—*Lonjéray Josiah Samadhi*
World Renowned Frequency Trauma Expert
Yoga Brain Life Coach
Meditation Guide

Dr. Jo Dee Baer is a blessing to this world. Her passion and dedication to humanity's well-being exude from every pore in her body. She is elevating her message to the world yet again with another health masterpiece: *The Essence of a Woman*. Every woman can live the secondary title that says, '*Unleash the Feminine Soul.*' Also, it is my recommendation that every man needs to experience this knowledge, too, for himself and the women in his life.

—*Josh Payne*
@joshbpayne
Financial Industry Leader

Dr Jo Dee, you never cease to amaze me!! After the unbelievable success of *Health-a-Pedia*, I was certain that lightning couldn't possibly strike twice…I was wrong. I just finished *The Essence of a Woman* and was blown away.

Leading the army of amazing women to yet another best-selling book that speaks right to the hearts of women is truly needed. In times like this when everyone is speaking about progressing (which is a good thing) we sometimes forget about the need to reflect on the past as well, so we can take the good with us.

As a doctor dealing with stress-related issues, I see women running successful businesses, running households, taking care of their husbands and children, and being great friend to those who need them every day. They do all of this and forget about themselves. With so many of life's plates spinning they sometimes lose perspective. With all the experts that you brought together to give insights this book is a game changer. It's the secret playbook that everyone should read, not just women but men who love them too.

I can't recommend this book enough.

—*Dr. Bill Janeshak*
www.yorbalindafamilychiropractic.com
@B_Janeshak

Dr. Jo Dee Baer is a remarkable human who truly cares about people's health and well-being. I got COVID recently, and Dr. Jo Dee jumped into action immediately and made sure I got exactly what I needed, overnighting me an all-natural healing medicine that she recommended created by Dr. Jim Marinakis, Co-founder of their company, Health-a-Pedia™. Their first book, "*Health-a-Pedia: Putting the Pieces Together in Foundational Health,*" was their first masterpiece. Now, they have focused on women's health: *The Essence of a Woman: Unleash the Feminine Soul.* For these reasons, and many more, she is on Traverse TV with their own channel labeled Health-a-Pedia. I could never thank her enough for her loving care. Now, this group of health author experts can take you to the next level; correspondingly enough, as you flip through the pages of this new women's health book, you will find more of a wealth of information for your health.

—*Tom Chesser*
CEO Rise Up Media and Marketing
https://riseupmedia-marketing.vcardinfo.com/

I met Dr. Jo Dee two decades ago and helped her through her healing with Stage 4 Melanoma. Since then, Dr. Jo Dee has become a partner of mine for 24 years, a fierce leader and health advocate, helping tens of thousands lose weight and optimize their health. Dr. Jo Dee has now elevated her message a second time with 40 other like-minded Alternative Healers and Advocates for a healthy lifestyle. Women, you're in for a treat because I know what heart and passion are inside of my patient-turned-partner to inspire more and widen the net for this healing message. This book is a must-read and will assist any woman or man in your next level of health and life of optimal health! Enjoy!

—Dr. Mike Van Thielen, PhD
CEO Biohacking Unlimited
Author/Speaker
www.mvtonline.com

Dr. Jo Dee Baer—You have changed my life. When I went through the most challenging health chapter in my life, and I experienced intense burnout, unlimited fatigue, and depression, your practices and natural prescriptions helped me overcome this difficult phase. What stood out the most was your love, commitment, and support; I have never experienced this kind of support from a health practitioner. My body's healing experience was amazing, thanks to you. You are truly a champion of health, and I am so grateful that you are in my corner—and in this case, walking together in *The Essence of a Woman* book—both in our high heel moments together. I know that countless other women will benefit greatly from this epic book.

–Blanca Perper
Founder
Laws of Life Platform
www.lawsoflife.shop

I have known and worked with Dr. Jo Dee for over 20 years. From her early days with "Team in Training" and the Denver Chamber of Commerce and running marathons to the latest chapter in her life working in Florida with her husband Bob. She has always been the consummate professional and leader in every endeavor she has undertaken. Her enthusiasm, drive, and focus have served her well, including the people on her team in business and coaching. Health-a-Pedia™, the company, is just another level of health and wellness on her journey for you. Now, the world has two books, and the latest is for all women.

—Bob Liebhauser
Action Coach
www.bobliebhauser.actioncoach.com

I have known Health Coach Dr. Jo Dee Baer for over a decade. I have learned so much from her and recommend her highly to others. If you are looking for someone who can guide you on your health journey and help you achieve your personal development goals, look no further than Health Coach Dr. Jo Dee Baer. As an international best-selling author, health coach, mentor, motivational speaker, and radio show host, Jo Dee has the knowledge, experience, and passion to help you transform your life and achieve optimal health and wellness.

As a radio show host, Dr. Jo Dee shares her knowledge and expertise on health and wellness with a wider audience. Her show, "The Health Coach Dr. Jo Dee Show," on Building Fortunes Radio, provides listeners with practical tips and advice on how to live a healthier, happier, and more fulfilling life. Her latest project and book on women's health: *The Essence of a Woman*, will bring more of the same, I assure you. Building Fortunes Radio is awaiting this new cadre of health expert guests.

—Peter Mingils
www.networkleads.com

At this time in history, we have so many tasks that we are facing and are challenged to deal with on a daily basis. I love this book and how Dr. Jo Dee Baer shows all of us how much she loves and cares for people. Dr. Jo Dee displays her intentional intelligence in two ways: One, she has created yet a second book that covers the Spiritual, Mental, Emotional, Physical, Financial, and Social parts of our lives. In this second iteration on women's health—*The Essence of a Woman,* she has also created a web of genius by bringing together 40 female experts and their expertise to advise us and encourage us in these highly challenging times. I strongly recommend you get two copies of this book today, one for you and a second copy to give to your best friend who always "borrows" your new book.

—Dr. Martin Pratt
Co-Founder Unidial Marketing

This latest book, from Health-a-Pedia™, *The Essence of a Woman*, is a treasure trove of expertise, bringing together a remarkable collection of female experts under one cover. It's an exceptional opportunity to access a wealth of advice and insights from such a diverse range of knowledgeable women. The book's unique offering sets it apart, making it a must-read for anyone seeking valuable perspectives all in one place for life and health.

—10g Colin Drummond
TMZ Entertainment

I have had the pleasure of being one of Dr. Jo Dee Baer's coaches for the last four years. I've witnessed her energy—passion not only for health, but for life. First, there was *Health-a-Pedia* and now with this latest project, a networking outgrowth of this passion, we have *The Essence of a Woman*. As the founder of Orphan to CEO Project and Network of Influence, I'm especially honored to read the message within the social pillar of health. I've seen the serving heart and how she's taken her level of influence to the next level for women's health. I'm so honored to read and enjoy the ride!

—Manny Lopez
Founder: Orphan to CEO Project
www.NetworkOfInfluence.com

Dr. Jo Dee Baer is a truly exceptional health coach and natural medicine practitioner with over 43 years of experience in her field. Round one as the author of *21 Days to Your Best You: Keys to a Life of Excellence*, was round one. She has postured herself with the medical icons and healers, first with *Health-a-Pedia: Putting the Pieces Together in Foundational Health*, and now the second book from Health-a-Pedia, *The Essence of a Woman*. I have personally worked with and seen the healing benefit from Health-a-Pedia™ Co-founder, most importantly, Dr. Jim Marinakis, ND, HmD, Acu.Phys. The level of expertise laid out in the pages of this book are one of a kind. It is a resource for all who want to commit to reaching their ultimate health. Let's call it a manual to instruct us all on WHAT to do and HOW to do it! Dr. Jo Dee and Dr. Jim are two of the best practitioners I have ever worked with and I am confident they have aligned with 40 other women who are the best of the best.

—Scott 'Rhino' Harris
President of Arcadia Integrated Solutions

As a Wellness Warrior for nearly two decades, I've had the profound privilege of immersing myself in countless teachings on holistic health, wellness, and abundance. However, every so often, a work emerges that captures the essence of wellness, expands its horizons, and redefines its very foundation. Health-a-Pedia's first edition, *Health-a-Pedia: Putting Together the Puzzle Pieces in Foundational Health* did precisely that. Now, they've elevated to another level for women's health with: *The Essence of a Woman: Unleash the Feminine Soul*. The women author's collection is extraordinary. As Dr. Jo Dee says: "Health isn't something you do; it's what you become along life's journey." Embrace it, amplify your light, and let these luminaries guide you.

—*Lindsaya VanDuesen*
Founder of the Wellness Warrior Collective

Prior to meeting and marrying my wife, I have taken numerous courses to understand how to not only be better with myself, but how to be better with women. Specifically, one woman, so I could be in a committed relationship, and deal authentically with upsets, miscommunications, and enjoy that sweet loving partnership we all desire. When I met my wife, I was drawn to values, her stories, her qualities for living well and successfully, and at the roots of her upbringing. All the things that I see women are revealing about themselves in *The Essence of a Woman* anthology.

Although this book may occur as being for women, it is absolutely for men. It is for the men who champion women. Who empower them from bedroom to boardroom. Who see them and honor their minds, their bodies, their creativity, their autonomy to choose and not 'fall-in-line', and honor both their partnership and leadership, without feeling challenged about their own masculinity or opportunities. If you are a man wanting to hold a more conscious and empowered space for women, then I invite you to read the stories and declarations from some of the world's leading women in *The Essence of a Woman* book created and anchored by Dr. Jo Dee Baer.

—*Chris Tramell, CEO, Executive Coach*
AuthorLaunch Pad
www.christrammelcoaching.com

I have witnessed the bird's eye view of Dr. Jo Dee's vision since she discovered the now infamous 1984 Goal Card in our home office filing cabinet. Watching her vision unfold into another mission and message to the world on health and abundant living has been, at times, exhausting, but more often than not, inspiringly emotional, and astounding. I've witnessed her daily dedication and am one proud observer because I get to witness it first-hand because I am lucky enough to be called her husband! Congratulations again to my wife, author, publisher, and world changer! Cheers to women's health: The essence of women everywhere.

–Dr. Robert H. Baer, PhD
Archaeologist/Author

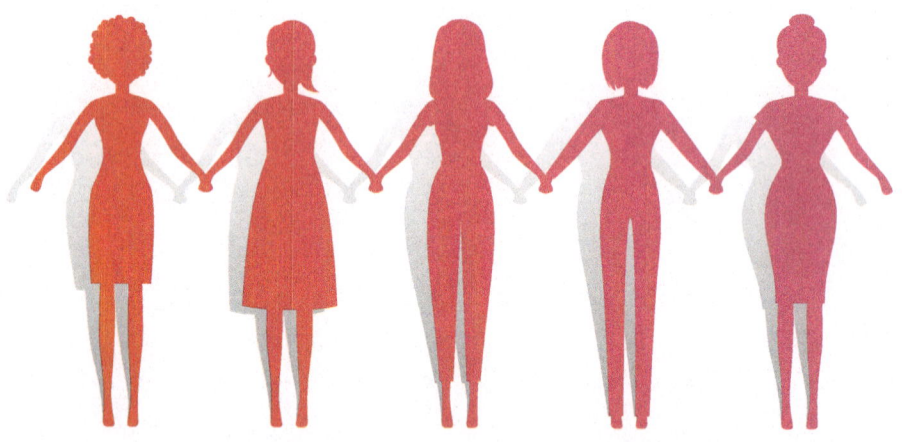

Preface

I've always believed that women are inherently community-driven, thriving on the social pillar of health. A woman at a dinner party or social event feels the necessity to go to the restroom. Unlike a man, who quietly disappears for this physical necessity, a woman will publicly announce it, extend a social invitation, and ask if anyone wants to come with her. This inevitably leads to a 'pack' of women converging for an extended social outing within a physical necessity!

Mentoring and mentorship are much the same social necessity within this of life's mastery. My manifest blessing was attracting the 20th-century iconic pioneer and naturopathic healer, Dr. Hulda Regehr Clark, ND, into my life. Finding her in Atlanta, Georgia, in 1983, was like finding a needle in a haystack. This needle wove the golden threads of healing and hope for my young son and myself as she mentored, created community, and empowerment for this then-young 29-year-old health coach. During these magical mentoring months, I wrote a goal card stating: "I will pen the Eastern Medical Version of the *PDR* (*Physician's Desk Reference*). Decades later, the Universe heard and delivered a sign to deliver and manifest this goal. Health-a-Pedia arrived in 2023 with our first edition: *Health-a-Pedia: Putting the Pieces Together in Foundational Health*—focusing on the Six Pillars of Health: Spiritual, Mental, Emotional, Physical, Financial, and Social. Now, our 2.0 Edition, *The Essence of a Woman: Unleash the Feminine Soul* focuses still on these Six Pillars of Health—written by women for women.

In a professional sense, Dr. Hulda Clark was the epitome of an empowered woman who truly desired to share her protocols, wisdom, and healing gifts in the community with the younger and thirsty soul of a fledgling health coach.

On a personal level, my Mother, the late Tillie K. Wruck, was also the embodiment of the 'essence of a woman.' So confident in her uniqueness that given the common girl's name of her era—Tillie—she always introduced herself as Tillie Katherine and always signed her name:

Tillie K. Wruck. Her explanation was clear: "The K and Katherine make me stand out!' Widowed at the young age of 36, she devoted herself to my sister Kathleen and me, sewed designer fashion clothes for us, and gave us unconditional love along with cultivating our goals and dreams into reality. She sacrificed to the nth degree to provide us with piano and voice lessons that ultimately led us both to the Concert Stages of the World—transmuting her essence and uniqueness through to her daughters.

The foundational Six Pillars of health: Spiritual, Mental, Emotional, Physical, Financial, and Social—their intrinsic nature and essence—are bestowed upon each baby girl at birth and evolve into womanhood through the following poem. I venerate each of you and your essence, empowerment, love, and community within these couplets:

The Essence of a Woman

The Essence of a Woman lies within her heart,
the capacity to touch others with her love,
All within the quiet resources of her soul.

The essence of a woman—just one woman—
can lighten the burden of one who is suffering,
or stir the hearts of millions, and change the world.

Just one woman can make a difference
when she believes in her Creator-given powers
and makes an effort to use them.

Within each woman is the desire to give joy to others,
to live her dreams and to love with all her heart.
This kind of power kindles hope, inspires faith,
and keeps the spirit alive within all of us.

The Essence of a Woman

is in her inner strength and character,

and is the sum of who she is as an individual:

It is in her values and the ways in which

she expresses those values,

It is also in the way

she perceives herself in the World;

How she carries herself, responds to others, and conducts her life.

Others will always be drawn to the woman

who is certain of who she is,

And She?

Who is unafraid to freely

express her true Creator-inspired nature.

This is the Essence of a Woman

—Dr. Jo Dee Baer, PhD

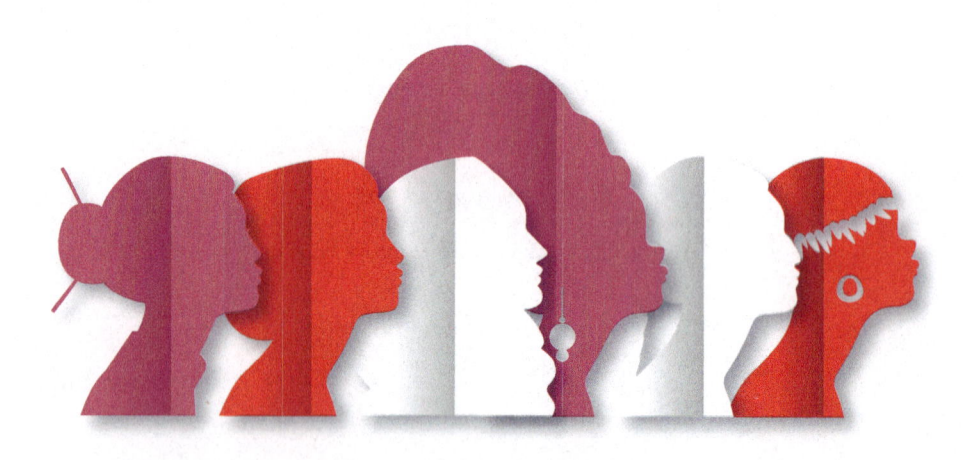

Introduction

The essence of a woman is—the perfect understanding of all things. However, it is impossible to examine this reality without comprehension, particularly of the meaning of 'essence' itself. Found in the French, Latin, and original Greek languages, in the latter meaning: "I am." As in the famous quote from the bible by the Messiah, Jesus of Nazareth, "I am" the "I am." Who also was quoted to say, "I am my father." Both of these expressions are by the Spirit and of the Spirit. One of the female principles, or 'essence,' the other of the male 'essence,' the father.

Essence is the one, the divine, the spirit, God, Allah ...

Everything that is—has its own essence.

In biological science, the *'birds and the bees,'* show both the mother and father are in all of us. Yet we are individuals due to the presence of the infinite "essence" in all things, the source of creation and understanding themselves. All sitting atop the three pillars of existence, Knowledge, Wisdom, and Understanding. 'The Holy Trinity' always united and identifiable only as accretions—one face of the infinite one God—before which there never was, after which, will never be.

What is Woman? The holy grail; Structure itself; The receiver; The nurturer; The manifestor.

Together with man, she becomes the bringer of life. The mother.

The essence of a woman: Is in everything.

—Dr. James Marinakis ND, HmD, Acu. Phys.

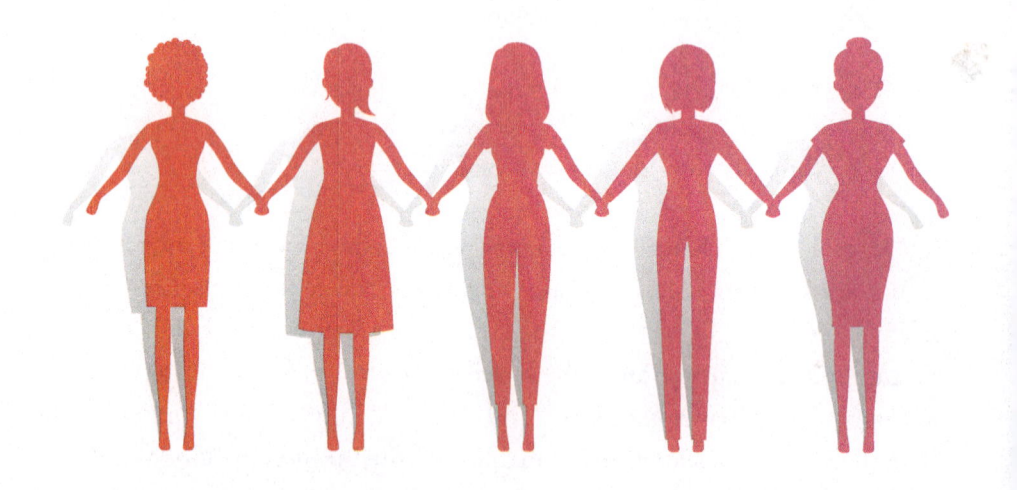

Disclaimers

The information provided on the pages of this book is for educational purposes only and is not intended as a substitute for professional medical advice, diagnosis, or treatment.

Always seek the advice of your physician or other qualified healthcare provider with any questions you may have regarding any medical condition. Never disregard professional medical advice or delay in seeking such because of something you have read in any media or publication.

None of these stories contained subsequently within this book have been designed to treat, mitigate, prevent, or cure any disease. These are personal beliefs and philosophies of each individual author.

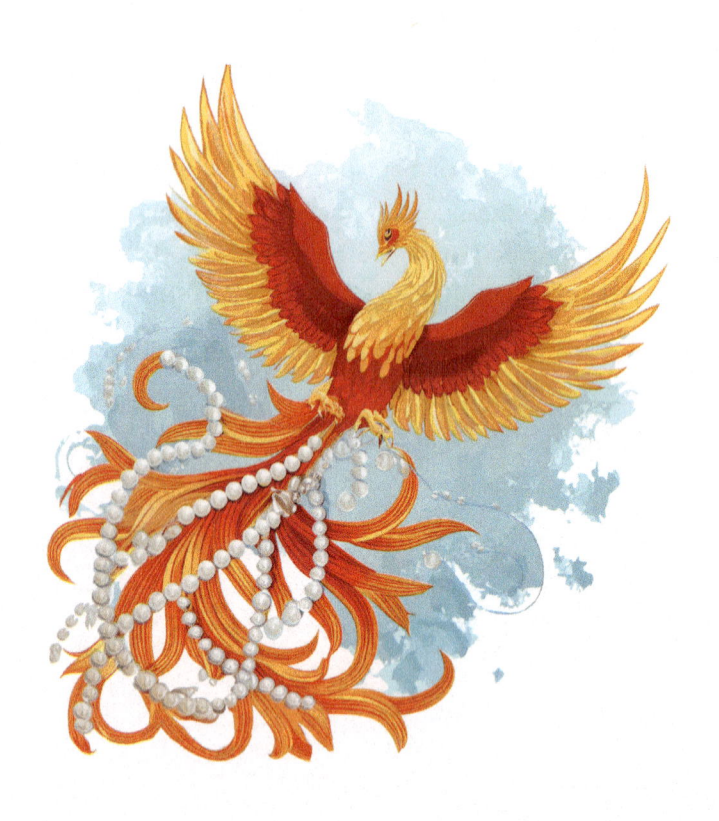

CHAPTER ONE

Spiritual Pillar

"You are not born with beauty; your beauty is created by who you are."
—Cindy Ann Peterson

"Beauty is not in the face; beauty is a light in the heart."
—Kahlil Gibran

"If you are humble nothing will touch you, neither praise nor disgrace, because you know who you are."
—Mother Teresa

"A beautiful woman delights the eye; a wise woman, the understanding; a pure one, the soul."
—Minna Antrim

"She is worth far more than rubies. Her husband has full confidence in her and lacks nothing of value. She brings him good, not harm, all the days of her life."
—Proverbs 31:10-12 (NIV)

"Your beauty should not come from outward adornment, such as elaborate hairstyles and the wearing of gold jewelry or fine clothes. Rather, it should be that of your inner self, the unfading beauty of a gentle and quiet spirit, which is of great worth in God's sight."
—1 Peter 3:3-4 (NIV)

"Grace is the power of God to help us in other areas in which we cannot help ourselves."
—Joyce Meyer

Dr. Khalilah Camacho-Ali

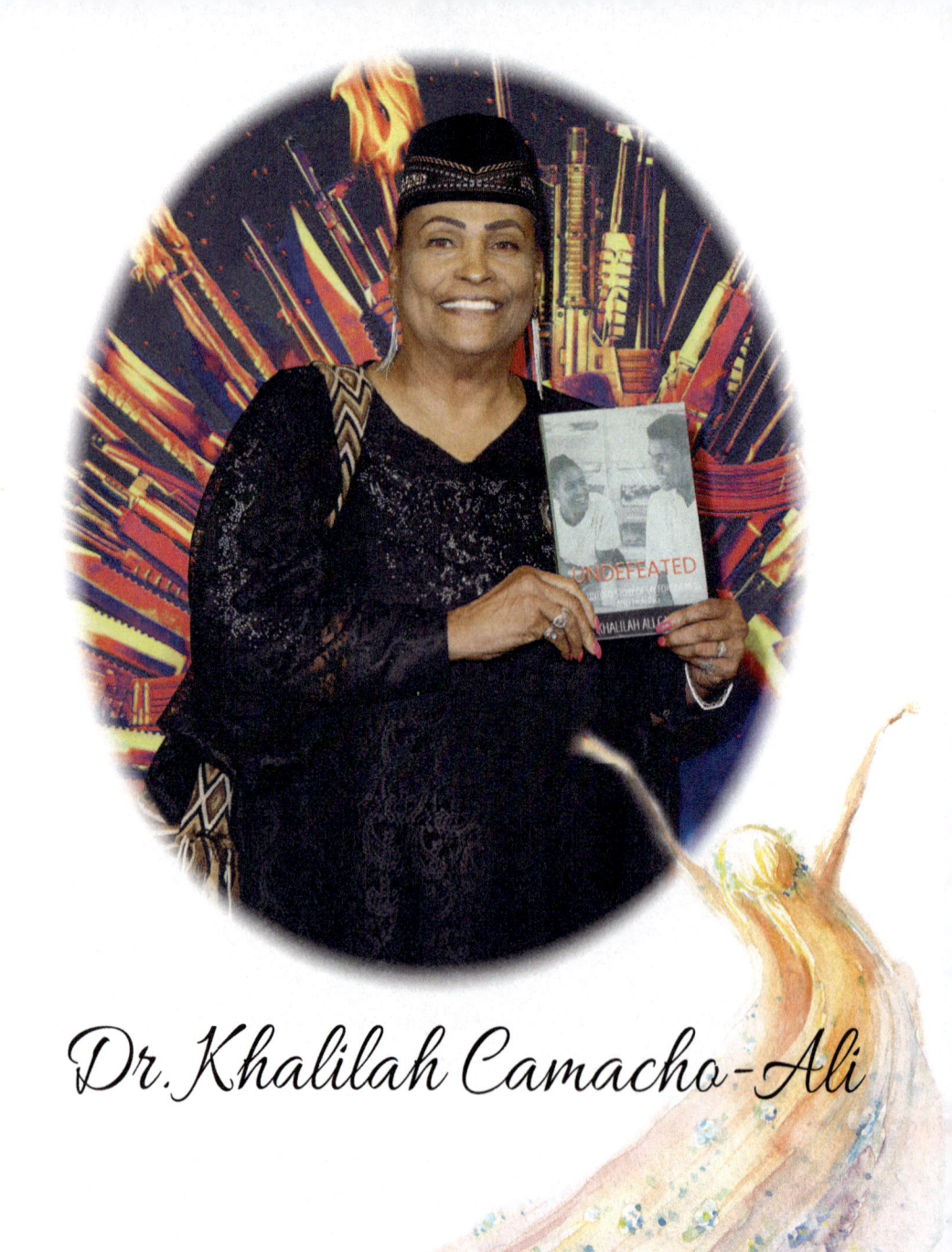

The Essence of Faith and Forgiveness

"Don't count the days—make the days count."

Intention:

When leading with faith and forgiveness, may you feel peace flowing through you as a woman. You may feel the love for your recipe: adding intuition to the recipe of faith and forgiveness to unfold your purpose.

Story:

Growing up as a young Muslim girl, my entire family, from my grandparents to my mother and father, always stressed character and the proper way of doing things. They always said: "Doing things the right way will make you a better person." They taught us all the 'little' things that you don't get in school: heart, intention, and mannerisms that instill excellence. These character-building essentials have been passed down from one generation to the next within my family. I spent a lot of quality time with my grandparents, and we were always together during holidays and vacations. Even these special times were interwoven with stressing what to do and the reason to do things the right way. Even as a little 10-year-old girl and now myself as a grandmother, character building has been the backbone and foundation to practice in my everyday life. I now teach my family members the same way. This old-fashioned, legacy-building way is tried and true.

When Muhammed Ali first came to our private Muslim School, he was the then Cassius Marcellus Clay. Whenever he spoke about the school, I was inspired to explore a vast amount of history as well as elevating the religious principles from that school, that would eventually assist the both of us forever. One intrinsic principle involves your name, and what and how you carry your name, becomes as good as gold. Your name truly tells everything about you. For example, in Latin Cultures, some names are given to them from their grandfather, and they attach that name to their name. They never drop it; they just keep attaching names onto it. Thus, some names become very long, because their family builds it up with this generational attachment. Similarly, in the Muslim world, when a person is given their name, it is not a made-up name. It always has significance and history behind it.

Any Muslim person becomes their name and who they are named by. You don't say the name, you wear this name, and it is as good as gold.

Usually, when you have a son by a man, who is the ruler of the family, the very first son always gets the name of the Father. Automatically, the very first son has to be named after the father. This is the Muslim culture. When the girl is born and with whatever the chosen name, they attach the father's last name to the girl. For example, my name is Khalilah, and my father's name is Sadru Din. Therefore, my name is Khalilah Sadru Din-Ali. That means that Khalilah is the daughter of Sadru Din. It tells you who you are and how you're connected. When you choose these names, it is purposeful and tells you about your whole familial history. If I'm a Muslim, I have a Muslim name. So if I marry another Muslim, it is best and wisest to do so because it's more harmonious not only in name, but spiritually as well. We then pray, do the rituals, and commune together as one instead of being separate. Muhammed is the *ace* name, because you are identified with the name of the Prophet.

I grew up learning the true essence of a woman, and I tried to give Muhammed the essence of a man. I believe you first have to have faith in yourself. And in turn, you have to always be kind to others. The gift for your future is always being kind. Kindness keeps you grounded for yourself and within society. Staying grounded wasn't part of Ali's upbringing, growing up in the South. He picked up a lot of qualities from me, along with the character building and manners. He simply wasn't taught the intensive way of being like I was taught. I would always be blunt and tell him straight out: "You KNOW you got it. You've got a gift and talent. But you can't do something this way, or be disrespectful." I was blunt and straightforward with these principles. I steered him away from greedy people who only saw the money. The people you communicate with and hold close in confidence are critical pieces to a fulfilled life. My faith and upbringing gave me that intuition for him, and I used my gift. He eventually learned these skills, and embraced this heightened way of living. Even as I taught him, he just marveled at how much I knew at such a young age. Growing up in a strict Muslim family truly gave me wisdom.

When I was in Muslim School, I was the hero or *she-ro* in school and very religious. I didn't back down from anything or anyone. I lived with my family's mannerisms and character. So, one day this guy comes into our school named Cassius Marcellus Clay. This formidable 18-year-old man got on stage to speak. I was only 10-years-old and only knew he'd just won the Olympic Gold Medal in Rome, Italy. I didn't remember anything he said or spoke about except that he said: "My name is Cassius Marcellus Clay, and I'm going be heavyweight champion before I turn 21. So, get your autographs now, because I'm going to be famous." He had enough confidence and proclaimed that with such swagger, that I considered him quite cocky. But I heard him out. He sounded so convincing, yet, at my young and impressionable age, I internally questioned myself. "How could he have figured that out? How does he know he's going to do that?" I concluded that he must know his art of this boxing thing that well and have faith in himself. After he spoke, he started giving out autographs to all of us in the school. His autograph said: Cassius Marcellus Clay. He gave it to all the girls and all the boys. Then he came to me. I was the last one in the room. He said, "Hey, little girl, here's my autograph. You will want to keep this, because I'm going to be famous. You're going to own my autograph with a famous name." He was proud of this autographed paper when he handed it to me. I did an about face and even at 10 years of age, I didn't back down. I looked at this paper and then at him and said: "Wait a minute. Wait a minute! This paper says: Cassius Marcellus Clay. You said, That's your name, right?" He said: "Yes, that's my name." Then I laid down the history of his name. "First of all, Cassius and Marcellus are both Roman names. Then, I proceeded to ask him: "Do you know what Romans did to the people back in the day? And lastly, how did you get your last name with the site clay, which means dirt? Clay is dirt that is molded into any shape any person wants it to be." Then, I quizzically spoke: "I am looking at your name and this autograph, my dear friend. It is nice and everything, but this is a Roman name like a slave. Until you have a name of respect and honor, with a Muslim name, you can take this piece of paper back." I tore that piece of paper into pieces, and put it back into his hand. Then, I concluded with my knockout faith punch; "Don't worry, I don't want it. You keep it." With that, I did an about face, and made an abrupt exit.

    He was truly in a state of shock! Before I got to the end of the doorway, he was screaming; "She taunted my name!" One of the other teachers consoled him and replied: "Man, she said don't worry about it. She was probably teaching you some kind of lesson. This girl is like a virgin with her intuition and knowledge of history." Cassius asked the headmaster: "Who is she?" The headmaster replied: "That's Elijah Muhammad's Princess of Islam. She's a karate instructor. She teaches security for the Muslim Girl's Training and Generalized Civilization Class and she's 10 years old." "10 years old! And she knows all this stuff?" With who my father was, Elijah Muhammed, and all I knew of martial arts, history, and the Muslim faith, he was impressed. He was influenced even then, by one so young.

This whole lesson and encounter bothered him for more than a minute! I was informed years later just how much. Three years later, while preparing to fight Sonny Liston, he would occasionally visit our school. I never spoke to him during that time, because I had said all I was going to say to him—period. All the while, I was studying him trying to figure him out. From my martial arts background, I surmised that he was a pretty good fighter and usually prevailed in his boxing matches. He even predicted when and in what round he would knock opponents out. I concluded that he was an accomplished athlete and boxer. He knew that I admired that, observing that he trained strategically. From my martial arts and karate training, I admired people who actually trained and were disciplined. My instincts told me that he truly had potential!

On the threshold of his Sonny Liston Heavyweight Championship Prize fight, the then Cassius Clay was in his prime. This confidence enveloped him, which was soon to become his trademark. He stopped calling Sonny Liston by his name and started calling him a nickname—'Bear.' Clay psychologically flipped the switch from fighting to playing, which was a tactical intimidation maneuver on Sonny Liston. The mind game became one whereby he was merely playing, yet his opponent was relegated to fighting. On another occasion, Floyd Patterson failed miserably in attempting to use this trademark tactic of verbal warfare and called him a 'Rabbit.' Muhammed toyed with the nickname, so when he got in the ring, he carried a bushel of carrots in his corner. At which time, he announced: "Eat this rabbit!" The intimidation for his opponent was as strong and resilient as the religious intimidation that I displayed years earlier. He always said: "When I do these little tricks, they don't fight straight. They just get upset. When you get upset with somebody, you can't think through the fight properly. Your training all goes out the window. Because when you're angry, all you are is *angry*. Anything is likely to happen. It's impossible to be on point or focused."

The rest of this story is recorded in infamy. Sonny Liston got on National TV for a pre-fight interview. During that time, he noticed that Cassius Clay was hanging around with a lot of Muslims. Sonny just assumed that he was already a Muslim, at that time. Sonny Liston proceeded to make a fatal verbal error, when during his televised interview concluded with this final statement. The knockout blow was soon to be delivered before one punch was even thrown. Liston disclosed: "I'm gonna knock that Black Muslim out!" Furious at Liston's statement on TV, I was offended and abruptly replied: "*Why* did he say '*Black* Muslim?' We're just Muslims. I didn't know we're now coming out with colors of Muslims." His statement made me angry when he profiled and pigeonholed us as Black Muslims. My anger turned into inspiration shortly thereafter. I just knew I had to do something to make 'Clay' as I called him, irritate this Liston. So, I wrote a poem for Clay hoping that I might see him again before the fight. My intuition and inspiration kicked in again, for I had never written a poem in my life. I shouted for someone to give me a paper and pen. A brown paper bag was thrust into my hand with a pencil and pen. I was writing with lightning speed. Within minutes, someone said: "He's in the building." When he came to the room, I shouted: "Hey, *Clay,* come here!" He said, "Me? Are you sure you want *me*?" I replied "Yes, you." As he approached me, I said: "Clay, I don't like Sonny Liston. I'm telling you that right now. I just don't like him! He calls us *Black* Muslims. I want to support you to win because I do not like him." I gave the poem scribbled on a brown paper bag to him, turned around, and walked away again. Later that evening, I was washing the dishes after dinner, pondering the poem I gave him. I wondered if Clay even read it or would do anything with what I had written, but I had peace about the fact that I did what my heart told me to do. I got the words out of my spirit and made the effort to tell Clay what I thought. At least I made the gesture to tell him.

Our household was a traditional Muslim home. My father was a very stern and insightful man—a serious Muslim. Whenever my father would summon one of his children into his quarters and ask a question, it was assumed that he already knew the answer. If you would ever dare to lie, you knew you were in *deep* trouble and there would be consequences. So, when my father summoned me into the living room that fateful night, I immediately panicked and thought, 'What *have* I done?' His piercing gaze penetrated into my soul when he asked me: "Did you or did you not write a poem for that fighter today and give it to him? Did you do that?" I was forced to acknowledge: "Yes, Dad. I did. Uh, huh. But how did you find out?" He continued: "Well, he said he got this poem from a little Muslim girl today. He's on TV and ready to read this poem right now!" Clay positioned the paper bag front and center of the TV as he proclaimed my poem on air to the world:

This is the legend of Cassius Clay.

The most beautiful fighter in the world today,
This fear fights great. He's got speed and endurance.
But if you try to sign the fight? Increase your insurance!
This kid's got a left, this kid's got a right,
Look at the kid carrying the fight!
The crowd is getting friended there's not enough room
They all lead Lords there's the boom!
That's the upgrade: Who would have thought when they came to the fight?
They'd see a spook satellite!
No one would dream when they put down their money,
They'd see a total eclipse of the Man named Sonny.

I was elated that he actually read it! He made my scribbled poem on a brown paper bag instantly famous. I counted that day, where our history and destiny first collided as one. I said to myself, "This guy is all right. He's obviously got potential. He truly listened to *everything* I said and showed a vulnerable side that day, when he seemed embarrassed with his simple remark, 'You mean me?'" I said to myself, "Oh yeah, He's in." Everyone congregated at the Mosque again, a few days before the fight. This time, he came to me, almost for approval, when he asked me: "You think I'm gonna win?" With boldness, I laid my heart and soul down before him in a short pre-fight sermon: "I know you're gonna win. You have all these Muslims praying for you. I'm praying for you. You can't lose. God will give you the power to win, because you have faith. You had faith in me to do what I asked you to do with my poem and declare it to the world. You did it. This is the price of these demands that we live by. So, if you have faith in me, I have faith in you and God will have faith in both of us. Never underestimate the power of our Creator, because if you're sincere in what you're saying, you're sincere in your belief, God is going to take care of it. That's all you have to think about. Don't worry about anything else. It's in God's hands. You just win and make this day count."

When that day came and he got into the boxing ring, with that decisive Prizewinning Title win, he was ecstatic! He proclaimed to me, "I know who the real God is." He continued, "You said, I'm the greatest. I know that God is *real*. He's the greatest!" How passionately excited, down to his soul he became, because Clay didn't even know how good he was until God put the power in his hands to win. He was instantly and undeniably convinced!

This was the next sequence of events for Cassius Marcellus Clay to become a Muslim and transform into the Icon Muhammed Ali. He proceeded to ask the leaders: "If I can be a Muslim, and if I become a good Muslim, will I be as smart as that little girl? Our leader affirmed that would be the case. Clay went on to inquire, "Can I always talk to her? I feel like I *must* talk to her. If you will give me permission to talk to her, I'm in. If not? I won't join." He got his permission, became a Muslim, and was drafted soon after.

With the Vietnam conflict escalating now to a War and in full display to America, a personal conflict arose within the now Muhammed Ali, who was then drafted. He didn't want to disrespect his country. This southern boy didn't want to go against his own religious people either. The military explained his special scenario: due to his status as the Heavyweight Champion, he would merely sign the formality of a paper, and be a part of the Army and the U.S. Military. They assured him that he wasn't actually going to fight in the War. They'd allow him to fight in the ring like Joe Lewis did in World War II. He pondered deeply about it, and concluded to himself he could do just that, but wanted to check these terms and conditions out with his Muslim Hierarchy first. Despite the Military's elaborate array of enticing options, thankfully he paused before he committed. He thought he also better call that little girl too, now a teenager, to inform her of his decision. His Muslim brothers dissuaded him as well, but I indignantly and unabashedly laid out our core faith and delivered his next life changing sermon. When he called, I explained what a conscientious objector was. Those were the real faithful Muslims. Whenever the Military comes to draft one of them, they reply respectfully and honestly. Simply stated, "I'm a Muslim and we don't fight in wars." He recanted with his personal caveat, that he wouldn't actually have to fight in the war. He would just join the Army and still fight like Joe Lewis did in World War II. He would just represent the Army by fighting in the boxing ring. Heavy, my heart and soul pounding, as though it was outside of my body, I emphatically replied, "Devout Muslims don't sign any document like that—Period! When you sign your name on that document, you must do whatever they tell you to do. It doesn't matter what they promised you, you have to do what they tell you to do. You have orders, and they own you. If they say jump, you say how high? Once you sign your name, they own you." Then I gave a jab-hook with my final TKO question: "You trust a white man for that? True Muslims when they come to the draft, they turn it down and reject it. Muslims don't join the army. They sacrifice themselves, even if they go to jail."

  Then the courthouse merry-go-round began for this new Muslim named Muhammed Ali. He appeared in court panicked that he would be thrown in jail. However, the government didn't put him in jail right at that moment. They took him to court threatening to charge him with a charge of draft evasion. If he lost this case, he would be sentenced to jail for 10 years, or pay a hefty fine between $5,000 to $10,000 which was a large sum of money in the 60s. He fought in court, and stated in his case that as a Muslim, he was a conscientious objector, and it was against his religion to take people's lives. Making a similar parallel-case to Jewish people, explaining that his decision was based on a foundational premise of his religion. I encouraged him to pray, and he would win his case. It will be just like when he prayed before he fought Sonny Liston. I felt it. With tears in my eyes, I said: "You're going to win because God is with you already. He already prepared a path for you to win this battle as well. Most importantly, you have to first stand up for your beliefs: I know you told me you wanted to be famous. Well, this is your ticket. Guaranteed. Once this is over, everyone in the world will know your name. Now, it's up to you to make the decision."

He paused for a moment still fearing the consequences of possibly going to jail. I reminded him that faith often demands sacrifice. I assured him that he wasn't going to jail because the Government just wanted that money. It took as much muscle, focus, and tenacity as being in that boxing ring. He had to be strong and resilient for all his other brown brothers in Vietnam. I reminded him of this small history lesson on how they made ancestors slaves, called you nigger, and burned their houses down. We prayed about it together, and he made his decision to follow his heart. It took tremendous faith and internal resolve, and recall and counted that day a blessing when they called him up and stripped him of his title, his passport, and license—everything that he worked, dreamed, and lived for. They stripped him of everything, except his dignity and convictions. The Government used him as an example because of his fame and Muslim faith. I admonished him throughout this traumatic ordeal to fight for all the people who needed to stand up for what they believed and fight for true freedom. They were banking on him getting out of shape and pitting everything against him. Since he wasn't going to fight for America, they decided to condemn him to an extreme verdict and fine. Only a convicted felon loses their passport. Muhammed Ali had not even committed an actual crime—only the crime of standing strong and firm in his beliefs.

I quickly evolved from preacher to motivator to assist him in seeing the big picture. They wanted to shackle him down in his own country to still be controlled by their beliefs. If he'd retained his passport, since he was so famous at that time, he could've gone to another country, lived like a king forever, and never come back. But he played the hand that had been dealt him and eventually won. He had said years prior that he was "The Greatest." Now it was time to prove it again.

I became his support and trainer, having my 9th Degree Black Belt in Karate. I knew that it was only a waiting game, and eventually, they'd give him his License back. All the nay-sayers were betting that he'd get soft and out of shape. I believe one of the reasons I audibly heard that still soft voice whispering in this little 10-year-old girl's ear "You're going to be in his life forever" was manifested for this time in our lives as one of those 'not just counting the days, but making those days count' moments which was now.

How we made those days count, as we immersed ourselves in our newly enforced vortex as I became his trainer. The Government and critics were all counting on him to get out of shape, lurking in the wings with an anticipated great White Hope to beat him. Then, they would be satisfied and vindicated. This standstill and arduous waiting game took three years, and during those three years, I focused on promoting him as the people's champ. My intuition kicked in once again: if public awareness and his subsequent popularity indeed elevated him as the people's champ, his detractors would see him out speaking and still being in top shape. They would aqueous and be forced to give him back his license. It was a perfect combination of my martial arts training, and his passion for boxing, that provided our training platform and focus.

Boxing as an elite sport is a true discipline and boxing was his entire life. He was already a talented and good fighter. Being in exile brought us into a closer and more eminent and lifelong dimension. It was then that we were married. In addition to our spiritual alignment, I was also called to support us financially; I was truly a Muslim entrepreneur, sewing clothing and cooking for our community. A few months into this holding pattern and process, an epiphany came over me with a dose of entrepreneurial PR (Public Relations). Feeling in my heart that they would give him his license back soon, our recipe was going on the road to different colleges. He would earn a little check for speaking and we would return home. The repetition of this road-trip and public speaking increased his visibility and popularity. Soon, it became the trend to join our crusade and fight for Ali rights. Writing some of his speeches, sewing, cooking, and driving was truly work, but I knew it would all be worth it when I saw my husband back in the ring, doing what he was destined to do.

Finally, our victorious day arrived! Living then in Philadelphia with our oldest daughter and twin baby girls, I was in the kitchen when that infamous phone call came. After answering the call I screamed from downstairs, at the top of my lungs, "It's Jesse Hill, from the Boxing Commission on the phone! He said you just got your license back!" Stunned and in shock he said, "It's a joke, right? Don't play with me!" I summoned him downstairs to the kitchen phone. Indeed, it WAS Jesse Hill. When Muhammed heard the news, he dropped to his knees and sobbed. Our day had come, and my faith spoke to me daily during those three years. I knew he would be reinstated. We both collapsed on the floor together, cried, embraced, and prayed in thanks to God. Redemption was ours. He won the case! Throughout his life, Ali remained thankful that I stuck with him, during this period of crisis. I believed in my husband, father, and professional boxer with my heart. Through this tremendous turmoil I evidenced the true power of a woman steering the wheel of marriage as we became closer than ever.

Instantaneously, after he won his reinstatement, the Commission announced his fight with Jerry Quarry. There was more to overcome during his expulsion than just a boxing license reinstatement. People misunderstood our religion and believed that he was turning his back on America and wasn't being Patriotic. Some Blacks even joined in, saying that he was weak and wasn't strong enough to fight for his own country. It was never about the lack of love for his country, but his predominant love of God. When the public found out that Jerry Quarry was to be his opponent, they immediately labeled Jerry 'The Great White Hope.' When Quarry was interviewed on TV, he was questioned why he even agreed to fight Muhammed Ali. Quarry's straightforward reply was simply: "He has every right in the world to fight. That's what he does. He was the Heavyweight Champion, and you never should've taken his license away." Jerry Quarry was such a classy professional, who supported us during our three year ban. Jerry just treated him like another fighter, and Muhammed in turn responded being respectful to him. This mutual respect was especially epic to observe, since the venue was in the Deep South of Atlanta, Georgia.

On fight night, racial tensions were extremely high, because a lot of people, especially white people, came out in droves protesting against Ali. Unfortunately, I couldn't be a part of this event for redemption, because of the heightened racial disturbances and ensuing unrest. We agreed that it was more important for me to take care of our daughter and our newborn twins. Ali won decisively and reclaimed his Heavyweight Title. However, basking in the ecstasy of his victory was fleeting, when I received a threatening phone call. This onerous male voice bellowed: "He won, but you all lose when the bomb goes off at midnight!" Frozen in time, I hung up the phone. Startled and shook, however, I moved into action and I immediately called some of our close friends to tell them the dreadful news. I resolutely gathered up my girls and headed to a safer haven in the city line of Philadelphia. Our friends panicked, but I remained calm. It wasn't logical that if someone was going to blow you up, why would they pre-announce the event and time? I wasn't in fear because I'd stared down cowardice in the face before. Muhammed Ali was a man who lived faith, his religion, and stood strong in both. Why would a person want to kill somebody for that? After I pondered my own unstated question, my own faith again rose to the surface, and I began to pray for him.

Belief:

That intuitive voice inside my heart that spoke to me the night of our bomb threat was that same voice that first spoke to me about Cassius Clay when I was a little girl attending that Muslim School in Chicago. When I first laid eyes on Muhammed Ali, then Cassius Clay, walking confidently down the hallway—the voice of destiny that whispered: "This man is going to be in your life for the rest of your life." The true essence of a woman is having that ultimate and intimate conversation and relationship with your Creator, yourself, that then transfers and transcends to your man. A woman's essence is compounded when she listens to her instincts. All women, especially, are born with that 'inner wiring' and gut feeling. Those feelings are reinforced, when we pray, and make our daily ritual of prayer—especially against the Evil in this world. Prayer is the spiritual martial arts magic that allows anyone to act in faith, unconditional love, and forgiveness. These three are a true TKO recipe for spiritual abundance and a fulfilled life. Add a dose of common sense, and prayer becomes a habitual practice and standard to live by. Feel your feelings. Your instincts are your instincts. With intention behind these instincts and feelings, The Creator will guide and connect more of your life together than you ever would imagine. Your faith becomes that connection to the blueprint and proclamation of life. No one can truly predict anything on a goose-bumpy feeling. More than a prediction, intuition with intention is the ultimate trust in Guidance from The Creator. Through this guidance, especially through the bumps in the road of life, the faith and forgiveness code becomes magic for any couple, when the woman initially listens to this intention. Then, any couple can draw closer, with deeper intimacy as husband and wife.

When you feel something, you should act upon it, for you already have a pre-ordained conviction that it's right and a right decision for you. Although you may count the days, initially listening makes the days really count. It doesn't matter the intentions of what you're striving for, God will always bless you. It may not be the way you envisioned it, for we never planned for three years of being banished from Professional Boxing. But it always is as boldly glittering as a Heavyweight Prize-winning belt adorned in sparkling glory. Trust that God puts these thoughts and desires into your heart and mind. Be sincere about your intuition with intention and elevate it with a dose and frequency of love.

The essence of a woman, especially with her man, is one of support, laying a feminine and secure foundation. In my case, my secure foundation was first based on Faith. Muhammed Ali was the first professional in sports to be called the G.O.A.T. (Greatest Of All Time). This new title was born out of the fact that he first proclaimed himself "The Greatest." Now, in my storied and colorful life, I've now been honored and referred to as the G.O.A.T's G.O.A.T. I smile and shake my head, with an inner knowing, reminiscing and counting back the days of how I made each of those days count. Supporting my Man, and especially in a TKO of *"Undefeated Faith and Forgiveness,"* has been the greatest gift in the world: My true essence of a woman.

Action Steps for Faith and Forgiveness:
- Keep your focus: Life's situations are all temporary.
- Listen to your heart and intuition.
- Never waver in your faith.

Dr. Khalilah Camacho-Ali
Author, Actress; Filmmaker, Motivational Speaker, Philanthropist
www.MamaAliToday.com
TKO2020@yahoo.com

Dr. James Marinakis,
ND, HmD, Acu.Phys.

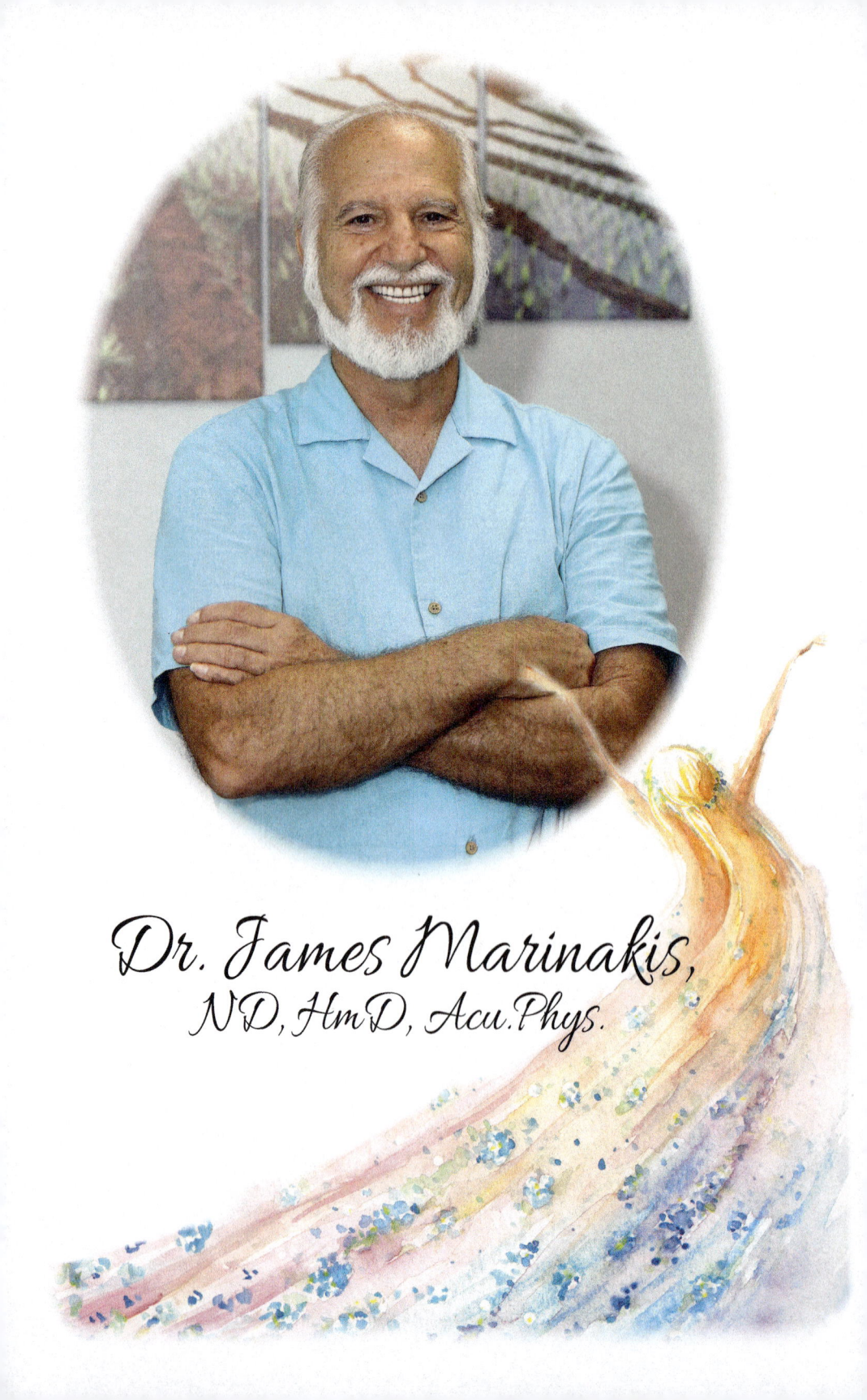

Humanity's Core

"The Essence of a Woman is in everything!"

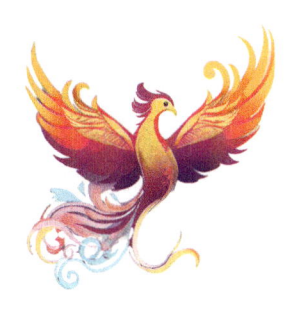

Intention:

The essence of a woman is almighty. Keep that in mind when you ponder the words, hell hath no fury, like that of a woman scorned. And put that next to all the funny, fuzzy little animals, like rabbits, guinea pigs, gerbils, and mice. She is severity.

Story:

Constantly observing and experiencing and learning from others, not only by what they did but also by what they didn't do. At age thirteen, I tragically lost my father. He was, a physically strong individual, about 6 feet tall and built like a line-backer with Herculean fortitude. He surrendered his life to a miserable bout of cancer caused by lead poisoning. Watching him waste away in the sterile hallways of the hospital, I had full awareness that my Dad didn't want to die. Peering at the sheer magnitude of the facility, and the doctors and staff bustling, it dawned on me that you needed something more, something absent in all of this magnanimity

The next thing that propelled me toward my destiny occurred when I was an athlete in high school and began to study nutrition and whole foods under the teachings of the world-famous physiocultopath Paul Bragg. I was able to gain a competitive edge despite lacking years in experience. My ascent to victory was very short-lived and a severe knee injury abruptly canceled my dreams of an Olympic gold medal. How could I have known that I was on a collision course with my own destiny.

I rejected the surgery due to horror stories from many athletes in various sports. The swelling subsided over time. The pain was only present when I fully extended the joint, but it was excruciating when I tried to bend and put all my weight on my knees in a squatting position. I walked normally, but my knee was unsound. In an unimaginable chain of events, after three years of lost dreams and ignoring the impediment, I came into contact with Dr. William J. Huls, a world-famous osteopathic physician, pathologist and scientist, who had ended a parasite epidemic in the Southeastern United States just after the turn of the 20th century. What I suffered with all those years, that guided me away from sports and into academics was all changed in seconds with one swift and precise manipulation of my knee. As I left the man´s office with no previous intention I inquired about where I could learn this not so unfamiliar manipulative therapy. Unbeknownst to me the only reason this 78-year-old physician had returned to private practice was to find his protegee, his progenitor. I carried on his work. However, I supplemented it with nutritional therapeutics and prescriptive exercise, organizing it into a profession which has come to be known by a word, called Myopractice.

Life continued to press ahead. Treating and seeing 30 to 60 people per day became my norm I worked in the clinic by day and taught by night. I incorporated the first school of Myopractice and graduated the first students. From there I departed to California continuing my practice and formerly studying Traditional Chinese Medicine at the first university, organized by the Sino-American Rehabilitation association as set up under the Nixon administration. I later worked for the State of California as an examiner for physicians to be licensed in oriental medicine.

Now, ten years and 35,000 patients later, my work spread purely by word of mouth to all corners of the world with patients coming from nearly every country and all walks of life. In the pursuit of the truth as to what else was needed which that hospital did not have to offer to my father, I left my comfortable and celebrated life with a 5,000-square-foot palatial home in Malibu California overlooking the Pacific Ocean, and headed East.

I had created an idyllic life: I married a would-be movie star of a wife and fathered two extraordinary children, a boy and a girl. With their Malibu birth certificates, a community that has no hospitals, I began my new life in Boca Raton, Florida.

Discussing a respite in the Caribbean while I was working as a consultant for a probiotic engineering group from California funded by Japanese partners, Ann and I instead were treated to a transformative healing weekend. The techniques experienced there involved reprogramming the biological computer using unique modalities ranging from vibrational healing and plant medicine to new techniques in neurolinguistics.

I reincarnated myself and over the next few years I established myself a global teacher. Over the next three years I traveled frequently to Rio de

Janeiro and the Bahamas, and later to other destinations throughout the region, mastering my craft. After three years of intensive studies, I planted myself at the Eastern edge of the Florida Everglades, finally. Born of the asphalt jungle of Boston, Massachusetts I acquired my first piece of heaven. I purchased a working horse farm on the outskirts of the prolific and lush wilderness at the edge of the Florida Everglades. Immersed in the natural habitat and surrounded by wildlife, I began my research and proving the many technologies. Some saw me as an egregious fanatic, others, a total visionary that was far ahead of the trends and on the cusp of something exceptional.

As part of my research, I used the opportunity to develop dogs that could immunize themselves to the most lethal virus known as parvovirus, without medications. Something that has come in very handy over the last few years especially during the pandemic. Had it not been for the ignorant but zealous county employees who destroyed the breeding program, the whole world would have known about it before the pandemic.

All those years of my schooling in multiple fields of naturopathy, homeopathy, and traditional Chinese medicine, in the end, amounted to knowledge mostly. Through innovation, I was fortunate and blessed enough to find myself emerging as a world-renowned, multifaceted physician at the apex of the true global healing phenomenon we now embrace.

Philosophy-Manifestation:

The Ten Commandments which transcend mere religious doctrine and embody a narrative of profound significance that intertwines with the essence of femininity. Moses begat this Divine message with the symbol of a flame—the heart of this narrative is the burning bush—a powerful symbol of divine presence and maternal care. This moment serves as a manifestation and representation of the Divine Mother, the quintessential essence of a woman, who nurtures, guides, and shapes humanity's moral compass.

The burning bush, from which God spoke to Moses, is a striking image that evokes the characteristics of the Divine Mother—the Divine Feminine. It is a manifestation of life, vibrant and consuming, yet not destructive. This paradox reflects the nurturing aspect of femininity—capable of both creation and transformation. Just as the bush burned without being consumed, the essence of a woman embodies resilience and strength, providing sustenance and warmth to all.

At any divine moment, any person can call on humanity and will receive a roadmap for ethical living, encapsulated in the Ten Commandments. These commandments serve not only as directives for behavior but also as reflections of the values traditionally associated with femininity: love, compassion, fidelity, and justice. They guide individuals toward a life that honors relationships and community, emphasizing the importance of caring for one another, akin to a mother's foresight to protect and nurture her children. This mandate is humanity's core which is embodied in the essence of a woman.

The essence of a woman transcends mere biological definitions; it embodies a profound understanding of existence itself. This essence, often characterized by intuition, empathy, and nurturing qualities, invites us to explore the deeper meanings of life and creation.

It descends into every woman at the moment of conception, remaining there for life to protect the new souls and spirits as well as the deliverer, the mother. However, to fully grasp this reality, we must first comprehend the concept of "essence" itself. Rooted in languages such as French, Latin, and Greek, the term carries significant weight, particularly in its Greek interpretation: "I am." This notion resonates with the biblical declaration of Jesus of Nazareth, who famously stated, "I am" and "I and my Father are one." (John 10:30). These profound assertions reflect a spiritual connection that transcends gender, encapsulating both the feminine and masculine principles inherent in existence. Beyond the spiritual core, the essence of a woman is in the physical core of all we as humanity are as human beings.

Essence can be understood as the fundamental nature or intrinsic quality of a being. It is the divine spark that animates all things, whether they are living organisms, objects, or abstract concepts. In various religious and philosophical traditions, essence is often equated with the divine, encompassing terms such as God, Allah, or the universal spirit.

In biological science, the interplay of male and female principles is evident in the reproductive process—the "birds and the bees." Each individual carries within them the genetic legacy of both mother and father, yet the presence of the infinite essence ensures that every person is a distinct manifestation of creation. This individuality highlights the importance of the three pillars of existence: Knowledge, Wisdom, and Understanding. Together, these elements form a cohesive framework often referred to as 'The Holy Trinity,' which represents unity and interconnectedness in the universe.

To ask, "What is Woman?" is to delve into a complex and multifaceted inquiry. Woman embodies the archetype of the holy grail—the ultimate source of life and creation. She represents structure, the receiver of life, the nurturer, and the manifestor of dreams and realities. As a mother, she becomes the bringer of life, nurturing not only her children but also the potential within every individual she encounters.

The essence of a woman is found in her ability to connect deeply with others and to foster growth and understanding. This nurturing quality is not limited to biological motherhood; it extends to the broader community, allowing women to serve as healers, mentors, and guides. The essence of womanhood is thus intertwined with the essence of humanity itself, as women play a crucial role in shaping societies and cultures through their compassion, resilience, and strength.

The interconnectedness of 'essence' reveals that both women and men share a commonality that transcends gender. Each individual, regardless of their gender identity, possesses the potential to embody the qualities traditionally associated with both the feminine and masculine essences. This interconnectedness serves as a reminder that we are all part of a greater whole, a reflection of the infinite one God. The essence of a woman, therefore, is not isolated; it exists in everything and everyone, manifesting in diverse ways across different cultures and contexts. Just as my father embodied such physical strength and character, my mother bestowed an emotional spiritual 'essence' and core for our family. An illustration of this was the mural that was painted on wall in the living room of our home which always displayed, in a billboard-size font, with the words of the Serenity Prayer:

"God, grant me the serenity to accept the things I cannot change, the courage to change the things I can, and the wisdom to know the difference."

She navigated the direction of our entire family with these words.

Just as I recognize my mother, wife, and daughter within these words, we, as men, recognize the essence of a woman as integral to the fabric of existence within all human beings. We honor the contributions and experiences of women throughout history. Women have been the backbone of families, communities, and nations, often sacrificing their own desires for the well-being of others. Their strength and resilience are testaments to the profound impact they have on the world, shaping the future through their nurturing spirit and unwavering commitment to life.

Women are humanity's core, similar to the Ten Commandments, which are more than a set of rules that represent a vision for a harmonious society. Each commandment resonates with the essence of a woman's nurturing spirit. For instance, the call to honor one's parents reflects the foundational role of motherhood in shaping character and values. The commandment against stealing underscores the importance of respect for others' boundaries and possessions, mirroring a mother's teaching of respect and integrity.

In a world often fraught with conflict and division, the Commandments offer a timeless framework for unity and understanding. They urge humanity to rise above selfish desires and to act with compassion—a trait deeply embedded in the entire human experience. The essence of a woman, as illustrated through these commandments, is a call to embrace empathy and to foster connections that transcend individual needs.

The impact of the Ten Commandments is an everlasting legacy and extends far beyond their immediate context; they resonate through time, shaping cultures and societies. This enduring legacy mirrors the influence of women throughout history—often the unsung heroes who have nurtured and guided generations. Just as the commandments provide a moral framework, women have historically been the custodians of values and traditions, passing down wisdom and nurturing future leaders.

Contemplating the Ten Commandments through the lens of a woman's essence reveals a rich tapestry of meaning that speaks to the heart of humanity. The burning bush symbolizes the Divine Mother, whose nurturing presence offers guidance and strength. The commandments serve as a roadmap for ethical living, reflecting values deeply rooted in the feminine experience.

As we navigate the complexities of modern life, the teachings of the Ten Commandments remind us of the enduring power of compassion, respect, and love—qualities that define the essence of a woman. In embracing these values, we honor not only the divine feminine but also the potential for a more harmonious world grounded in the principles of empathy and understanding. The legacy of the Ten Commandments, emanate from the essence of a woman, is everlasting, guiding humanity toward a future filled with hope and promise.

The essence of a woman is a powerful and multifaceted concept that encompasses understanding, nurturing, and the divine connection to all of Creation. As we have unearthed the depths of what it means to be a woman, we uncover the intricate relationship between essence and existence. Ultimately, the essence of a woman is indeed found in everything, illuminating the path toward greater understanding and unity in our shared human experience. The essence of a woman is in everything!

Action Steps for a Woman's Essence:
- Embrace your multi-faceted gifts as a manifested being. .
- Acknowledge your core gifts and contributions to the world.
- Reach deep to discover the Divine Mother in you!

Dr. James S. Marinakis, ND, HmD, Acu.Phys.
www.vitalessence.com

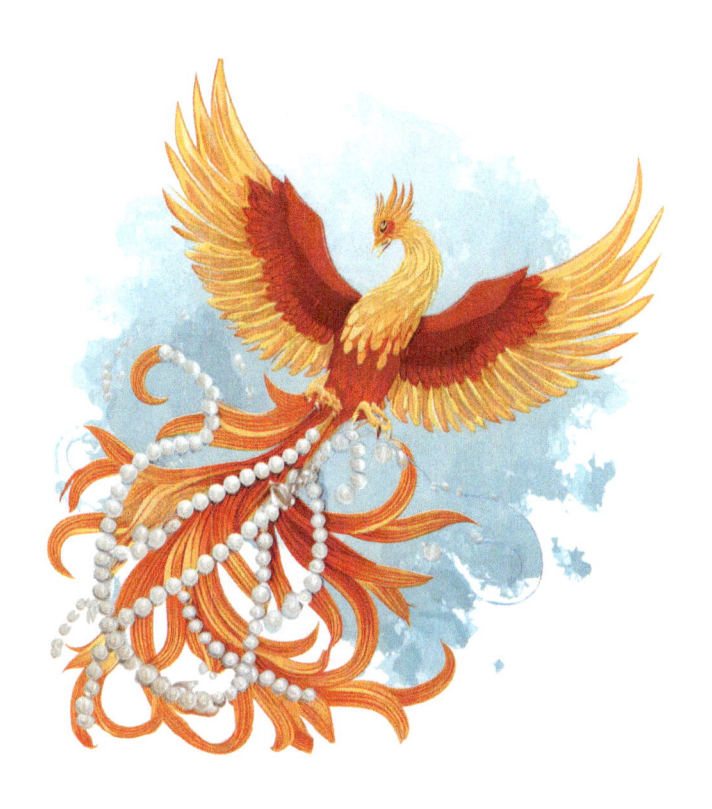

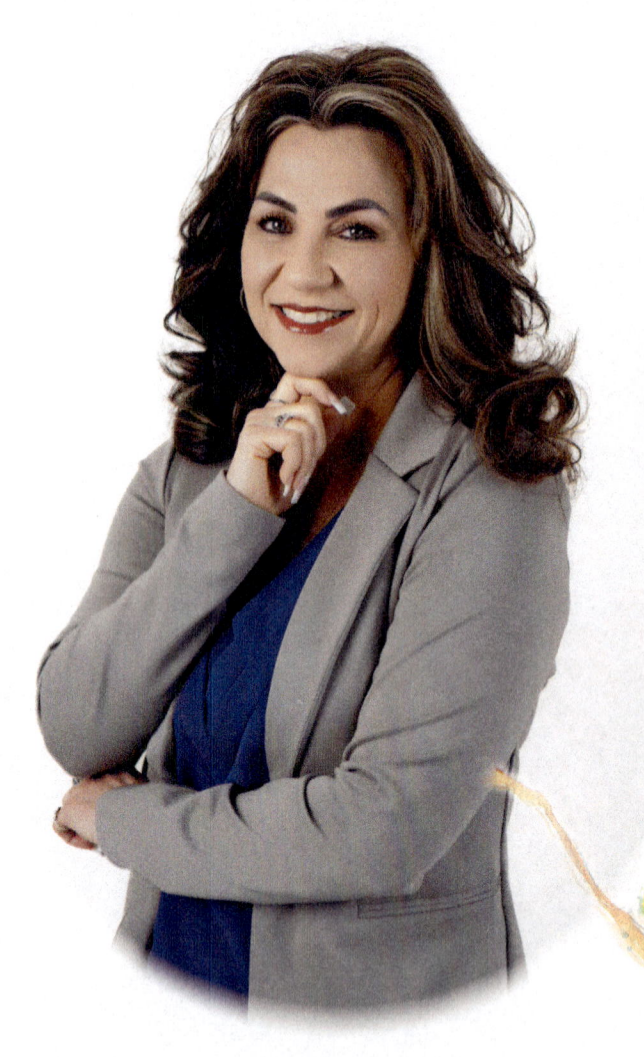

Shannon L. Roper, FNP-BC

The Virtuous Path of a Family Nurse Practitioner

*"Redirect your desire for control:
Live in the peace and joy God intends for you."*

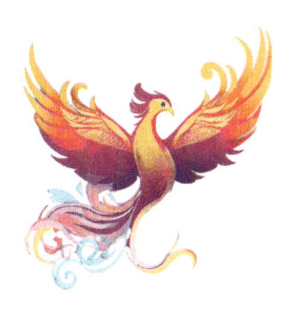

Intention:

All too often, we fail to live in the moment and completely dismiss the importance of what God is trying to show us. We worry about what we should have done yesterday or will need to do tomorrow and miss the blessings of today. Worrying is the work of demons acting to divert our attention away from our spiritual journey. Ultimately, it deprives us of the love and devotion we should be giving to and receiving from our Lord Jesus Christ. May you reflect on my words, as worry dissipates from your mind and soul, and may you be filled with peace.

Story:

Women are often expected to embody the qualities of love, grace, joy, and peace. How do we become women of virtue and be willing to submit to the life God wants us to lead without a proper role model or guidance? First, we must understand and firmly believe that virtuous women must walk in humility, love, and forgive one another without carrying grudges or ill feelings toward those who have offended us. These are not natural attributes. They must be observed, nurtured, and implemented into our daily routines until they become a normal part of who we are as women. We must also strive to avoid drinking negative energy into our mind, which turns into a diabolic poison that degrades our spiritual well-being, our relationships, and our physical health.

The phrase *'Fear Not'* is mentioned 365 times in the Bible. Everything happens for a reason and it is no coincidence that this number is equivalent to the number of days in a year. God is encouraging us to trust in Him, reminding us that no amount of worry can add a single moment to the length of our lives. We spend countless hours worrying every single day, mostly over things we have ZERO control over. I am encouraging you to give your concerns to God, early, often, and daily.

My personal path that led me to the peace and joy that I experience today required daily devotion and acceptance of God's Word. I put a personal line down in the sand because I was done pretending I was truly satisfied with my life. I decided I was done choosing to live in fear of the unknown with the "what if" mindset any longer. I began to pry open the door to self-examination—which is painful and never an easy task, but essential for progression through a true spiritual health transformation. I instituted journaling as a method of self-analyzation to try and determine my inner issues so that I could begin the healing process. I also incorporated reading self-help books and praying A LOT! Through these activities, I retraced my childhood wounds which were never addressed, and continued to infiltrate my adult life.

As a Practitioner, I was so focused on making everyone else healthy and happy, that I never took the time or put forth the effort to heal myself. My transformative examination was liberating as I lifted the mask of who I was trying to portray, and began to *make sense* of my life. Weaving a fictitious web of lies and living under false pretenses, I uncovered the destructive self-talk I was using for survival. I was unhappy in my personal life, which infiltrated into a definite lack of discipline in my spiritual walk. I was dedicating every ounce of energy to my family and my patients, resulting in a lack of love and respect for my own self-care. One of the most significant obstacles I uncovered was my unending desire to be in control of everything. The demon of control was literally affecting every aspect of my life! In my mind, if I was in control, I could prevent any potential failure. By overthinking, analyzing, and anticipating ALL potential variables, I thought I could control the outcomes. I pray you will resonate with this concept and understand the level of exhaustion it produces.

I was raised to believe in God but was not faithful in attending worship services. One of the most beneficial things I learned during this time was how pleasant and soothing it was to pray. I was hurting from traumatic past experiences including the death of my grandmother as a child, to the death of my nephew ten years ago. Unfortunately, these events are still plaguing my family today. So, I started praying every night for Jesus to help me out of the crater I had grown accustomed to as normal.

I had never spent much time alone as an adult. I needed to be in a relationship in order to "fix" someone or something. During the time I was trying to heal, I forced myself to be alone in order to get to know myself as an individual. I spent lots of hours praying, shed countless tears, and many sleepless nights. It was painful but worth every second for the growth I achieved in my mind, body, and ultimately my soul. Once I reached the milestone where I understood who I was as an individual, I began to pray for a strong man to come into my life who put God first and would lead me forward by his example.

Soon thereafter, I met a wonderful man named Robert who gently grabbed me by the hand and guided me through all the necessary changes I started to make. Just like me, he had issues from his own past he was working on, but God was speaking to him as well. He could see the trauma in me and even though his defense mechanisms were telling him to run, God was telling him he had work to do. I am very thankful he not only listened but heard and obeyed Him.

Within weeks, our spiritual growth together began when he asked me to attend a charismatic Catholic Conference in Alabama with Father Jim Blount. The conference was sold out but a friend of his was unable to go and graciously offered her ticket to me. It was My *"Golden Ticket"*! Her misfortune was life-changing for me and I will forever be grateful to her for allowing me the opportunity to attend. I was a little nervous going since I was not a member of the Catholic faith but I knew it was what I was supposed to do. After three days of prayer, testimony, and education, my spiritual desire was ignited! I wanted to know MORE! I met so many genuinely caring and inspiring people while we were there and their love of God was contagious.

On the final day, Father Blount took a moment to bless each attendee individually. The auditorium was full with more than 500 people so it took several hours for our turn. I was so nervous to go up to the front and sit down. I watched each person and what they did so that I would know exactly what to do before it was my time in the spotlight. He would anoint the forehead with holy oil and then exhale to drive the demons away. When it was my turn, after the anointing with oil, Father Jim's eyes grew as big as saucers as he stared into me. He exhaled and then exhaled again and then he smiled as he looked off in the distance behind me. My body was overtaken by a warm sensation, full of emotion, and I felt as if I had lost 20 pounds immediately. When it was time to stand, I was unable to stand on my own.

My legs were weak and shaking. I was tearful and scared. I knew Father Jim had just saved me from the demons who had been ruling my thoughts for so long. Robert assisted me out the side door supporting me so I didn't fall. That was the most powerful experience I've ever had and it set the stage for my new future! At that point, I realized God was speaking directly to me, and it was not too late to seek Him. I was the stray who on that day He sought out when He left the other 99 sheep unattended to come find ME! Why? Because I am worthy of his love and forgiveness.

When we returned home, I began reading various books about the Catholic Religion and decided to join the Church. In September, I began the Rite of Christian Initiation of Adults (RCIA) classes. This is the process through which non-baptized men and women progress through the curriculum in order to enter into the Catholic Church. We met every Thursday evening for 2 hours to learn, explore, ask questions, and grow spiritually together in our faith. Most of those in attendance had been raised in the Catholic Church and were there to complete the sacrament of confirmation. As an adult convert, I was learning all the things they were exposed to through their education as children. I was digging deeper into the meaning of the different rituals while they proceeded to just go through the motions. There were times I had questions but was afraid to bring them up during class. As a degree practitioner in life, I didn't want to look dumb personally asking something everyone else knew the answer to. Towards the end of our classes, I figured out they appreciated my questions because looking at things from an adult perspective versus how it was presented to them as a child was very insightful.

Recently, I was baptized and received communion for the first time, and I was confirmed into the Catholic Church. I now appreciate the essence of life itself, with purpose, peace, and joy. I no longer struggle with the need to fill my life with objects to feel complete. Identifying worry at the outset and relinquishing the things out of my control have become a miracle in a daily life of peace and joy.

Philosophy:

Living many years as a people pleaser, I prided myself on the health and well-being of those patients who entrusted their lives to me as a Board Certified Nurse Practitioner. It became even more clear to me that the majority of society is consumed with worry, stress, and a lack of self-awareness. All of these unnecessary activities result in producing inflammation which leads to chronic disease. I make it a point with every patient, every day, to remind them of the importance of perspective. God says for us to *Fear Not*. Now, it is even more prevalent in the scope of care, to provide them with ways to redirect their focus on those aspects worthy of their energy consumption.

Chaos and confusion are not fruits of the spirit. The demons of guilt and shame are designed to divert our attention away from our spiritual journey. We have choices. We can choose to surrender our will and our obstacles and live in love. We can release fear. We can decide we want to live from the spirit of giving: receiving our love and guidance from the Lord Jesus Christ. I have done my initial healing and am so grateful and fortunate to have a wonderful support system and a man of faith walking beside me to navigate the growth and transition. I no longer feel like I have to battle life on my own. God continues to provide guidance and has opened doors I never would have attempted to enter.

Through prayer, education, journaling, and LOTS of practice on my communication skills, I discovered many details about what guides how we all respond to trauma. For 30+ years, I dedicated my efforts to the healing process of others as a nurse, educator, and then a provider. I have experienced the essence of true joy by assisting my patients in removing barriers to their spiritual growth. I find this extremely necessary in order to allow themselves to be genuinely loved—so the real healing of the whole person may begin.

Fear has many meanings to individuals and may vary depending on one's current circumstances and past experiences. As I shared earlier, I experienced the loss of my grandmother who was a significant part of my life when I was five years old. As a result, I discovered that I began to live in fear that those who were important to me might be gone at any given moment. This fear became disabling and spilled over into every section of my life as I grew. The fear of losing something important to you leads to the development of people-pleasing behaviors, emotional eating, and dysfunctional relationships. Recently my own beloved mother went to heaven on the same day as my grandmother so many years ago. PAIN and sorrow? Yes, but it no longer has control over me.

Living a life in fear causes women to become aggressive and controlling. This cumulative trauma response results in the day-to-day functioning in survival mode which is just existing instead of living! This type of activity is not what God intends for anyone. By embracing my Savior, I gave my life to God and do my best to follow His Commandments. I am so thankful that this allows me, and can allow you, to exhibit strength through the power of your role as a Christian woman.

This virtuous path has been extremely therapeutic and beneficial, and I am thankful for all the support I have received along the way. I look back at the person I was a year ago and have a difficult time recognizing her. I look at photos taken recently and also find it difficult to identify who I have become. Change is inevitable and necessary, but not easy. If you have found yourself lost, anxious, sad, or feeling unworthy, please don't think you must deal with it alone. Start doing the daily work. The real, actual work to strengthen your faith and your relationship with God. That means getting real with yourself and deciding to dedicate your time and effort to growth! Not the fake, behind-the-scenes, cover story that makes you look good on the outside but doesn't get the job done in your soul. Take it from the master of *"I'm fine; everything is fine."* I have discovered the word FINE is really the ultimate masque for insecurity and neurotic emotion. You cannot do this alone.

Proverbs 31:26 — A Virtuous Woman Speaks with Wisdom and Kindness

> *"She opens her mouth with wisdom, and the teaching of kindness is on her tongue."*

Be that virtuous woman: Live in peace and joy.

Action Steps:

- Value your worth: Challenge yourself daily to self-reflect through the eyes of Jesus.
- Love yourself first: So you can properly love others.
- Spiritual mindset: Being truly loved by God is better than any type of medicine.
- Choose confidence and love: A woman's finest accessories to adorn her beauty.

Shannon L. Roper, FNP-BC
Family Nurse Practitioner
Roper's Health Oasis
www.ropershealthoasis.com
shannon_roper@ropershealthoasis.com

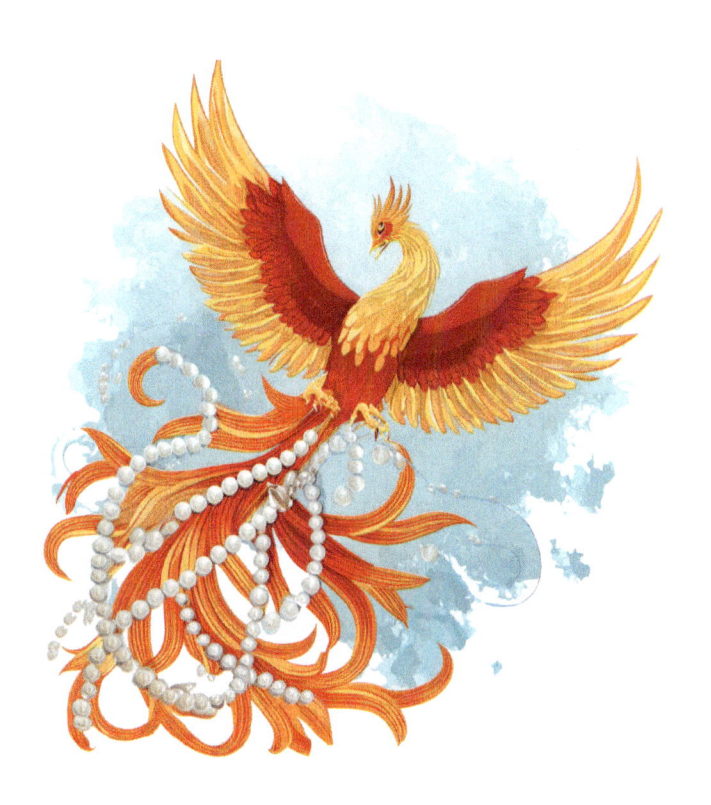

Shannon L. Roper, FNP-BC | 37

Dr. Nephetina L. Serrano

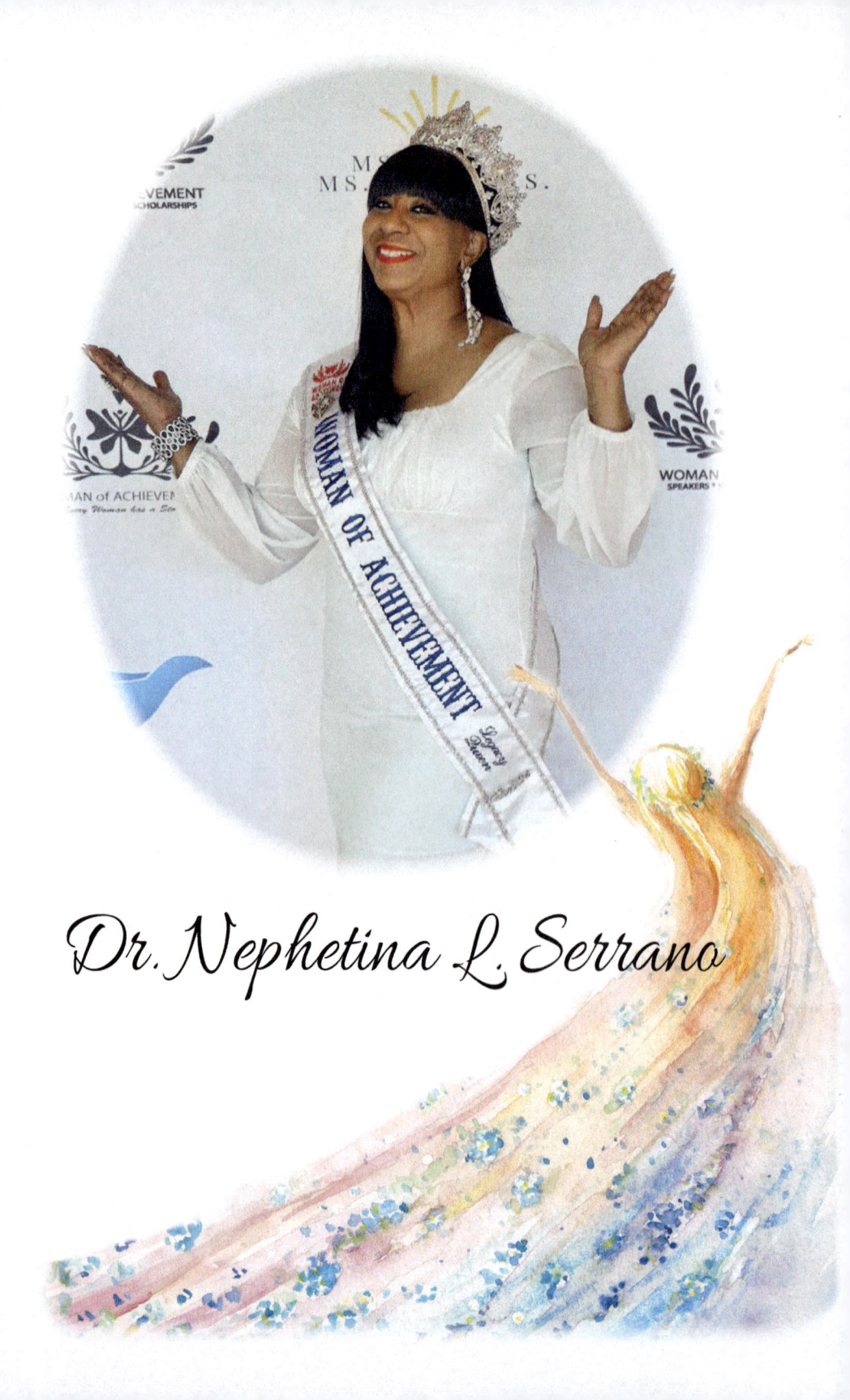

My Dream Personified—
A Woman's Spiritual Mandate

*"Woman; Thou art awesome and wonderfully made,
and in thy loving and nurturing energy lies
the key to divine light."*

Intention:

This is a mandate statement to remind you that you are a beautiful queen molded in the perfect image of your Creator. As you move boldly forward on this path of self-discovery and empowerment, wipe away the tears of regret and embrace the dawn of a new day.

Story:

Right from the outset, I recognized that, as a woman, I had a spiritual mandate to fulfill. I knew I was on a journey to become a dream personified. A pivotal moment arrived for me at the age of sixteen. I was faced with making the toughest choice of my life. Afraid and alone, and just emerging into womanhood, I walked away from my family. I left my younger siblings and my home to be on my own, and to pave my own path in life. I left them to be with people I had only recently met in an unfamiliar neighborhood. My conflict was real. I could no longer tolerate a situation that was inimical to my well-being. My trust in those who were supposed to protect me was shattered. There was no turning back. Overnight, I was transformed into an adult woman. Destiny was calling me to a higher place. I could feel God even though I could not see Him. I heard God whisper, *"I got you."* That gentle, yet powerful voice gave me strength, tenacity, and hope.

Leaving home was a truly frightening experience. The emptiness I felt was unimaginable. As I filled the black trash bag with my personal belongings, I wondered if this was the right thing to do. Who would look out for my siblings? Yet, I was convinced that this was a season of discovery in which I had to tap into my divine destiny. I drew strength of purpose from my self-confidence, my innate abilities, and my faith in the God who had promised never to leave me or forsake me. No matter how I was treated, or what I went through, I knew God would see me through. I kept the words, *"The fight is fixed, and you have won."* I was taught the power of prayer as a young girl and had learnt to talk to God a lot. God gave me the strength I needed to pack my bags that night and escape. I use the word *"escape"* because my mom would have never let me leave, and my dad would have had a fit. My siblings would have cried their eyes out. Yet, I had to leave to rescue myself. By the time everyone woke up in the morning, I would be gone. Although I had no definite plan for how I was going to chart a new course for my life, and although I knew only too well that I desired to see my family again someday, I was determined to make it on my own.

Life had prepared me for independence from an early age. I had been working since I was fourteen, buying my own clothes and paying my own way. However, stepping into the unknown with a trash bag full of clothes and a few personal items was a whole new level of independence. It was around this time that I met Richard, the man who has been my husband and partner of thirty-five years. His kindness and support were a crucial part of the journey to becoming my dream personified. I persevered to finish my last year in high school, with the hope and desire of going to college, which for me was never a question of *if*, but *when*. Yet, my sudden relocation put me at a temporary disadvantage as I had to leave school for one school semester in order to care for myself and my needs. I was in a fight for my divine purpose as a woman, and I was committed to that fight.

Philosophy:

God had given me a spirit of discernment to be able to separate those who were not for my greatest good and those who were. Were that not the case, I may not have been married to the wonderful man who is my husband today. As a woman, I have always worn my spiritual armor as described in Ephesians 6; The *belt of truth* protected me from the deception of the enemy; the *breastplate* of righteousness protected my heart from the enemy's accusations; my *shoes* of the preparation of the gospel of peace readied me to walk in tranquility in all my dealings; my *shield* of faith created a barrier against my trials; my *helmet* of salvation protected my mind from thoughts that did not serve my greater good; the *sword* of the Spirit allowed me to take an offensive stance to slay my goals with grace and elegance.

I believe that the essence of a woman is comprised of many parts. While her physical beauty is immediately apparent, her spiritual beauty lies within. She is under an obligation to care for the combined well-being and intellect that contributes to her overall beauty in order to nurture her power, beauty, and love. She was created in God's perfect image, as a living example of His character, and a crown to His glory. The woman is a light, and a force to be reckoned with on Earth, both reflecting her lasting influence and divine purpose in life. She allows her light to shine before others, such that they may see her good deeds and glorify her Creator in Heaven (Matthew 5:23). Women are powerful, unique, and beautiful. As the Proverbs 31 woman, we are the walking, living, and breathing dream personified.

I subscribe to the *essence of a woman* as exemplified by the scripture in Hebrews 10:24. As women, we can spur and encourage others toward love and good deeds. We become stronger when we understand that we are not in competition with others. We should eliminate conflict, and flow in the beauty of purity, for we recognize that the "iron" in us sharpens the iron in those around us (Proverbs 27:17). The divinely-connected woman has access to supportive sisters who possess those traits that she wants to exhibit in her own life. Her tribe of sisters cheers her on, offering resources and guidance, while keeping her aligned with her divine purpose. Her community will listen to her, encourage her, and affirm her, but also question and challenge whenever necessary. She recognizes that meaningful resistance offered in a safe space of love promotes growth. Naturally, she contributes her own quota to this tribe while continually pouring into and mentoring other women into their own greatness. She should always find herself doing something to help someone else, whether it is in educating, encouraging, uplifting, or inspiring other women to be more, do more, or grow more.

There is a God-ordained path that is laid out for us as women, which we must take in order to reach that place of the fulfillment of God's promises for us. We must meet certain expectations and attain certain standards, exhibiting exemplary and imitable behavior. We journey to fulfill this purpose by rising up to it, acknowledging that we have been given the gift of life that we must utilize in a meaningful way. We must submit to God and make our paths straight with Him (Proverbs 3:6). We have an obligation to God to trust His Word, to believe Him, to walk in faith, understanding that there is work that we have to put into life, because if we put nothing in, we can get nothing out.

We must continue to seek the Divine on this path so that He can rejuvenate, refill, and strengthen us in our walk, talk, and way of being.

In this way, we are receivers, first receiving from Him so that we can process our experiences in understanding, and then giving back in such a manner as to positively impact and influence others. As the epitome of the Proverbs 31 woman, we should speak with wisdom, and with faithful instruction on our tongue *(v26)*. We should walk in the integrity, and in an understanding of the law of the land. We can then use what God has given us in grace, humility, and class. In social circles, we should be friendly and inviting to others. How we treat others and interact with them matters a lot, if only because we are the true influencers, and the original "content creators."

Women are innately purposed and designed to be receivers, birthers, and nurturers who learn to love others by loving themselves. They thrive in collaborative relationships, as they are co-laborers with God who have been designed as helpmates to their husbands. Also, they are always ready to support other sisters on their own journeys. Enlightened women recognize that they are not in competition with their sisters, brothers, or partners. They also do not constantly play the blame game, attributing and imputing negativity to others in such a manner as to deflect responsibility from themselves. The enlightened woman recognizes that the enemy is not her sister, or the woman next door. The enemy is simply the enemy *within*, and the power to overcome that enemy lies *within* them.

We receive so that we can birth children. Whether these children are physical children that we naturally birth with our bodies, or ministries, or dreams and goals that we birth creatively and spiritually, we are to nurture them, giving guidance, leading by example, and providing instructions to ensure the sustainability of our legacy. The woman protects the legacy of what she births because as she abounds in the work of the Lord, she is well aware that in Him, her labor is not in vain (1 Corinthians 15:28).

Women are nurturers by nature. We take what God gives us to birth and nurture to maturation. In that way, we are tremendously resourceful. Through our brilliance, we are impactful. We are the ones who others want to listen to, as we give advice and guidance. However, in order to nurture others, we must first love and nurture ourselves. We are powerful, graceful, anointed, and highly revered. But we must look in the mirror, looking past our exteriors to look deep within, excavating and treasuring our intrinsic value, loving ourselves first, in order to impactfully love others. Likewise, we lead ourselves in order to effectively lead others. As Matthew 22:39 affirms, we should love others as well as we love ourselves. The common adage is, *"We can't pour from an empty cup."* This rings true for women who recognize that they first need to seek God to fill their cups in order to overflow goodness into the lives of others. That is why our prayer should be, *"Lord, I ask that your blessings might cascade into my life, and fill it to such overflowing that it pours into the lives of those I encounter by Your Special Grace."*

As born leaders, women both love and lead by example. In order to lead from that space, we must be thoughtful and intentional with how we coordinate and utilize our resources. Our dealings should be well-planned, making our intentions plain and simple. We must also be diligent with our hands and intentional with how we flow, educating ourselves on how to learn, grow, and inspire others. The Proverbs 31 woman worked well with her hands, and because she was intentional in her dealings, she laughed without fear of the future (v25). The essence of a woman lies in fulfilling her God-given purpose walk, and not allowing distractions to take her out of alignment, and out of the place and direction in which she is supposed to go. She may walk through the valley of the shadow of death, but she will not have to fear or succumb to others' beliefs of what they think is right because she believes what God says about her. She can do all things through Christ that strengthens her (Philippians 4:13). In that way, she is unstoppable. She trusts in the Lord and leans not on her own understanding (Proverbs 3:5). In that way, she remains focused. The work that God has begun within her, He will also see unto completion (Philippians 1:6). The enemy's devices cannot stir her. She dresses herself in the full armor of God (Ephesians 6:10-18), allowing opposition to prompt her into action, further igniting the authority that she knows she has, so she can walk in dominion and serve faithfully on Earth. She is the woman who knows how to rise above the ashes and move forward.

It's probably no coincidence that in the story of creation, it was when man was put to a deep sleep that woman was birthed. Is it be possible that woman was the dream; a long-awaited desire that, when paired with his, would turn the world on its axis, allowing humanity to take true dominion and authority on Earth, and in the divinity of God's image? In this way, woman, her etymology combining the words *womb* and *man*, becomes an incubator for birthing greatness and a legacy for humanity. She truly is the living, walking, and breathing dream personified.

As a light on Earth that inspires others to fulfill their legacy of greatness, the woman's social mandate reflects the Light of the Creator, her God-given ability and her divine purpose. *"In the same way, let your light shine before others, that they may see your good deeds and glorify your Father in heaven."* (Matthew 5:16, NIV). Not only is it important that she fulfills her purpose, but it is equally important how she fulfills that purpose. She is clothed with strength and dignity, (Proverbs 31:25), always being gracious to those around her in kindness and in a willingness to be an example of triumph for others. She has been divinely comforted, so that she might comfort and divinely illuminate the life of others. In order to attain this state of consciousness, she must look deep within, recognizing her authenticity, excavating her purpose from deep within, and make actionable and intentional decisions towards that purpose.

Action Steps:

- Look at the woman in the mirror, and ask yourself these questions:

    What are my strengths?

    What makes my spirit beautiful?

    Who do I see as I see myself?

- Stand in front of your mirror and affirm to yourself as follows:

    I am fearfully and wonderfully made.

    I am the head and not the tail.

    I am above only and not beneath.

    I am a lender and not a borrower.

    I live in health and wellness.

    I live in the overflow of wealth.

- Write down your primary life goal; your major definite life purpose. Identify your divine calling.

- Commit to nurturing whatever you have birthed into greatness.

- Continually review the action steps above as a daily exercise in your life journey.

Dr. Nephetina L. Serrano

U.N. Global Ambassador for Peace, Relationship Expert, The Marriage CEO

Covenant Rescue 911 501c3

E-mail: drserranoministries@gmail.com

www.marriageCEOs360.com

www.covenantmarriagesinc.com

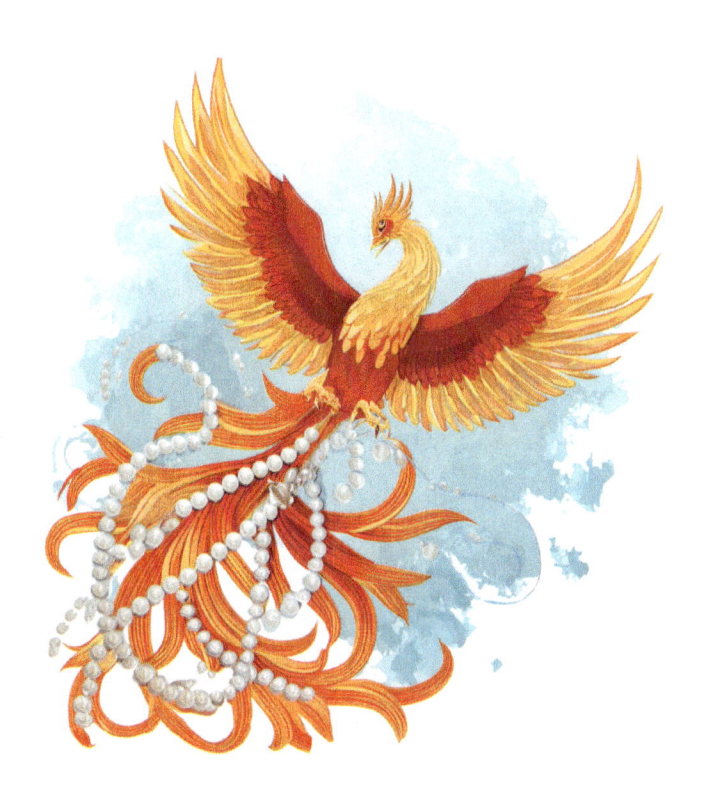

Debbie Morales

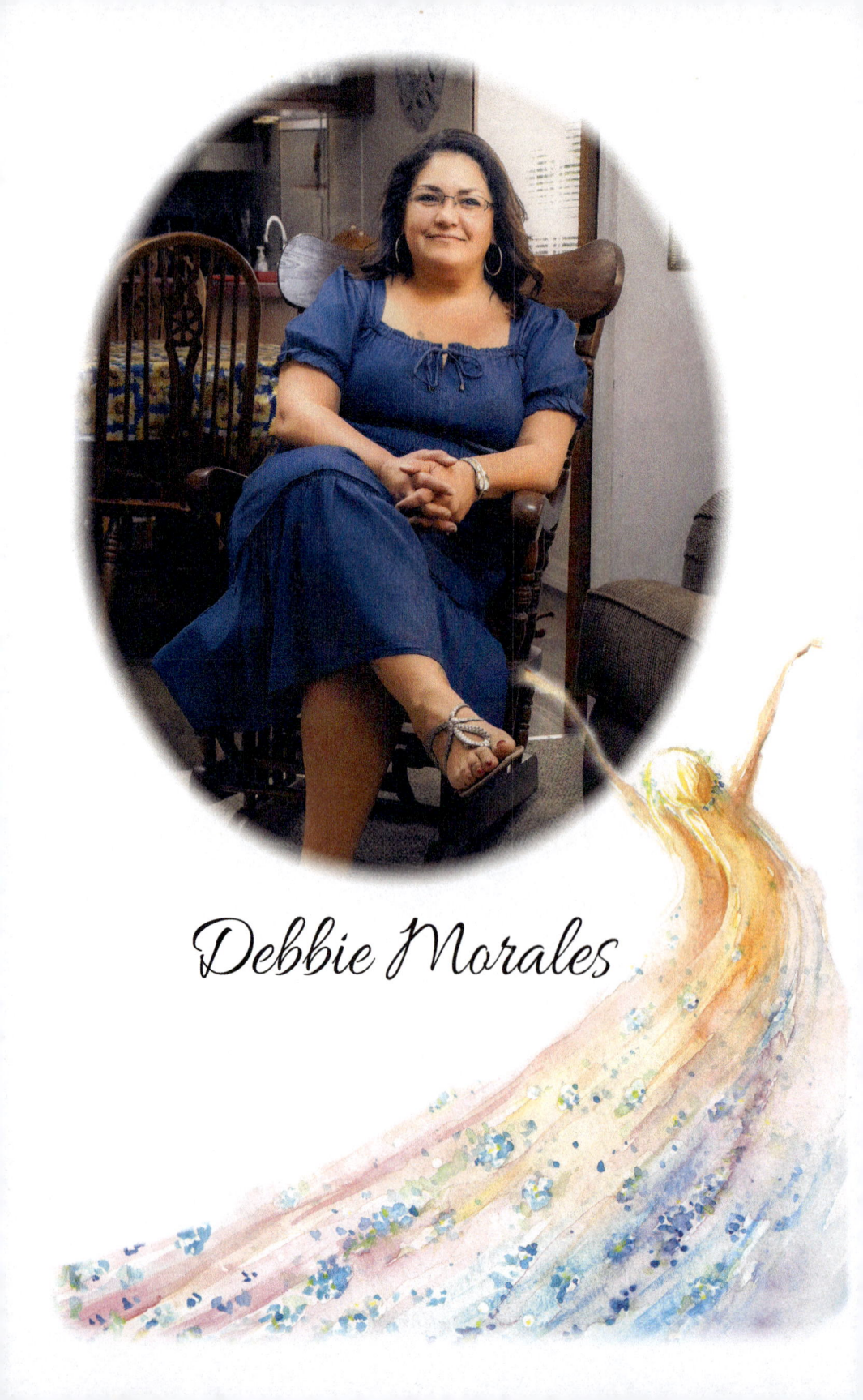

Love's Formula: Forgiveness and Healing

*"Love does not define God.
God defines love, defining me."*

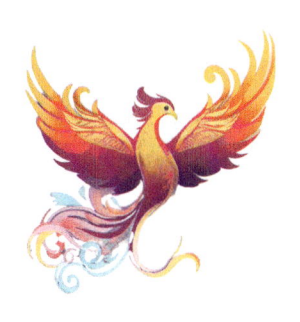

Intention:

My journey towards healing and life begins and ends with the God of the Holy Bible. May my words be used to help others better understand and experience the restoring love and power of God in a personal and practical way in every season of life.

Story:

Like many, I was introduced to Jesus at a young age. Though the atmosphere in my home was dysfunctional, to say the least, my parents still took me and my siblings to church. I did not understand much of what was being taught, yet God pierced my soul as a child. The message I walked away with from those years in the church was that Jesus was crucified on a wooden cross for my sins. That message eventually brought me to my knees and thankfully defined me.

Examining my history was essential to understanding where certain beliefs and behaviors began to develop. This practice is beneficial to everyone.

My parents divorced when I was eleven years old. The streets became my primary dwelling place as this is where I found acceptance and what I interpreted as love. I ended up pregnant at age sixteen and living in a homeless shelter in Ft. Lauderdale Beach, Florida.

Randomly, I would take the city bus to the church with my baby boy and sit in the back pew when God intervened and a couple I knew from this church offered to care for my son until I got on my feet. Initially, I declined the offer. Weary after eight months of homelessness, I accepted their offer and my son went to live with them.

I began working extra jobs in an attempt to get my son back when *a certain crowd* entered my life. Drugs are seductive, which started as a social thing and spiraled down rapidly. I was bound by the chains of addiction for a seemingly eternity of fourteen years. Everything I held dear vanished in the midst of this addiction. I was in and out of jails, hurting myself and those I loved—I was empty. Drugs were my escape from reality.

I knew there was more to life than this—this could not be it. I tried everything known to man to conquer this monster that consumed me. I admitted myself into rehabs, and detox centers, and attended too many meetings to count.

Due to my upbringing in the church, I was aware of God's presence throughout this mess. From time to time, I would pray and ask God to forgive me—yet I would whirl back into the abyss of destruction. Until one fateful night, God intervened and gave me the grace to understand my need for Him as my Savior. I will never forget that night. In a drug-induced high state of mind, I walked down a dark road on a mission to talk to God. I begged God to take me away from everything and everyone I knew. I wanted to live, I just didn't know how or where to begin.

One week after that prayer, I woke up in St. Augustine, FL, 280 miles away, with no memory of how I got there. I woke up in a hotel room in Northeast Florida and found myself, once again, going to jail. I was sitting in a holding cell when I was reminded of my prayer on that dark street that night, and I knew God heard the cry of my heart.

I had a choice to make. I could go back, but what did I have to go back to? That road was well-worn and lifeless. Or I could trust God with my life from here on out, a road of forgiveness not traveled. In that jail cell, I decided to trust God and began seeking *Truth*. I requested to speak to the Chaplain concerning God and His Word. I wanted to know this God in whom I was putting my trust. I desired to know this God who claimed to be loving and forgiving.

This is when God brought Joan Clements into my life. She was the Founder and Director of the Women's Refuge of St. Johns County, St. Augustine, FL, which I entered upon my release from jail.

The Women's Refuge of St. Johns County is primarily a discipleship program. It is an intensive twelve-month residential program where women can start over with a true understanding of God's love, purpose, and plan for their lives. At the Women's Refuge, we become students of the Word of God. We are engrossed in daily studies and counsel. In addition, we address and work through every emotion and area of life: traumas, fear, anger management, codependency, boundaries, forgiveness, and so much more. We walk through an individual's entire life, taking the resident woman deep into their past. The method of walking through one's history is critical to the healing process. I learned how my upbringing, time in the streets, and addiction shaped me.

It was only when I fully surrendered my life to *the* Savior, Jesus Christ, and in becoming intimate with *the truth* of God's Word that I truly was set free, breaking the chains that held me captive for so many years. Have you heard the saying, "The truth will set you free?" It is scriptural and true. I'm living proof. I have been set free! Words are not sufficient enough to explain, Jesus must be experienced.

> *"If you abide in My word, you are truly my disciples, and you will know the TRUTH, and the truth will set you free."*
>
> —John 8:31–32

Why does our Creator offer us eternal life? Because of love. God defines love. Love does not define God. It is crucial to have a deep understanding of love. We are all on the search for love until we are restored to Love.

There are numerous recognized forms of love. However, the scriptures narrow it down to four base forms. Understanding each form of love encourages the ultimate love journey, providing insight into the freeing, healing power of our sovereign Creator.

- **Phileo love**: The emotional bond found in deep friendships.
- **Storge:** The natural love shared between family members.
- **Eros**: A sensual or romantic love.
- **Agape love:** The perfect, unconditional, sacrificial, and pure form of love. This love was displayed on the cross, where in the verse:

> *"God so loved the world that He gave His only begotten Son, that whoever believes in Him should not perish but have everlasting life."*
>
> —John 3:16

Circumstances, human logic, and emotion separate all other forms of love from Agape Love. Emotional and circumstantial love is conditional, which leaves room for discard. The love of God is faithful, eternal, and unending, and does *NOT* reject the seeking heart!

> *God's greatest gift to mankind is Himself, for "God is love."*
>
> —1 John 4:8

> *"God was in Christ reconciling the world to Himself, not imputing their trespasses to them."*
>
> —2 Corinthians 5:19

Until we are restored to Love, we have a love deficit, which leaves us on the superficial, never-ending search experiencing temporary satisfaction. God's love displayed through Jesus provides eternal healing, forgiveness, and wholeness, meeting mankind's greatest need.

> *"But God demonstrates His own love toward us, in that while we were still sinners, Christ died for us."*
>
> —Romans 5:8

I did not deserve to be forgiven. Yet again, God's love does NOT leave room for discard. The love of God forgives, heals, and restores the yearning heart back to life.

Following Jesus does not mean that a magic wand is waved and we are now exempt from trials and temptations. Tragedy struck my life when within a mere three-month period, my younger sister passed away in her sleep, and my only son lost control of his truck and went to Heaven. I am so grateful that God restored my relationship with my son after I became sober and saved. These memories I hold dear and sacred in my heart. Then, my Godmother and mentor, Joan Clements, went to be with Jesus, and her husband soon followed, which deepened the hole in my heart. Shortly thereafter, grief struck my family once again and threatened to rip it apart when my sister-in-law passed away leaving behind my brother and four kids.

The grief grew heavy. All this trauma was breaking me as I tried to navigate through my own emotions and life. I felt obligated to hold the pieces together and be strong for everyone. I felt alone, the grief was almost too heavy to bear and, this time, I turned to temporary counterfeit solutions for comfort. I thank God for not allowing me to get too far. His love allowed me to experience a small taste of where I was headed if I stayed on that road.

In my grief, my vision became blurred and I was unable to recall God's Word. I could barely see or hear Him. At first, I was angry at the world and my circumstances. I was confused and hurt at the rejection I faced from people who claimed to love me. At times, I was even angry at God but I never stopped loving Him. Once again, I was ridden with shame and condemnation. The liar whispered in my ear, *"You see, you are still that old person, you haven't changed."*

Holding on to shame, anger, and unforgiveness was preventing me from healing. God used my inner circle of faith who helped me realize that shame had no place in my grief and that grieving did not mean that my faith was weak. Furthermore, God used a speaker at a conference, Sheila Walsh. Her testimony helped me identify what I was experiencing, and I grabbed her book, *Holding On When You Want to Let Go*. The profound message I received was that God had not abandoned me and no matter what, *hold on!* Seeking wisdom from someone who can relate to what you are going through is a powerful instrument in the healing process.

I began practicing forgiveness by laying myself and others at the feet of Jesus, along with my circumstances. As I did this, I began to hear God speak to my heart, telling me to go back to the beginning and recall all that I had learned saying, "Debbie, you know Me and I know you. You are Mine. Abide in My Word." So, I turned to what I knew to be true—His Word.

His promise in James 4:8 says,

"Draw near to God, and He will draw near to you."

I knew I needed to draw near to Him more than anything. Jesus was not only my Savior when He died on the cross and rose again three days later. He is my Savior every single day that I breathe.

"Therefore, let that abide in you which you heard from the beginning. If what you heard from the beginning abides in you, you also will abide in the Son and in the Father. And this is the promise that He has promised us—eternal life."

—1 John 2:24–25

Sometimes, we need to go back to the beginning, and it is ok.

"I will sprinkle clean water on you, and you will be clean; I will cleanse you from all your impurities and from all your idols. I will give you a new heart and put a new spirit in you; I will remove from you your heart of stone and give you a heart of flesh. And I will put my Spirit in you and move you to follow my decrees and be careful to keep my laws."
—Ezekiel 36:25–27

"Though your sins are like scarlet, they shall be as white as snow; though they are red like crimson, they shall become like wool."
—Isaiah 1:18

"In all these things we are more than conquerors through him who loved us. For I am sure that neither death nor life, nor angels nor rulers, nor things present nor things to come, nor powers, nor height, nor depth, nor anything else in all creation, will be able to separate us from the love of God in Christ Jesus our Lord."
—Romans 8:37–39

God's Word began bubbling up in my heart and soul reminding me of who He is and who I am *in Him*. I was reminded that my identity is not found in my circumstances, my poor choices, people, or my feelings, but rather in the truth of God's Word.

We will experience challenging seasons. Though we try, we will not always make the right decisions, but these times do not define us. We are valuable and loved in the eyes of our Creator. Pick yourself up when you fall, learn the lessons, look forward, and keep walking with Jesus.

"For I know whom I have believed and am persuaded that He is able to keep what I have committed to Him until that Day."
—2 Timothy 1:12–14

Currently, I am blessed to be the Director of the Women's Refuge of St. Johns County, working with women coming from places where I have been. While positioned as a lay counselor for many years; I will soon graduate from Liberty University in Christian Counseling where I can further assist women on their journey toward healing and life.

Belief:

I am thankful for every mountain top, every valley, and each lesson. I am thankful for God's Word and for a true faith family who are emblematic of love and forgiveness. I am thankful for the saving power of agape love and grace, praising God daily for who He is and the essence of the Spirit-lead woman I am ever becoming.

Action Steps for Healing:

- Admit your need for healing, hope, and life, and be determined to go after it. *Do not be afraid to ask for help.*
- Know what you believe. Seek truth for yourself. Do the study required to gain confidence in your faith, but also be willing to walk by faith when it is called for.
- Walk through the tough journey of your past with Jesus, and preferably another trusted person(s) of faith.
- Approach everything in prayer.
- Forgiveness is crucial to healing. Practice forgiveness where necessary. Look to Jesus for the motivation and strength to forgive yourself and others.
- Look closely into your life, examine and learn what shaped you. This process will help you discern the healthy from the unhealthy.
- Practice being thankful, pray, learn the lessons, study, laugh, fellowship, cry, rejoice, and abide in agape love.

Debbie Morales
Executive Director
Women's Refuge of St. Johns County
www.womensrefugeofstjo.com

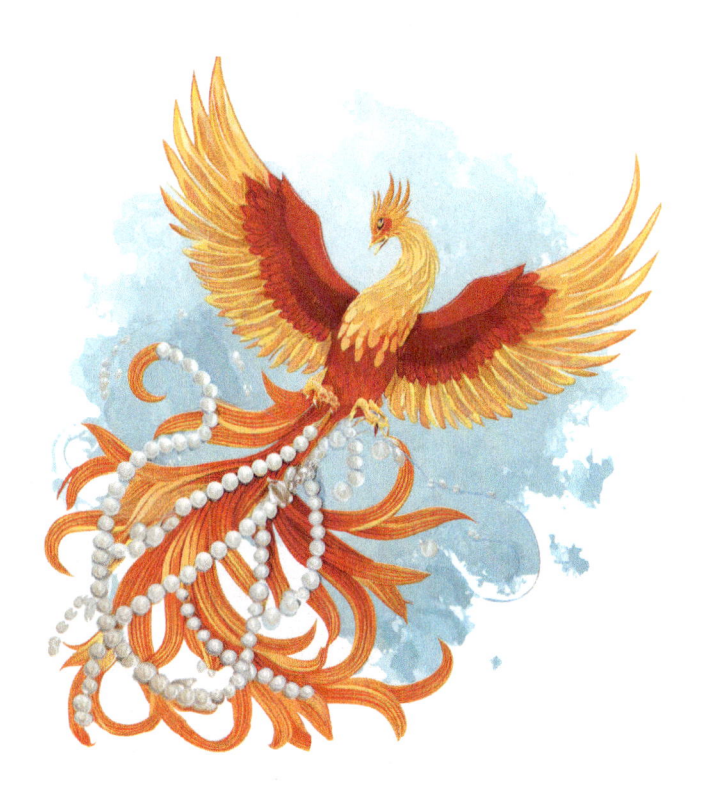

Desiree Peacock

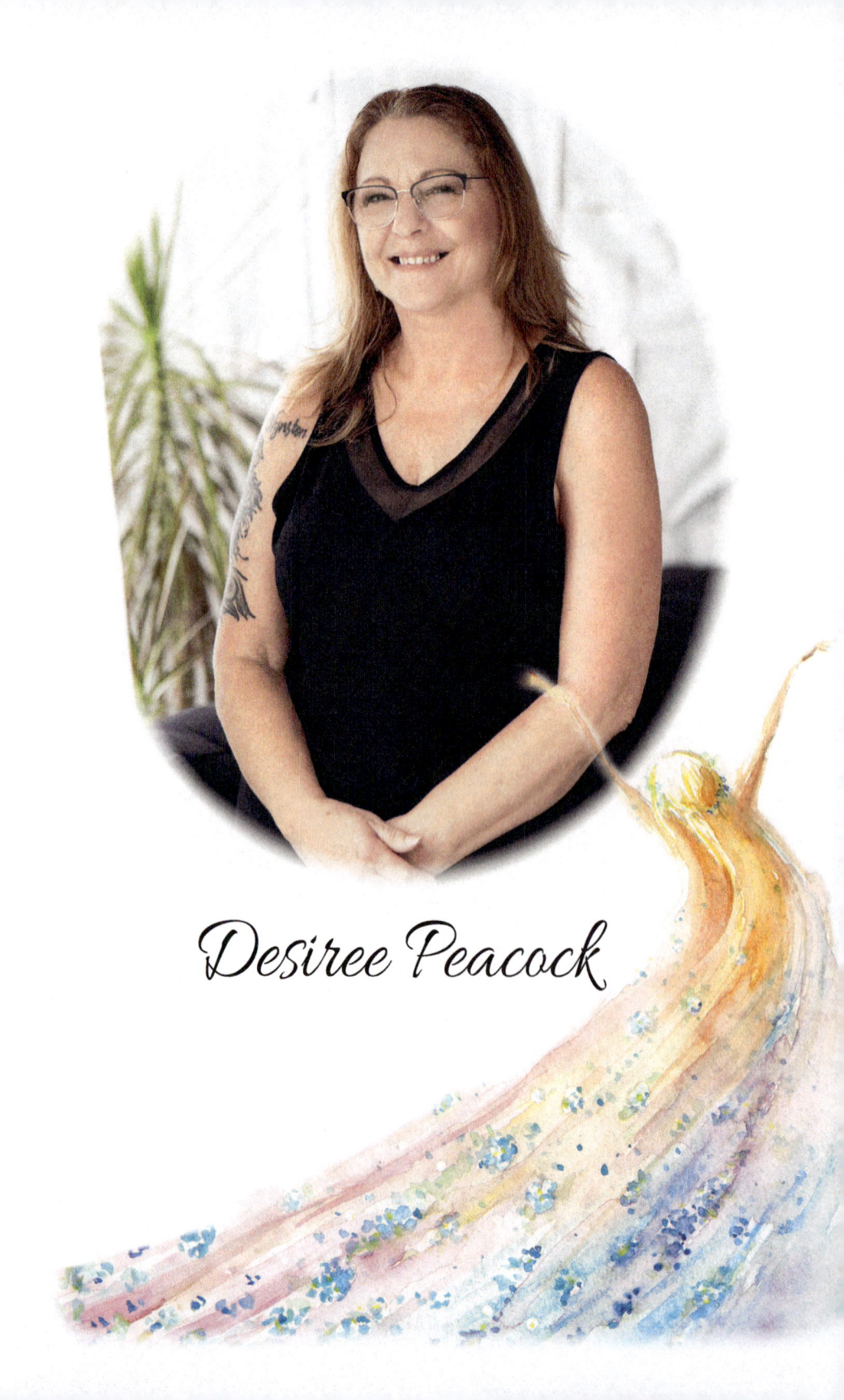

Finding My Identity

"The Pursuit of Happiness is Within."

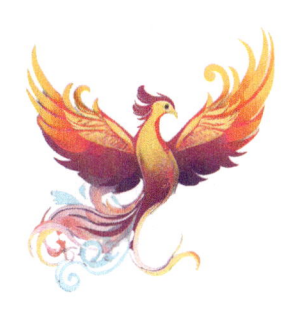

Intention:

By sharing my story and the journey within myself, I hope others will come to understand and experience who they are in Christ. My desire is to enlighten others that the lies and deception about yourself and others do not have to leave us in a prison of unforgiveness with no hope. The war that wages in our hearts and minds can be overcome, and with the sword of the Spirit, we can all have freedom. A ray of light penetrates through the darkness in our souls, revealing the enemy, the guard to the fortress built, facing ourselves and realizing that we are our worst enemy.

Story:

As a child, my family always made jokes about me working in the film industry. I loved to pretend and display what I thought others would accept, hiding behind a mask not to show my feelings. It allowed me to pretend I was someone else, but shame seemed to engulf me like a wet blanket, shaping my life into something I was not.

My parents were divorced when I was just a toddler, still in my most vulnerable and formative years. I spent most of my time with my so-called dad because my mother was always drinking. I did not know then, but she had alcoholism. My mother's absence left me exposed, afraid, and vulnerable to being sexually abused by my stepfather. Abandonment, fear, and unloved emotions made me take on responsibilities and burdens that were not mine to carry. My mother passed away when I was ten years old, leaving me angry and alone. At this time I found out that my so-called dad was not my biological father, leaving me with another missing piece to the puzzle—who was my real dad? This added to feeling unloved and unwanted. My aunt indeed became my advocate and fought for custody of me, severing my stepfather's rights. During this time, it was unpredictable, and I was sent away to live in foster homes and be hidden away in another state, leaving me confused and distant from the only thing I knew: my stepdad. This plunged me into a wall of protection to hide my hurt and distrust towards everyone, including myself. My life was turned upside down, and I blamed myself, which made me angry, and I became very rebellious. At fourteen years of age, I began seeking love in all the wrong places, being promiscuous at an early age. This gave me a way of escaping the guilt and shame by self-medicating through sex, drugs, and rock and roll. Life was uncertain, and I had no answers. I was overwhelmed with the pain of feeling rejected, abandoned, and alone. All I had was an immature childlike reasoning of believing that I was lacking, not good enough, and unloved. I was a misunderstood child unable to explain myself. My family's remedy was to move me from one family member to the next believing they had addressed my problems. Living in their deception that time would work everything out, I decided I knew what was best for me; I got pregnant with my first child at sixteen years old and was forced to have an abortion, making me feel under the ultimate thumb of control. Everyone was working to correct my behavior, but with each attempt through schools, programs, and detention centers, I became a master manipulator. The mask of deception kept me in the prideful prison of showing others I could do it myself.

The journey and highway to hell was an exhausting struggle involving drugs, men, and a battle of my mind. The recurring feelings and behavior left me in a pit of hopelessness. Everything I tried failed; marriages, jobs, even being a mother, and I became worthless in my own eyes. I have three living children and two that are not living. I had taken their lives by having abortions. I was full of pride born out of hurt, and it would have killed me, but Jesus intervened.

A life-altering miracle occurred when, in 2008, I attended the Women's Refuge of St. John's County. The other altar was presented to me when I was introduced to a God of love for the first time! I had grown up Catholic and believed that by breaking one commandment, I was damned to hell and that God perpetually punished people. The seeds of truth were sown into my life as I was a resident at the Women's Refuge, and I believe that is where God became something other than the angry father to me. Unfortunately, I was still performing to be accepted by others, only to be disappointed. So, the path of destruction continued, and I was in and out of jail for drugs and fraud until 2018, when I was sentenced to thirty-eight months in prison. I was alone, pushing my children, family, and friends far away. The wall for protection was no longer working and the things I used to survive were now suffocating me. All I wanted to do was die. I had nowhere to run, and I had to face the enemy within myself.

Until then, I fought to survive, but now, I surrendered, and I have learned to thrive. I felt in my soul that something had to change, and the Spirit brought back to my memory the Women's Refuge and the studies in the Bible. I was content and showed love differently from Joan Clements and Linda Huff, two women who facilitated this program. I began reading my Bible in hopes it would make a difference. I prayed and became brutally honest with God about my beliefs and relationships and how I was consumed by fear. I never thought I would be here today, but Jesus intervened.

My physical problems from car accidents, domestic abuse, and drug addiction had me in pain, a perpetual reminder of what I had done to myself. I had begun to take responsibility for my choices and stopped blaming others. I started seeing how I hurt other people because I was a wounded bird. I stopped internalizing the hurt that was done to me. This was the beginning of my spiritual awakening. The darkness that consumed me started to lift, and God's mercy was given to me while I was in prison. I had to die to myself, which was the beginning of my new identity.

"I have been crucified with Christ; it is no longer I who live, but Christ lives in me. The life I now live in the body I live by faith in the Son of God, who loved me and gave Himself up for me."

—Galatians 2:20

Three years later, I was released from prison, and I was truly free for the first time in my life! I moved into a transition home in St. Petersburg, Florida, run by the Pastors of Seminole Community Church. As God opened the first door into my new life, things started to evolve slowly, at a pace I could embrace. The job I had from being on work release, I was able to sustain and become responsible for working from home. Yet in my newfound independence, my prideful spirit returned with a vengeance; I was still broken from the inside out. The lack of self-esteem plagued me, and I felt insignificant.

My past was littered with regrets. Because of previous bad choices, I had to endure three surgeries in a year, which put me in a walker. It took the mercy of God to walk freely again. The Lord's intervention was another miracle with my physical pain. Today it is gone. Even after successfully regaining my ability to walk, my frayed emotions remained a challenge telling me that I was unvalued. Believing the lies, I resumed my previous survival coping mechanisms or flesh patterns of pushing love away. Thankfully the **Holy Spirit** faithfully visited me, helping me to renew my mind, body, and soul.

> *"Therefore I urge you, brothers and sisters, by the mercies of God, to present your bodies as a living sacrifice, holy and well-pleasing to God, which is your rational act of worship. And do not be conformed to this world, but be transformed by renewing your mind, so what the will of God is, that which is good and acceptable and perfect."*
>
> —Romans 12:1–2

I made another life-changing pivot when I enrolled at Liberty University to get my degree in Christian counseling. This enhanced my relationship with Jesus and built a relationship with who He is and what He says about me. Staying foundationally planted gave me opportunities to grow into who I am today. I am a blessed and forgiven child of God. This new chapter of grace in my story brought opportunities through Seminole Community Church. I have been able to be counseled by a Christian woman and have been able to work through the trauma in my life using *theopoetics*, meaning God's light. As I journeyed within the Pandora's Box of my soul, revealing these lies, God replaced them with His truth. I was going through my recurring feelings, dredging up the past, allowing the Holy Spirit to show me the walled fortress of lies that held me in bondage. I chose to surrender and allow the Lord to break down the deception I had held so tightly and replace it with the truth. Each layer is like peeling an onion; sometimes, it's a putrid smell and makes me cry tons of tears, but the cleansing transformation of the Holy Spirit regenerated me into healing and restoration. It has changed me from running away from God to running into His loving arms daily. The more intimate I become with God, the more He shows me who I am—my true essence of a woman.

> *"For you died, and your life is hidden with Christ in God."*
> —Colossians 3:3

I have become a dove instead of a peacock, choosing to be submissive to God's word and be at peace—still in the midst, I can display my peacock feathers. I am mindful and grateful daily that a heart of stone is being replaced with a heart of flesh. Trusting in Jesus has given me the ability to trust Him and then rely on my intuition. Choosing to rid myself of rage, malice, slander, and obscene language from my mouth has stripped off the old self with its destructive practices. I continue to practice love, righteousness, and forgiveness, renewing myself in the actual knowledge of the image of Jesus, who created my new self.

> *"When Christ, who is our life, appears, then you also will appear with Him in glory."*
> —Colossians 3:4

When I began to embrace and believe the reality of my feelings truly, my empowered behavior became a reality. The battle of my mind was designating where my soul was going to end up: defined—either in heaven or hell. Forgiving myself was the most challenging thing I've ever done. I knew what was done to me and what I had done to myself and others, and it was ugly to look at. How God makes everything beautiful in His time. I stopped striving for perfection and accepted my imperfection with a willingness and peace to rest in God's sovereign mercy.

> *"Be still and know (recognize, understand) that I am God."*
> —Psalms 46:10

I have become deeply rooted in Christ, overcoming degenerating fears and replacing them with rejuvenated faith. I have been given the miracle of using my voice to communicate, resolve conflict, and speak the truth in love to the best of my ability. My life within has transformed me with wisdom and discernment to follow in Jesus's footsteps with a passion for helping other women become free from captivity, as I am! As I continue along this path, God is restoring what the locusts have eaten. Seeing the changes in my life and the bountiful fruit of my choices, some family members, including my son, have even returned back into my life; I am moving forward with my education at Liberty University. I have accomplished more in my life during these last few years than I ever dreamed or imagined; all through the help of Jesus. It does take time for the promises of God to appear, which is not always easy, but so worth the wait! The wet blanket of negative emotions that engulfed me has been swept away and replaced with the soft velvet fabric of joy, giving me the strength to expand my colorful peacock wings to soar. The missing pieces to my puzzle are being filled in daily as a masterpiece of God's glory.

> *"Therefore, as you have received Christ Jesus the Lord, walk in Him having been deeply rooted and now being continually built up in Him and established in your faith, just as you were taught, and overflowing in it with gratitude."*
>
> —Colossians 2:6–7

Belief:

My daily focus and mission are revealed in Philippians 4:13:

> *"I can do all things through Him who strengthens me."*

That strength is my inner soul, and it can be yours just for the asking. This truth is the key to success, life, and true abundant living. The overflow begins with receiving God's forgiveness, forgiving yourself, and transferring this renewed message of life to others. This basic human condition is understanding that we *all* fall short and need a Savior. The resilience and perseverance to willingly accept and walk away from what you think is right in your own eyes, and being dependent on the Lord and his word will redeem you to a path of restoration. The Holy Bible will transform anyone who humbles themselves, no matter what the cause or transgression, to lay down their life, accept and receive the free and priceless gift of salvation.

The truth will liberate anyone—just for the asking! I am secure, I am creative, I am significant, I am loved, I am holy, and I am righteous in Christ Jesus. Your pursuit of happiness and true identity can radiate inside of you too. Become my last name with me—Peacock—a new creation in Christ, soaring in peace like a Dove.

Action Steps to Spiritual Peace:
- Look within yourself daily.
- Depend entirely on God in all your decisions.
- Receive the Lord's forgiveness, forgive yourself, and then forgive others.
- Be vulnerable with child-like faith.

Desiree Peacock
Christian Counselor
Liberty University
peacockdesiree4@gmail.com

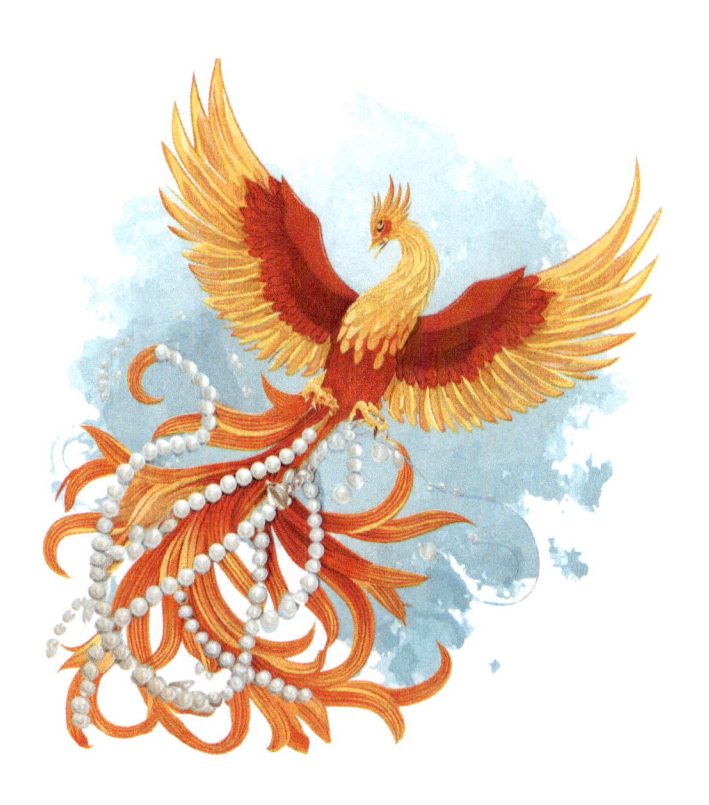

Dr. Nitikul Solomon,
MD, MSHM, ABIHM

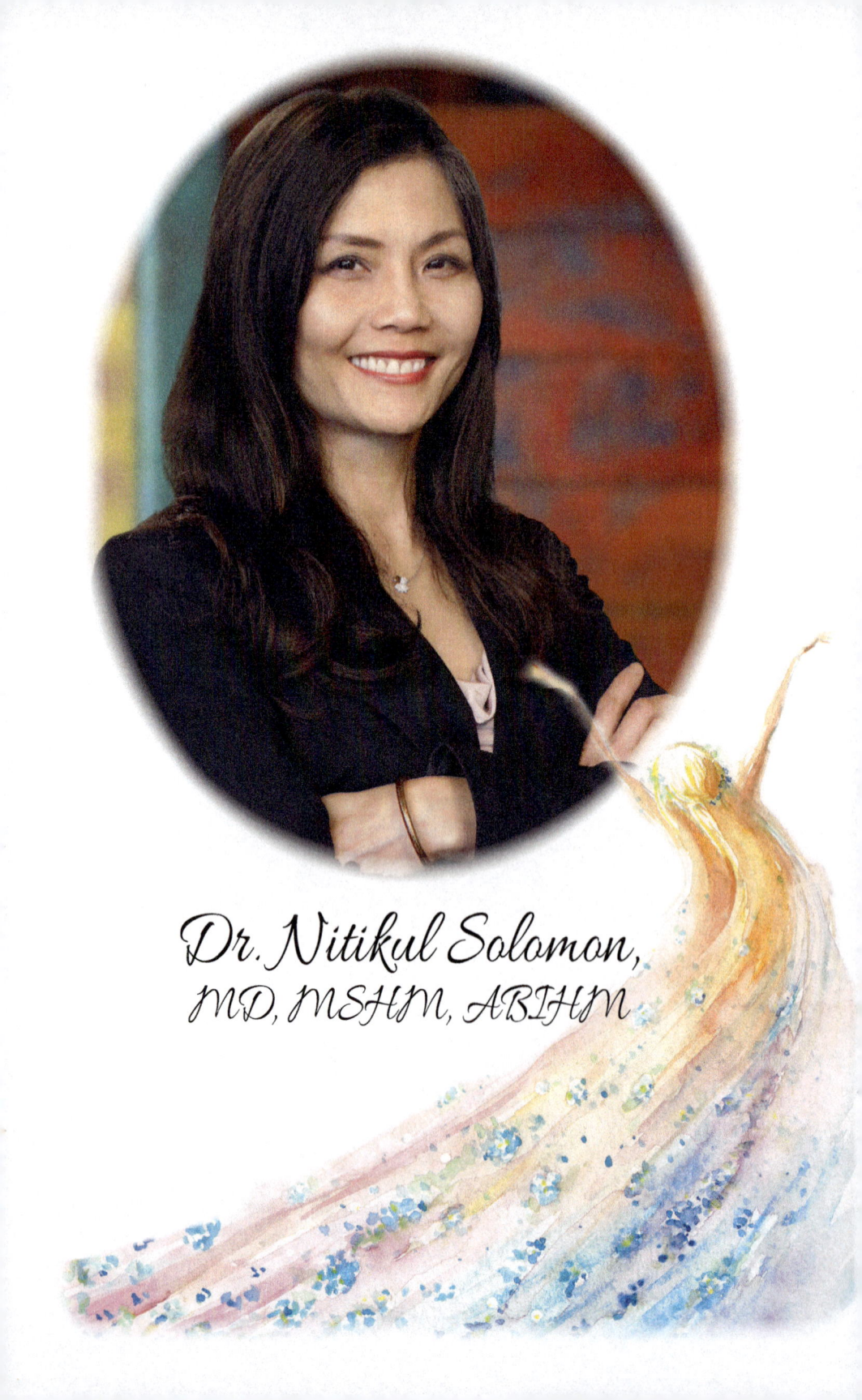

The Divine Feminine Essence

"Spirits always seek joy and ways to express love."

Intention:

Think oneness rather than separateness. This is truly the Divine in all of us. Every human being has a feminine and masculine side—physically and spiritually. May you embrace both the feminine and masculine inside of you to truly live purposefully and divinely.

Story:

The physical and physiological aspects of males and females only depend on cellular receptors to express the seemingly vast differences in quality. We are more alike than the *Men are From Mars and Women are From Venus* concept—a Worldwide Bestseller by Dr. John Gray.

By nature of design, women tend to take on nurturing roles. They tend to put others' needs before themselves, which can lead to the burden of a lack of self-care. Focusing on self-care is essential for women to avoid depleting themselves from their destined caretaker role. Collaborating, connecting, and communicating with other women, the similar passion and purpose can be beneficial and rewarding, especially for women's well-being.

The Divine feminine and masculine are within all of us. We are all one. We commonly think of men and women as separate and different, calling the other gender 'the *opposite* sex.' As a woman who has been living in this body for over five decades, I am still learning about how magnificent and fascinating my beloved body is: we are the continuum of one another. Even the word "woman" has "man" in it.

I truly experienced Mars and Venus on the brink when I was married to the father of my only daughter. Relocating to Portland, Oregon, after living in Thailand for 2 years to fulfill my immigration requirements. I was presented a few challenges, including unavailable childcare and the competition with me obtaining a job. The local medical school graduated thirteen pediatric residents annually, making it hard for me to find a job. The "default" caretaker role would fall on me without question. The consequence of this period is a "gap" in my resume, which usually warranted an explanation by the potential employer and likely made my candidacy less appealing.

Amidst the divorce and my ex-husband fighting not to fulfill his financial or parenting obligations, I realized how difficult it must be for other women to deal with such life agony. Wouldn't it be divine for women to unite in solidarity and propel themselves toward graceful existence? However, I survived the ordeal that nearly killed my body, mind, and spirit. When someone who used to be your life partner can intentionally hurt you mercilessly, it was soul-crushing for me. Tears well up in my eyes even now, sharing my past. I desire to shed light upon the subject at hand and to let go to move forward fearlessly with dignity. I have overcome that phase of indignity when I reduced my power. It was my own doing of blind devotion to a man without performing regular self-care. The result was me with a devastating self-image and self-worth—not knowing who I was at the time.

The deeper story was that I was beaten up as a child by my father, who displayed his anger frequently towards me. Feeling unworthy led me to be even suicidal in my teens.

Tragically, as I approached my 20s, I repeated the same behavior as a child, related to men with self-punishment, and picked my ex-husband unconsciously because of the energetic familiarity.

I have gone through healing phases about my family and my failed marriage. Needless to say, what doesn't kill you makes you stronger. I am happy to survive and come out in one piece. Truly the Divine *'yeah'* in life!

To add to my Mt. Everest life experiences, I was stricken with a health crisis, including surgery and a cancer scare which inspired me to follow my divine calling further into holistic medicine. My transformative lifestyle assisted me in obtaining a holistic board certification in 2009. As a holistic physician who went through these physical challenges and circumvented the rejuvenation of my health again, I know from my expertise and experience the importance of a personal, self-focused daily lifestyle.

Navigating experiences within my divineness has assisted me with great compassion for the families I serve and concurrently empathize with and expand my capacity to help and support patients suffering from depression. The personal discovery of my Divine balance in life, I have forgiven myself and anyone involved with graceful gratitude to embrace its invaluable lessons. Each person served the purpose of my learning and has made me who I am today. I have elevated my awareness as a woman with more compassion and physician-heightened skills to uplift and heal even challenging juveniles. The power of the Divine Feminine and Masculine lies within all of us. We are all here for one another, seeking joy and love.

Holistic medicine and healing embody energy as a life force. There's a systematic way to explain the subtle energy shapes by our breathing, emotions, movements, feelings, and intelligence. The system can be explained as multiple organized, energetic centers called 'chakras', or spinning wheels or energy disks. Chakras line up in order similar to rainbow colors. Imagine the purple color at the crown of your head, followed by indigo, blue, green, yellow, and red at basic or base chakra of your pelvis. Let's delve into these in detail:

- #7 Crown Chakra *(Sahasrara)—light purple, indigo, or white*: The only chakra outside the body is considered a spiritual body: associated with higher consciousness.
- #6 Third Eye Chakra *(Ajna)—deep purple*: This chakra regulates pineal and pituitary glands, the ears, and the nose. Located between the eyes, it represents wisdom, intuition, and imagination.
- #5 Throat Chakra *(Vishudha)—blue*: The hypothalamus, thyroid, throat, and mouth are organs associated with this chakra, which involves communication, truth, and creativity.
- #4 Heart Chakra *(Anahata)—green*: The chakra is located near the heart and is associated with the circulatory system, heart, arms, and hands.
- #3 Navel Chakra *(Manipura)—yellow*: This chakra is located by the belly button and corresponds with willpower and assertion. Organs associated with it include the liver, pancreas, and stomach.
- #2 Sacral Chakra *(Svadisthana)—orange*: Located by the sacrum and connection with emotional balance and sexuality, which respond to our reproductive organs, prostate, and bladder.
- #1 Root Chakra *(Muladhara)—red*: This chakra represents survival needs and grounding. Associated organs include the spinal column, colon, kidneys, and legs.

Modeling after the color patterns of the rainbow, one can imagine wellness, understand the energetic body, and weave and move the energy and frequency to course correct using our emotions as guidance. Movements, breathing, thoughts, and cognitive functions can temper the ups and downs of life from moment to moment. Therefore, meditation, breath work, physical activities, journaling, and gratitude practices can dramatically affect and improve the outcomes of the physical and mental planes. These practices help uplift and raise your vibrations, enhance your sense of self, and foster creative ability. The sense of feeling grounded is essential for a person to possess the ability to adapt and achieve wellness by having a good night's sleep and using cognitive ability without feeling loss in the ether. Self-acceptance and self-acknowledgment can also stem from having a solid foundation in this practice. Too much focus on the lower chakras, though, can cause stress and lead one astray from a heart-centered way of thinking and being. On the contrary, if one is in higher energetic centers and is ungrounded, living an abundant day-to-day life can present friction from the inability to relate to current conditions.

We are spiritual beings in the human experience as long as we think along the line of togetherness instead of focusing on the separation due to our differences, which is the "opposite" or counterpart. Seeing ourselves as a continuum of personal and internal marriage vows from one to another, 'to have and to hold for better or for worse,' is essential for Divine Feminine REALIZATION. We are eternal and made from the essence of love; everything else is only an illusion.

"There are only two ways to live your life. One is as though nothing is a miracle. The other is as though everything is a miracle."
—Albert Einstein

Philosophy:

Don't be disillusioned. We are not going to be perfect all the time. Life is a huge roller coaster—we have all, at some point, fallen off the bandwagon. I remember that suicidal teenager in despair. Life is a natural and effortless spiritual experience in the Chakra flow. We evolve and aspire to be spiritual beings having a human experience.

In truth, our current reality is a simulated experience—a virtual reality game of life. This frequency results from our love and conscious awareness, raising the vibrations for the planet and for us all as a whole.

Imagine throwing a pebble into a pond. You hear a slight splashing, soft water sound, yet the ripple effect can extend to the other side of the body of water. The lasting impact of our thoughts and actions can be profound and expansive, like the ripple effect of the pebble. Because we are all connected, carrying a net below on the trapeze of life.

When we are in alignment with our higher self, we possess clarity. We can then make loving choices, furthering our consciousness and enhancing our compassion. However, without this compass guiding and illuminating the path, our souls have fewer resources to support and advance. The union's balance can be achieved by allowing the energy to flow fluidly with love and compassion.

The Divine *NATURE* leverages love by bringing us into that ultimate place of compassion or selflessness. The fingerprint of individuality is to serve our purpose and to fulfill our own needs as well. The integration of who we are has love as our core essence.

Love graces us with divine presence and never fails to illuminate our spirits. Until we embrace the unity of our beings and embody the light toward our spiritual journey, the emergence of divine feminine and divine masculine will unite as one upgrading a mundane biological phenomenon into a higher form of beings. Adding a dose of visualizing goodness and heartfelt blessings can propel us toward the ultimate of loving unconditionally.

By consciously balancing the Seven Chakras of the Soul Energy, this embodiment will lead you to enter the door of life and abundance to receive and embrace your divine counterpart. The interpretation of feminism as asserting oneself to do it all without masculine assistance can result from an emasculated perspective, which impedes the integration of the union to create oneness. The World needs love to go around, and to keep peace on earth, we have to be able to get past the illusive separations.

Loving oneself unconditionally is the foundational key to achieving a heightened sense of invincibility and limitlessness. Self-compassion and kindness to ourselves serve as the compass for navigating and threading the water to the Eternal Source—the true Source of Oneness. Self-care is crucial in leading women into their essence and power.

Cultivating self-love and self-compassion are the keys to achieving a state of empowerment. The purity of our intentions must lead us to this energy. Then, a wealth of satisfaction in living a meaningful life can flood one's being with happiness and fulfillment.

However, when presented with the burden of everyday living and the occasional dissatisfaction with life, how does one go about keeping balance? Maintaining the integrity of being grounded is critical based on your current circumstances. In other words, you do not have to be stuck in your head or in 'la la land,' just remain heart-centered.

Everything is within us. Each of us is a Universe within herself. Inside every woman lies the innate wisdom and ability to tap into The Source—born in all of us. Stay open to unite and thrive together. Leaving the tendency for isolationism behind, togetherness prevails and is the spiritual abundance of a life worth living.

All of us are relational human beings. The wave of connectedness summons up the alluring beauty of human-dom and womanly grace.

The clarity to manifest and maintain the perfect connection is obtained by starting with the connection to our feminine goddess energy. Deep down, we possess this goddess quality innately.

Our feminine inner power exists as our natural resources to tap into when situations call to our attention. We are powerful beyond perception. We are interconnected without question. Let's become superHUMAN by being superFUN. Relationships serve as reflections of our inner world. This can be utilized to enter the Kingdom of Heaven and uplift our spirits and vibrations toward our enlightened self. Embodying childlike hope and faith and taking stock daily as a rebirthing and renewal experience is essential to awakening your divine self. The ray of sunshine confirms and reassures that well-being is definite and infinite. The sun rises every morning without us conducting the procedure or controlling the circumstances. It's a sure thing. We can **trust** in the well-being of the Universe to have our backs.

When we can embody the rekindling playful connections and embrace the opportunity to elevate our beingness that was miraculously conceived and brought into existence at birth, The Divine appears and perpetually reappears. Giving and receiving constructively to center oneself by: Believing-Knowing-Praying are essential. Thus, we reach the stars and expect brilliant outcomes in return. Imagine this World so heavenly and illuminating! We can only sustain this by projecting our love toward one another…toward our beloved planet—Mother Earth. *Welcome Home.*

Action Steps to Embodiment of the Divine Feminine:
- **Practice Mindfulness:** Count 1 to 3 when breathing *in* and 1 to 6 when breathing *out* with Pranic breathing. Count to 20 when chewing each bite of food before taking another bite.
- **Regular Self-Care Check:** Balance your chakras daily and embed these practices utilizing a Gratitude journal.
- **Self-compassion:** Consistently catch your thoughts in action, especially ones regarding YOU. Self-Actualization: Do activities that bring you JOY daily.
- **Love:** Realize and cultivate this grand aspect of ourselves from moment to moment.
- **Self-acceptance:** Acknowledge and appreciate where you are and practice self-forgiveness regularly.

Dr. Nitikul Solomon, MD, MSHM, ABIHM
Doctor Niti
www.DoctorNiti.com
Nitikuls@hotmail.com

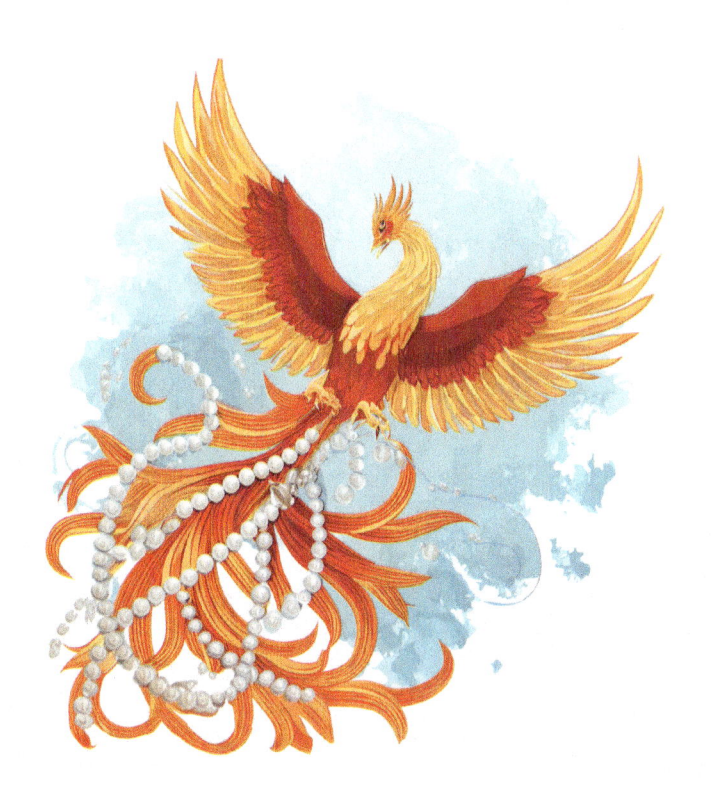

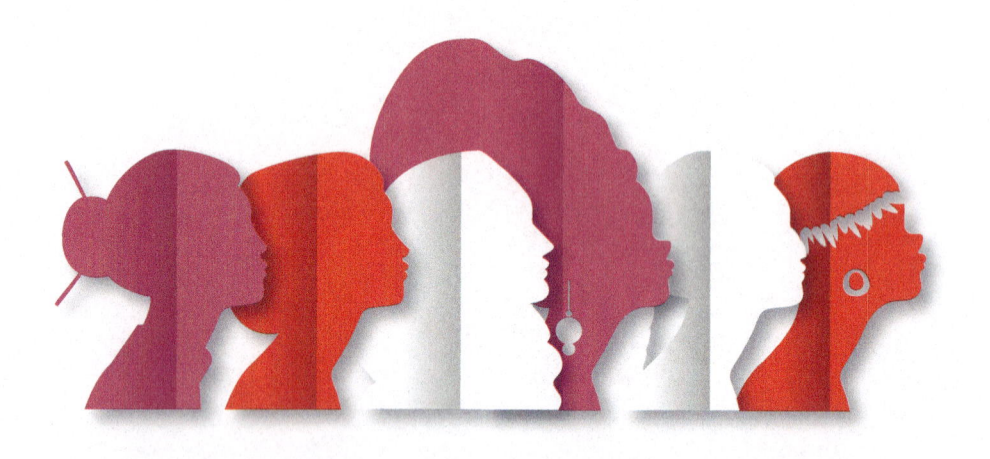

CHAPTER TWO

Mental Pillar

"A strong woman is a beautiful woman."
—Kirsten Dunst

"Passion first and everything will fall into place."
—Holly Holm

"The best part of beauty is that which no picture can express."
—Francis Bacon

"There is no cosmetic for beauty like happiness."
—Maria Mitchell

"Beauty begins the moment you decide to be yourself."
—Coco Chanel

"The beauty of a woman must be seen from in her eyes, because that is the doorway to her heart, the place where love resides."
—Audrey Hepburn

"Beauty is not flawless; it shines even through your flaws."
—Unknown

"People often say that 'beauty is in the eye of the beholder,' and I say that the most liberating thing about beauty is realizing that you are the beholder."
—Salma Hayek

Jennifer Louise Kerr

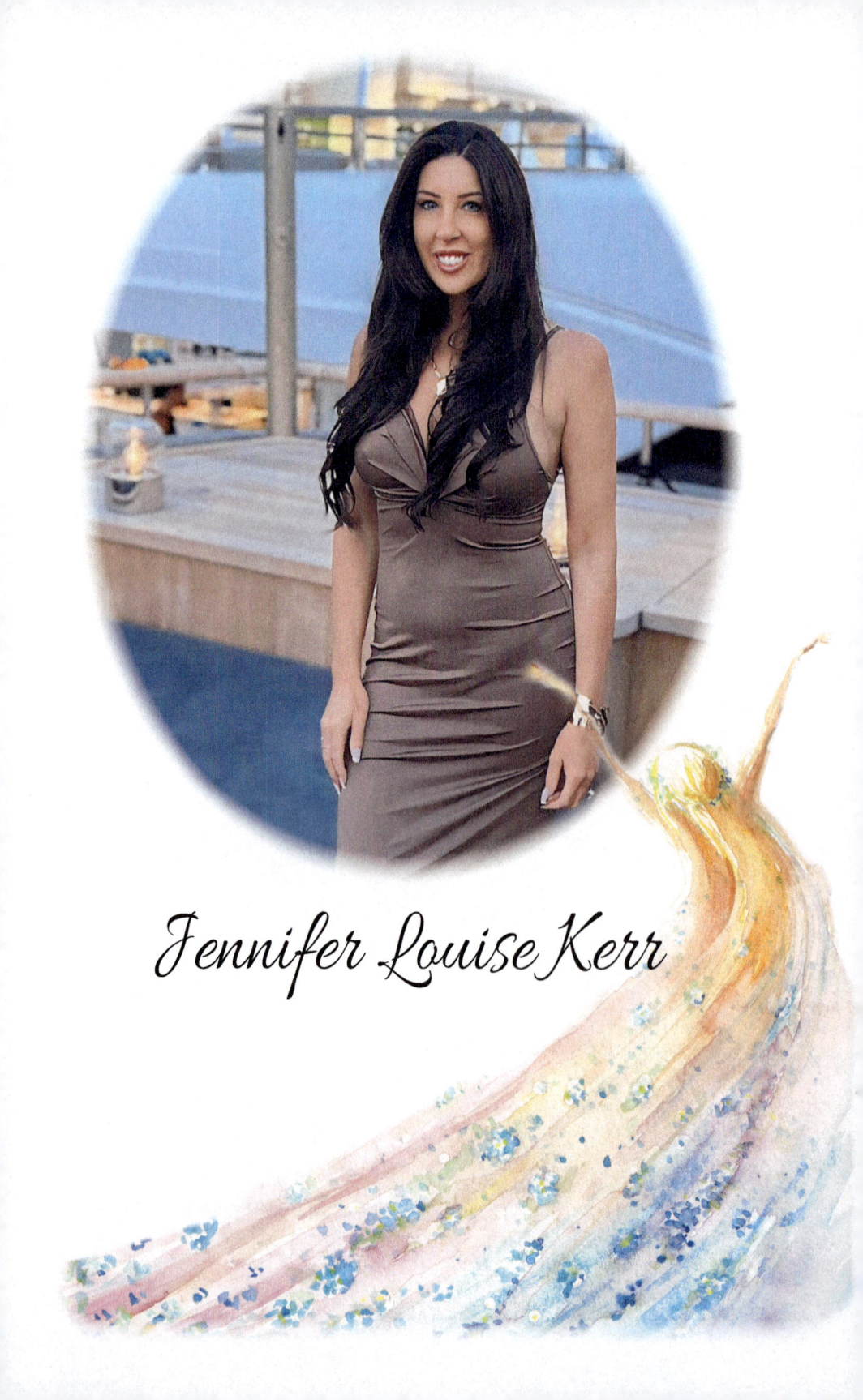

You Versus Your Armour

"True strength is not found in the armour we wear, but in the courage to shed it to embrace -our authentic selves."

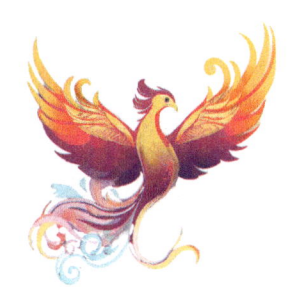

Intention:

Dedicated to the lifelong lessons of shedding the burdensome armour we have built and learning to trust in the divine protection that has been freely given to us, let us explore the process of dismantling our self-imposed barriers and stepping into a life of freedom, vulnerability, and authentic connection.

Story:

From the earliest days of our lives, we begin to construct an armour—a protective shell forged from experiences, defences against the world's harsh realities. As children, this armour is light, almost imperceptible, a mere whisper of protection. But as we grow, so does our armour, becoming thicker and more complex, layer upon layer of defence mechanisms meant to safeguard our hearts and minds from pain, rejection, and fear.

I have built a powerful yet heavy armour in my own journey. It has shielded me from many storms, providing a sense of security and resilience. This armour has been my steadfast protector, guarding my vulnerabilities and allowing me to navigate a hostile and unforgiving world.

Yet, as the years passed, I realized that this same armour, once my saviour, had also become my prison. It saved me from so much but deprived me of even more. It kept out the hurt, but it also kept out the joy, the connections, and the profound experiences that make life truly rich and meaningful. My armour had become useless, a relic of a past that no longer served my present.

Learning to strip away this armour has been one of the most challenging and liberating experiences of my life. It requires me to confront my deepest fears, to acknowledge the parts of myself that I had long hidden away, and to trust in something far more significant than my own strength.

Instead of relying on my heavy, self-made armour, I am beginning to embrace the invisible armour that God provides. This divine protection is far lighter and infinitely more powerful. With one arm extended, I hold the shield of faith, deflecting doubts and negativity. With the other, I wield the sword of the Spirit, the word of God cutting through limiting beliefs and illuminating my path with truth and love.

I was so consumed with battling the relentless pain that assaulted me from every direction, transforming myself into a woman who would never need anybody. I fortified myself with layers upon layers of self-sabotaging armour, forgetting that when someone came along who truly loved me, they could never access my heart until all those layers had been stripped away. Tearing off each layer is a daunting task; it hurts even more, as if it's glued to my skin. It's like the instant pain of ripping off a plaster, a sting that lingers in memory. When they say, "Love hurts" is this what they mean? Surely not!

I want you to understand that you are NOT your armour. Take a moment right now to say it out loud: **"I am not my armour."** Find a mirror, look at yourself with love and compassion, and repeat: **"I am not my armour."**

You are what lies beneath it all. Your armour is what you present to the world, but your true identity and personality exist behind that shiny metal exterior. Imagine, if you will, a tiny person sitting inside an army tank, driving it forward into battle. That tiny person is warm, loving, and full of hope, dreams, goals, achievements, fun, and love. Yet, from the outside, the world only sees the tank—your armour. The world takes the tank at face value: hard, dangerous, and scary.

The little person inside the tank is scared to come out, so they sit there, day after day, missing the beauty of the world outside. They believe that the war that made them retreat into the tank is still raging when, in fact, it ended years ago. The land has regrown, and the air is pure again. But the little person remains alone, scared, in survival mode, and slowly starving themselves of life, letting precious days pass by.

To truly thrive, you must begin to dismantle your armour and step out into the world. Recognize that your strength does not come from the protective layers you've built but from the resilient, loving person within. By doing this, you allow yourself to experience the fullness of life—the connections, the beauty, and the joy that await you beyond the confines of your self-imposed fortress.

My armour, in many ways over the long, hard years, has served a purpose. The desire to work hard, achieve my goals and high standards, provide for my two children alone, keep myself strong, fit, and active, and run a business for 20 long years are all admirable qualities. BUT when the obsession over working long hours, proving myself to anyone within a mile of me, having an inability to slow down and rest, and frequently running myself into the ground begins to surface like a persistent pimple, is the armour worth it?

Is the weight and heaviness in our heart and soul desirable to us or anyone else? I fear not. We were never meant to feel this heavy; life was never meant to feel this heavy. The qualities that once drove you to succeed have now become burdens that weigh you down. It's time to recognize that your armour, which once served you so well, is now a hindrance.

We need to shed this armour, to lighten our hearts and souls, and embrace a life that feels as free and joyful as it was always meant to be. Let's allow ourselves the grace to rest, to slow down, and to live without the constant pressure of proving our worth. Life is meant to be lived fully, with a light heart and an unburdened spirit.

This Armour is Heavy

Imagine walking around for a day carrying an extra 10 stone (one stone is equivalent to 14 pounds or 6.35 kilograms) in a backpack. Most of us couldn't complete an hour, let alone an entire day. And to the woman who just thought, "I can do that,"—girl, put that load down. You don't need to be carrying that any longer. I've got you.

The armour we put on is heavy. The stronger it gets, the heavier it becomes, and the less we can move freely. It restricts us, making it harder to truly deal with life's challenges. The stress grows bigger, almost addictive. Small issues start to seem monumental. The fun and lightness creep out of our souls, only to be replaced with darkness and a deep sadness that only we can feel.

Ladies, your armour has served its purpose. It has protected you, but now it has become useless. It no longer holds any value, and it no longer holds you captive. It's time to let go of the weight.

Let's strip away the layers, embrace vulnerability, and step into the world unburdened. Free yourself from the constraints of your armour and experience life with an open heart and a liberated spirit. You deserve to move freely, to feel joy, and to connect deeply with others. It's time to live fully and authentically.

When you understand that choosing fear over joy out of a false sense of security is holding you back, you will find the courage to trust that there is another way—a softer, more feminine way. Give yourself permission to let go, trust, play, laugh, and love life again.

If you need just a little more encouragement to take that huge leap of faith, know this: I was once too busy building walls of armour, determined to never need anyone in my life again. I had forgotten that when people walk into walls, they get hurt.

And so, the breaking down of the layers began, one chainmail link at a time. Some days it felt like it was taking forever. Some days I could see the progress and could feel proud, and other days I would get scared and add a few more links back on. With each layer removed, life became less heavy, more joyful, and a little more loving.

Steps to Dismantle Your Armour

Not wanting this to feel as frustrating as an Ikea flatpack, I have outlined the steps to take below. Documenting this journey in a journal will help you see how far you have come and make sense of your thoughts and feelings along the way. The energy and passion you give to project "Unarm" is the energy and passion you are choosing to give to your new life. Choose wisely.

Don't skip any steps. Stick with it on the hard days. Remember, feelings do not last forever. By changing your state of mind through meditation, going for a run, or doing something that brings you joy, you can quickly come back to yourself and move forward once again. *I wish you all the love in the world.*

Belief:
   Now Let's shed our armour and Let's Get Naked!
   1. **Self-Awareness and Acceptance:**
      - Begin by acknowledging the existence of your armour. Reflect on the experiences that led you to build these protective layers.
      - Practice self-compassion. Understand that your armour was necessary at one point, and it served to protect you. Acccpt that it's okay to start letting go.

- Decide on a joy-filled activity that you will use to reset your mind and energy fields during this journey when everything feels a little too much. By having this ready you can escape and quickly come back to yourself easily while feeling you have massive progress under your belt.

2. **Gradual Exposure:**
   - Start small. Allow yourself to be vulnerable in safe, controlled environments. Share your feelings with a trusted friend or family member.
   - Practice mindfulness and grounding techniques to stay present and reduce anxiety when you begin to feel exposed.

3. **Build a Support Network:**
   - Surround yourself with people who are supportive, understanding, and non-judgmental. Seek out relationships that nurture and encourage your true self.
   - If you have unsupportive people around you that you have to spend time with set yourself clear boundaries, i.e.: I am only going to spend half an hour with them, I won't engage in negative talk with them, I will go for a walk on the beach (or something you love doing) as soon as I leave them to rebalance my energy.

4. **Reframe Negative Beliefs:**
   - Challenge the beliefs that keep you in survival mode. Ask yourself, "Is this belief still serving me?" If not, work on reframing it in a more positive light.
   - Replace self-critical thoughts with affirmations and positive self-talk.
   - When meditating write down the negative thoughts that keep coming up to see where you have work to do.

5. **Embrace Vulnerability:**
   - Understand that vulnerability is not a sign of weakness but a display of courage. It's through vulnerability that we connect deeply with others and experience authentic relationships.

- Practice vulnerability by sharing your true feelings, even if it feels uncomfortable at first.

6. **Celebrate Progress:**
    - Recognize and celebrate your progress, no matter how small. Each step towards dismantling your armour is a victory.
    - Keep a journal to document your journey. Reflect on how far you've come and the growth you've experienced.

The goal here is not to become entirely armour-free, as some layers serve a true purpose. We build up four types of armour:

1. A layer to block out unwanted feelings.
2. A layer to keep a distance between us and other people.
3. A layer that hides who we truly are.
4. A layer that keeps us from growing spiritually.

The aim is to work each day toward a better version of yourself—a lighter, more love-filled version. There will be people and situations that challenge you along the way. The real goal is to reach a place where you no longer react to others' bad behaviour or life's problems, but instead tackle each day with love in your heart and light in your eyes.

Perfection is unattainable; no one is ever perfect.

Use these prompts to guide your reflections, dig deep and uncover the true, unburdened self that lies beneath your armour. Embrace the journey and celebrate each step toward a more authentic and fulfilling life.

I want to take these final words to pay homage to a man of distinction—a man who cares deeply enough to see the pain in my eyes yet holds me to my higher self. Often, he receives the childlike backlash of my tongue while steadfastly helping me remove my armour, even on the days I cling to it, kicking and screaming.

Like you, I am human and sometimes hurt this man as he tries to pull little Jen out from within Big Jen's armour-wearing grasp. While his coaching style can be harsh, I know deep down that he believes I can do better.

This is a lifelong journey of continuous improvement. From now until forever, I wish you a light and armour-free life.

Action Steps: Reflect on Your True Self:

Embark on your journey to a lighter, more joyful life with these journal prompts. Play with them, sit in a park or on a beach pondering them, and answer them often. Break through your limiting beliefs to embrace an unlimited life. Learn to love yourself again.

- What are some of the beliefs that are holding me back?
- How would the person who loves me the most see these beliefs in me?
- What is one thing from my past I need to let go of to take a layer of armour off?
- What's one thing I can do today to start to let that go?
- How will I know I have truly moved on from that one thing?
- How will I celebrate myself knowing I have finally let it go and removed a layer of armour?
- Name five areas in your life that letting go of that one thing will positively impact.
- What different choices can I make if that one thing ever turns up in my life again to stop me from adding another layer of armour?
- How will I feel as I start to see the layers coming off?
- What will this mean to me?
- What will this mean to the people around me that I love?

Jennifer Louise Kerr
Co-Founder at MindKite Wellbeing | Mental Health First Aid Trainer
Expert in Mindset & Performance Coaching
www.MindKitementalhealth.com
Jenniferlouisekerr@gmail.com

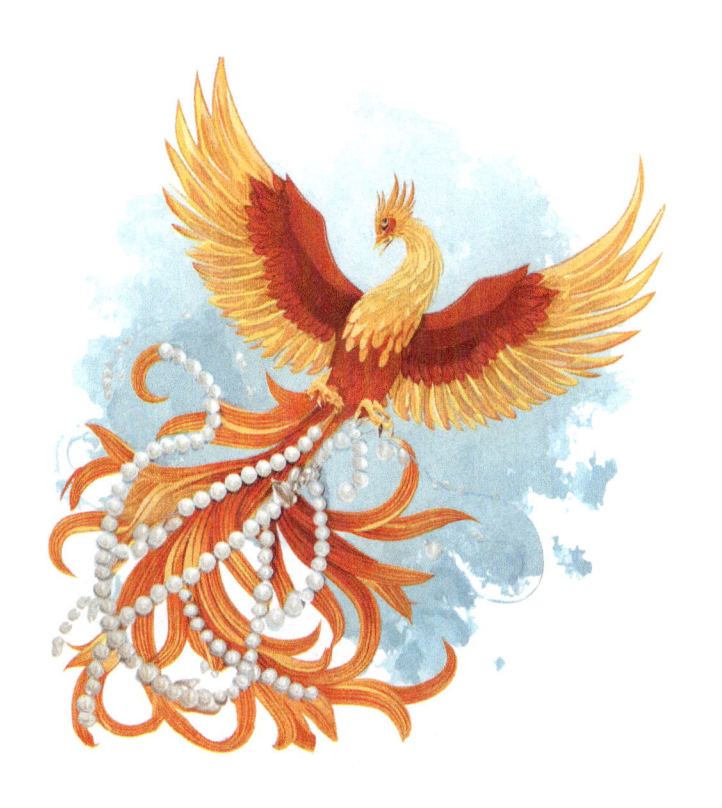

Jennifer Louise Kerr

Kathy Strauss, CCFC

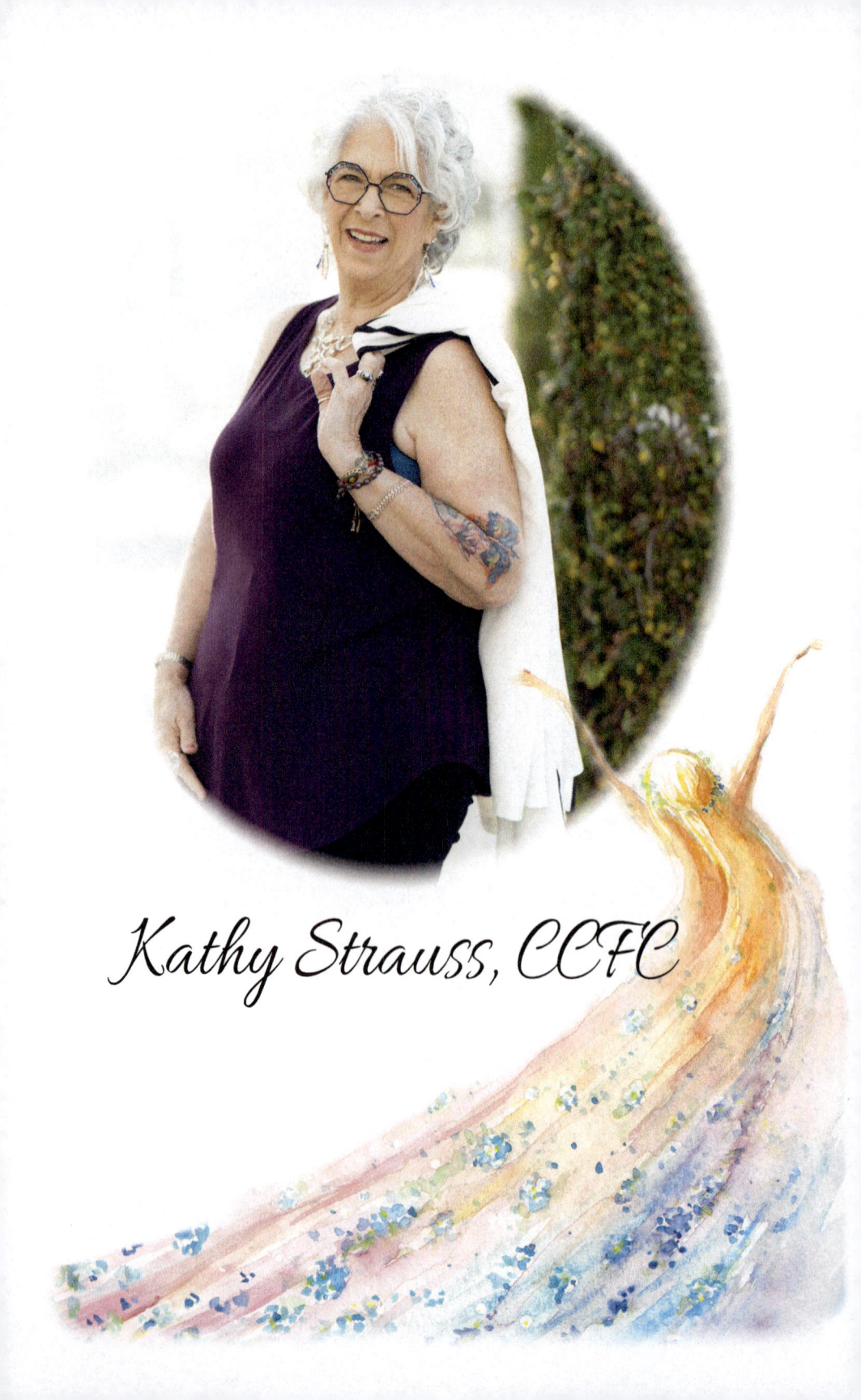

The Transformative Power of Creativity

"In the canvas of life, creativity serves as the brushstroke of healing."

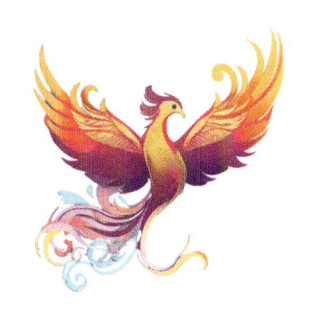

Intention:

Every action we take in our lives affects all living things. As human beings, we share our environment, community, attitude, and knowledge—individually and together, each aspect influences who and what we are. If we act negatively, our actions create negative happenings—when we act positively, we create a ripple that affects our lives in a positive manner. For every action or thought, there is an equal or opposite reaction, and as we know, thoughts become things. I like to frame it as "we are the artists of our lives."

Story:

Creativity is not merely confined to the realm of artistic endeavors; it is a potent force that permeates every facet of our lives, including our relationships. When we embrace creativity as a means of expression, we open ourselves to a world of possibilities. At its core, it encourages us to delve into the depths of our imagination, unraveling the layers of our innermost thoughts and emotions. This journey of self-exploration is instrumental in fostering a deeper understanding of ourselves and our partners.

I create my current life, using a proverbial brushstroke. I am an artist—creative—doing my best thinking outside the box, and seeing everything around me in full color. This wasn't always the case. Even though I took the creative path to make a living and teach it, I had doubts that I wasn't good enough. I compared myself to others and had the *'doubting mind'* always popping up in my head. I was allowing myself to be guided by thoughts that didn't serve me and though I put on a good front, I let my "left brain" rule most of what I was doing or thinking. It was as if I had an imaginary character sitting on my left shoulder named "George" who told me to judge everything or take things personally. Looking back, it wasn't until I started diving into creativity fully to de-stress that I realized "George" was directing a lot of my life. As I did, I found myself becoming more mindful of everything. Creativity became a guiding force and a teaching tool, "George" even learned to step away when I needed him to. Of course, when I need his logical guiding voice—I let him back into my life.

One of the most profound ways creativity influences us is through its ability to promote clear communication. In a world where words often fall short, art and design have become a universal language through which we can convey emotions, ideas, and feelings. Whether it's a heartfelt painting, a soul-stirring poem, or a melodic composition, creative expression transcends linguistic barriers, allowing us to connect with each other on a deeper, more soulful level.

Creativity serves as a powerful tool for navigating conflict as well as overcoming adversity in relationships. When we face challenges or disagreements, it can be easy to succumb to frustration or resentment. However, by channeling our emotions into artistic expression, we create a safe space for dialogue and introspection. Whether creating a painting, writing a poem, or composing a piece of music—we express our feelings in a way that is clear to ourselves and others.

Early in my career, I was employed as a senior graphic designer by the World Bank, which to me was a very left-brained environment. For each project I took on, my coworkers would give me data to translate and then design business presentations, graphs, charts, and/or publications. They needed something that would get their message across simply and easily. By using my creative "brushstroke" the process looked like this: boring numbers in, work my magic, and out would come a masterpiece bright and colorful. Yet I wasn't always that way, when I was in junior high—I marched to the beat of a different drummer. Art didn't inspire me, and it showed—I flunked art in 7th grade! It wasn't that I didn't like art—I did! Creativity was a part of my youth. I took music lessons, danced, journaled, and doodled when I could. I remember clearly that my teachers kept telling me I had that spark, I just didn't know how to tap into it fully.

In 8th grade, I had an art teacher who recognized my hidden spark—he challenged and encouraged me to think differently. I had other teachers who influenced me too, but it was art that became something I did, enjoyed, and even wanted to teach. After college, I dove into a graphic design career. I loved my colleagues, and I made the work as colorful as I could, yet I wasn't truly inspired.

Unlike the beauty of my design career, my first marriage was an abusive one—it lasted 14 years until I took charge of my life and screamed "Enough!" The relationship was rocky from the beginning, but looking on the bright side, it taught me strength and resiliency. One of the stories from that relationship was our daughter had discovered the love of competitive dance. Her classes and costumes cost a lot of money, and even though we could afford it—her father didn't see the value in it, refusing to help financially. He preferred to spend freely on all his sound and music equipment rather than encouraging his own child. I saw the value and joy that dance brought her and used my hobby of designing and selling jewelry to pay for everything that supported her. There were other struggles with the marriage that included both verbal and physical abuse. The strength I learned from that relationship showed me that life partners should build up, care, and support each other. What I experienced taught me that creativity and forgiveness were the sparks that helped me to think differently about my situation. Creativity became the art of my strength.

Shortly after my divorce, I met my second husband. He was my twin flame, my creative sounding board, my greatest teacher, and one who reflected images of my life through a different lens. When we met, it was a moment of synchronicity. We were both attending a creativity conference—where I was one of the instructors. When we met, I was captivated by his soft brown eyes, his chipped front tooth, and his sharp wit. We spent five days together, immersed in creativity, weaving our connectivity together. We knew instantly we would be married. The unfortunate part was he lived in Spokane and I lived in Washington D.C. and we were three thousand miles apart. Staying connected through early morning long-distance phone calls, we got to know each other by sharing stories and feelings. By the end of six months, he told me he was moving east to be with me and my daughter. That was the happiest day of my life!

Once he moved east and into my daily life, we did our best to establish a rhythm for our new blended family. We also promised ourselves we would always keep the line of communication open. It became an integral part of our relationship. We were both graphic designers and specialized in branding. Part of our old full-time jobs was helping our clients design and refine their message. We both had a dream to start our own company and with our knowledge and experience, we did! The challenge that some people might have seen is that we had just started living together, got married, and now we planned on working together! Our new business was a success and I'll attribute some of that to the tools, strength, clear communication, and forgiveness we shared with each other. My attitude of creative resilience simply taught me how to roll with the punches and our relationship flourished.

Approximately ten years into our relationship, my husband started to experience some serious health issues. When they first started, I only thought it was a "one-off" illness. What I didn't realize was how serious it was. All of the ailments built one on top of the other. I kept telling myself I was a creative, not a medical professional, I was totally unfamiliar with this medical world. Little did I know these lessons would support me through a conventional maze called health care.

His health issue avalanche started a medical education that I refer to as "learning by the firehose method" or in creative terms, I took my paintbrush, loaded it with paint, and started painting on the canvas of my husband's life. The doctors didn't have an immediate diagnosis for his first ER visit. The myriad of three or four different reasons for his nausea and severe pain made my head feel like a ping pong ball. They eventually sent him home to "get over this 'virus,'" Tragically, he never got better—only worse. That led me on a journey of taking him to see doctor after doctor until he collapsed in one of their offices. Over a four-month period, it was a nightmare of diagnoses, countless doctors, two surgeries, and three hospitals. By the time we were in our third month of his medical hell, he landed back in the third hospital for what we thought was a stroke. That wasn't the core issue, my poor husband was finally diagnosed with chronic Lyme Disease—now they added strong antibiotics to the Heinz 57 mix of medication, which led to complications due to allergic reactions. To this day I say that had the first hospital and doctors done their job and diagnosed him properly, we could have prevented a lot of anguish and frustration.

During that time, I kept notes of essential details and conversations. They allowed me to learn and keep track of everything—they also got me appointed to a hospital family/patient advocacy board. How did that happen? The gift was I was able to present the misdiagnoses and poor care to one of the hospital's leadership, and with my guidance and stories, they were able to share case studies of ineffective care as lessons with their medical staff. I was proud of myself as I felt deep down, I was onto something—using mistakes as a way of learning.

My real creative lessons started when I began sharing his nightmare medical stories on Facebook. Doing this, helped alleviate some of my stress and I didn't feel like I was alone. After that initial nightmare, my husband started to experience other ailments on the disease menu: type II diabetes, congestive heart failure, kidney failure, Lyme disease, white matter brain disease, seizures, and a whole host of allergies and sensitivities to his mound of pills! As time went on, he relied more and more on me—I didn't stress out as I loved and was committed to him in every way. I kept records of what was going on including his ever growing or changing list of medications by using apps on my cell phone. As my medical self-knowledge grew, I felt empowered to stand up to what I intuitively felt was a lack of care or mis-care.

At the same time as the size of my husband's healthcare story grew, I found myself tapping more and more into creativity to keep myself centered within the chaos. Through creative thinking, I learned to navigate the bureaucratic system regardless of the lack of communication. My head spun as the doctors would toss out treatment after treatment, and eventually, his doctors finally opened their minds to the fact that I was the person to talk to about the mounting concerns around his health and treatments. If there was a lack of communication, I knew how to get their attention until we got our answers. Regardless of the care or the facility, the rabid patient advocate was born inside of me to be the best one possible. The core component and most important thing about us was—we believed in each other. There was trust, faith, and tenacity to know no matter what, we would always get to the bottom of what was happening and solve any crisis together.

Belief:

My growth of knowledge in the healthcare world or in other words, my husband's medical issue "world," pushed me beyond my own comfort zone. What I didn't know then was that my general artistic training had trained my brain to take on a superhuman trait—knowing how to think outside the box. Even though I was doing my varied art forms as my husband's health challenges continued, I personally struggled with my own stress levels managing my roles as caregiver, patient advocate, business owner, wife, and mother. It was at this time, I found the Creatively Fit™ coach training that changed my life. The tools in the program re-taught me to learn to paint for fun, doodle, craft, and most of all, meditate. Each simple creative activity allowed me to soothe my stress and help me center. I had found an inner strength and it helped me grow.

Creativity influences everything we do. It's the "how we see the world," its boundless force transcends the confines of artistic expression and can even extend its transformative power into the realm of healthcare. As I navigated the intricacies of my husband's healthcare journey, I found that creativity emerged as a guiding light, illuminating pathways to healing, connections, and holistic wellness. It kept me centered and calm. I took the time to quiet my left-brain "George" chatter by playing music, spending time in nature, and meditating. I created art for myself by exploring new techniques or materials, doodling, going out on a photo jaunt, or slapping paint on blank canvases. When I stressed I consciously spent time in a creative space. Practicing this new way of being, I began to think clearer, concentrate more, and was told that I had become a "nicer person" after doing such.

Creativity can infuse relationships with a sense of joy, spontaneity, and playfulness. When we embrace its spirit, we start experiencing a sense of wonder and curiosity. It also can heal a person in times of pain, heartache, or disease. The simple act of artmaking offers solace and comfort, serving as a beacon of hope amidst the darkness. Through creative expression, we can process our grief, mend our broken hearts, and emerge from adversity with renewed strength and resilience. It is a transformative force that has the power to enrich, heal, and elevate our relationships. As we navigate the intricacies of human connection and relationships, let us remember in the canvas of life, creativity is the brushstroke that colors our relationships with beauty, authenticity, and love.

Action Steps:

- **Explore creative outlets:** Experiment with different forms of artistic expression: painting, writing, music, or dance.
- **Share your creations:** Be vulnerable and open and share your creative endeavors proudly.
- **Realize your freedom of choice:** Just like you choose the color you put on the canvas, and the shape of your brushstroke, so do you choose your life experience.
- **Use creativity to navigate conflict:** When faced with challenges, channel your emotions into creative expression to facilitate dialogue and resolution.
- **Find joy in creativity:** Embrace the spirit of playfulness and adventure by engaging in creative activities.
- **Harness the healing power of art:** Use creative expression for processing emotions.

Kathy Strauss, CCFC
Creationeer
www.imagewerks.net
kathy@imagewerks.net

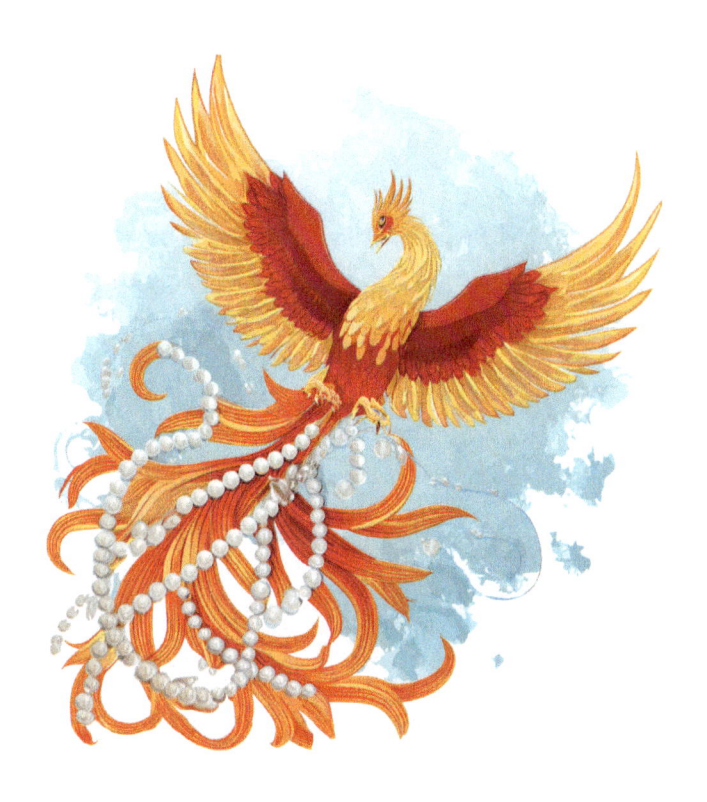

Kathy Strauss, CCFC | 99

Lorina K. Sanchez, MSN, RN

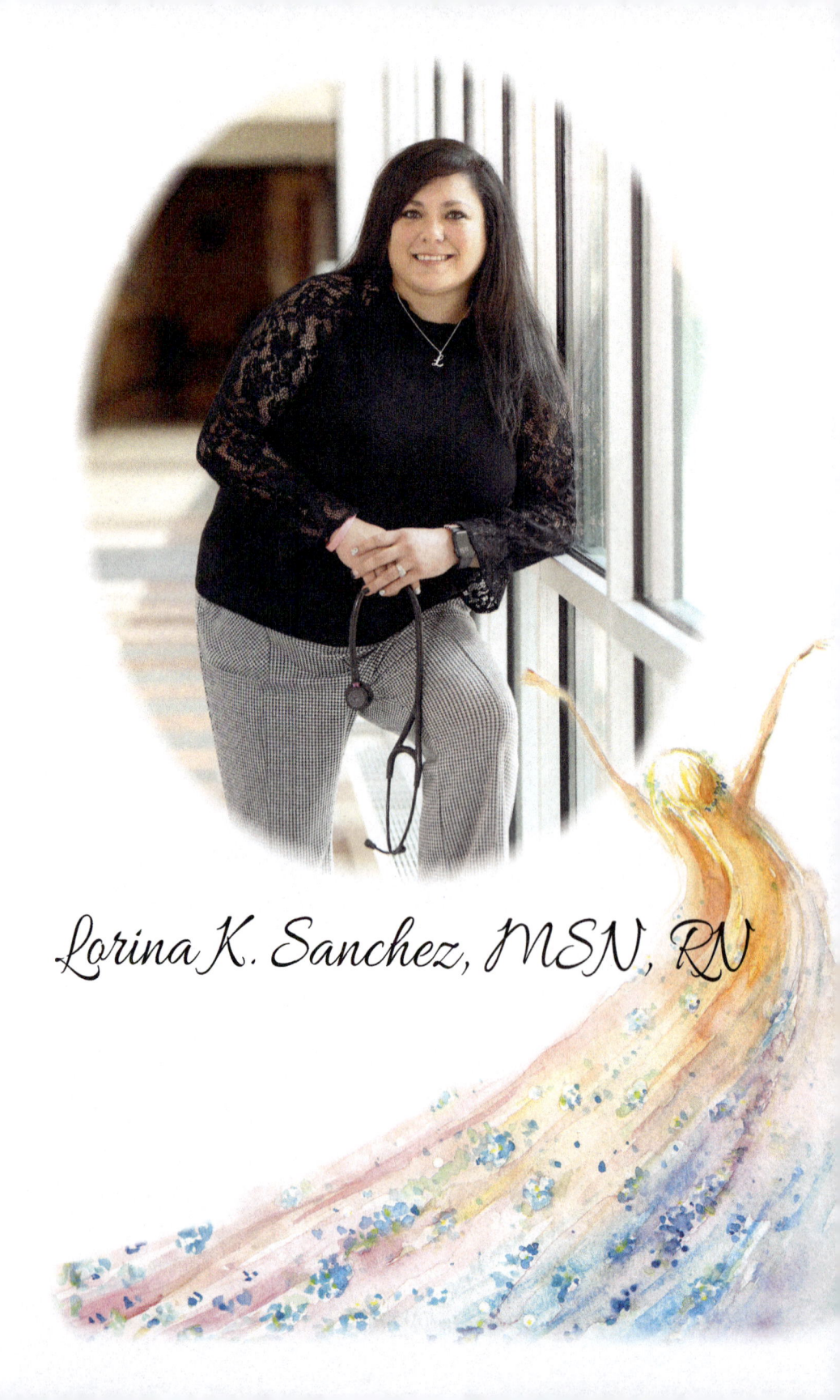

From Fear to Faith:
Becoming a Forensic Nurse

*"The courage you have been searching for,
has been within you all along."*

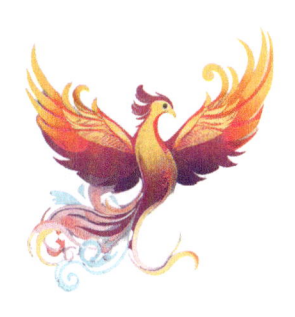

Intention:

Sometimes we experience things that we do not feel strong enough to conquer on our own. However, the women in my life have taught me otherwise. By sharing, may you find support and courage to continue moving forward. For any woman, she will not have to look too far, for the courage she needs has been within her all along.

Story:

It's easy to paint a perfect picture of what life is supposed to look like. We begin to compare our lives and experiences to those of others, including things such as our careers, relationships, and overall life. However, some of the most influential women in my life never had it quite that easy. In fact, most of them had to overcome emotional quandaries at some point in time. Their trials and tribulations led them to be strong, empowered, resilient, independent women, myself included.

Growing up, I had parents who dedicated themselves to making sure that my brother and I had everything we needed or wanted. We were both very active in extracurricular activities. We were fortunate enough to have these opportunities to no avail, trusting that we were the typical suburban, picket fence family. They were at every game or school event; the proudest in the crowd.

Then life '*lifed*' on me. The anvil of a hammer hit my heart, and at fifteen, my parents got divorced. Overwhelmed with a whirlwind of emotions, feelings of helplessness, hopelessness, and guilt all flowed over me. My brother had moved off to college and I felt abandoned and left alone to pick up the shattered pieces. Aloneness, however, became the apex of how I became the woman that I am, today.

The typical teenage divergence of leaning toward social temptation, I began to venture off in hopes that I would find something to numb the pain of my parents' divorce and all of the negativity that came along with it. The mind-boggling judgment from other kids became overwhelming. They didn't know what divorce entailed. They wouldn't understand. They didn't have to. They weren't going through it. Losing relationships with people that I considered family, simply because, let's face it, everyone thinks they have to pick a side. Why not just pick me? Eventually, it was easier to disengage than to attempt to explain or reach out to any of my family or friends. The trauma of divorce is always messy; regardless of the circumstances.

I primarily lived with my mom and although I knew how strong she was, it was in that moment of our life that I learned her true strength. I also learned the significance of the family support she had from my grandparents. My mother also had to pick up the pieces, pieces I never saw. Now, she had to work a full-time job, put her feelings aside, and hold it all together for my sake. She always tried to make me feel like eventually, everything would be alright again. Essentially, we were both experiencing the same aloneness. The life that she had known was over, and she was left to figure out how to do life on her own, all while raising a teenage daughter. I jokingly say that I am the reason for most of her gray hairs, with the reality of understanding that the statement has more connotation than we both thought. I found myself hanging around with the wrong crowd and making choices that were out of character for me but seemed to be the most alleviating at the time.

I saw her tears, frustration, and fear, but couldn't relate to all she was processing for herself. I didn't realize then, that she too had her entire world flipped upside down and had to begin her life again. She did it, though; like Velcro. She accomplished the heroine's feats flawlessly. I admired her strength, her resilience, and her authenticity; some of the core values that she instilled into this sometimes-wayward teenage girl she was raising. The shame of divorce—was the same shame I acted out.

Sweet sixteen wasn't very sweet! Life came crashing down on me— the victim of sexual assault (SA). Terrorized and traumatized, I did not say anything. I was terrified. I was afraid of retaliation and the judgment that would follow along in the next weeks, months, and years to come. It overshadowed any joy of life that was left. It stalked and haunted me for years to follow. It became a dark cloud that wavered above, but it was only raining on me. I projected my self-hate and loathing of myself onto the rest of my relationships: romantically, socially, family, and most importantly, with myself.

When I graduated high school, I ran away from everything and everyone that I knew. I ran as fast as I could! I moved to Carlsbad, New Mexico, and started nursing school. Those running steps, however, were the beginning of the beautiful transition that changed my life. It was the start of some of the most beautiful connections that I made with others. Although I was making progress in my dream career, I was still stagnant and hollow underneath with the agonizing thoughts and feelings that accompanied that dark cloud that was still lingering above my head. I still found myself attracting toxic relationships. It was then that I learned that abuse comes in many forms; in fact, it doesn't always have to be physical. The actions and words of someone else hit me like a whip, dropped me to my knees, and all of it just seemed to cement the feelings I kept secret since that night at sixteen years old. I felt worthless.

By the sweet grace of *Almighty God*, I eventually ended up moving back home. Living with my mom again, however, was bittersweet. I was thankful that I had somewhere to go, but I was an adult now. I was not supposed to live with my mom anymore. I was supposed to have it all together. The shame and secrets could no longer stay hidden and came billowing out of me. Dreading the conversations that were ahead of me, I finally had to muster up the all strength within me and tell my mom everything that I had experienced; sexual assault and intimate partner violence were the hot topics of that night. I feared that my mom, a woman mounted on the highest pedestal, would see me in a different light. I had previously heard about so many other victims' horror stories of being blamed and told they were lying or at fault. I never understood how it was any of their faults. But I had somehow convinced myself of that lie.

In retrospect, there was tremendous heartache and uncertainty that followed. Now, I can honestly say that I am thankful for it all. Had I never moved back in with my mother, I never would have had this spiritual, mental, and emotional cleansing that was necessary for the continuation and healing of my life. I felt and experienced what true unconditional love was. Through my mom's example, and deep understanding—a strength and anchor grounded inside of me.

Whenever a soulful conversation is had, each individual involved may have different interpretations or memories that transpire. Through the tears, anger, anxiety, and frustration, my mom sat and listened to me with an open heart. She let me tell my side of the story that I had been holding onto so tightly for so many years. The accumulation of mental warfare that took place was finally being acknowledged and combated, once and for all. My mother's spiritual insight into this cleansing process: "I am so sorry that this happened to you." As a victim, the first response from someone when you finally let your walls down is crucial. For many, it will determine how a victim moves forward with his or her testimony, or if they ever get to have one.

Healing wasn't as beautiful as it sounds. My emotions were *all over* the place! Thankfully, my intimate circle was supportive and knew all of the right ways to show me my way back to me. The simplest gestures went a long way. All of this support compelled me to accomplish my main goal. I was able to follow in my mother's footsteps and finally become a nurse! Once again, my mom became a beacon of hope and a shining example. During all of this turmoil, my mom ended her career of twenty years to "do something more helpful for others." Once again, I was reminded of how astonishing this woman truly was.

Finishing nursing school was like climbing my own Mt. Everest! I put my stake in that mountaintop of who I was, and all that I had overcome, and enjoyed the panoramic view and vista below. I was exhilarated with accomplishment and pride!

When you open your heart and allow your journey to move from within, making connections with people will lighten up the world; inviting you to enjoy it with them. A few years into my nursing career, I was introduced to a nurse who expanded my knowledge of a program that I didn't even know existed. She told me that she worked with the "SANE" program of Otero and Lincoln counties; SANE stands for Sexual Assault Nurse Examiner. SANE grants victims of sexual assault the opportunity to receive medical and forensic care after being sexually assaulted. This includes assessing patients for any critical medical emergencies, DNA collection, photographed/documented injuries, a history of his or her events that occurred, sexually transmitted infection (STI) prophylaxis, and most importantly, resources to assist patients to justice and support.

A flood of emotions overcame me, now knowing that there was a possibility of helping men and women gain back the life that was so senselessly ripped away from them, like mine was from me. Soon, I completed a 64-hour training for a pediatric, adolescent, and adult SANE program. To say that I was ecstatic is an understatement! Two years later, we expanded our program to help patients involved in Intimate Partner Violence (IPV), previously referred to as Domestic Violence. To date, I am trained in SANE exams for the entire lifespan, trained in IPV cases, and am a certified expert in strangulation. I have completed and attended numerous trainings and conferences throughout this time and continue learning the best practices I can utilize in the care of every single person I cross paths with. I guess Mom's example of helping others truly rubbed off on me.

I have absorbed the characteristics of all of the strong, empowering, and incredible women in my life and I am now passing on this wisdom to my patients; 'The courage that we need to get through any difficult time has been within us all along.' You don't have to go looking for it around you or in others, it is within your very core. I can now proudly say that I am no longer a victim. I am a *survivor*; I am a thriver; and so are my patients!

Philosophy:

One in three women (33%) have been subjected to sexual or physical violence worldwide, according to the most recent data collected in 2018 (World Health Organization (WHO), 2024). IPV includes any physical, sexual, or psychological harm related to physical aggression, sexual coercion, controlling behaviors, or arbitrary deprivation. SA (sexual assault) is defined as any actual/attempt of sexual actions, regardless of the relationship between the victim and offender. Physical force or coercion utilized in penetration of one's private parts (penile, digital, or other body parts/objects), attempted sexual assault, unwanted sexual touching, along with other non-contact behaviors are RAPE (WHO, 2024).

Do I think that one in three is an accurate statistic? I do not. I think that the vast number of women falling victim to physical or sexual violence is MUCH HIGHER! One in three is a REPORTED statistic of sexual or physical violence. Why wouldn't someone report this if it "really" happened to them? Here are a few fundamental examples.

Lack of knowledge. Victims may not understand that ANY form of violence is abuse: physically, sexually, emotionally, or mentally. Victims may not be aware of the resources available to them or how to obtain them. Victims have a right to report/not report their case, acquire a Victim Advocate, a SANE/IPV exam, and counseling, along with other resources.

Consent. Victims may not understand the demands that consent requires. "No" means no. Some victims will blame themselves because they finally "just gave in." This isn't consent. This is coercion. If a person does not undoubtedly say "yes," then it should be assumed that it is a "no." If a person is exhibiting signs of an altered mental state related to drugs, alcohol, or any other factor, then they cannot legally give consent. This should also be taken as a "no."

Fear. Trauma to this degree strikes fear into anyone. The fear of retaliation from the offender, not being believed or understood by their family or friends, or the stigma that is wrongfully placed on a victim of sexual or physical violence. If a victim is given the slightest idea that their report won't be taken seriously, chances are, they aren't going to speak up about it, ever again! Acknowledgment and empathy go a long way for a victim who so courageously musters up the strength to confide in you about the abuse.

The trauma associated with SA or IPV has many effects on victims, short- and long-term: physically, mentally, and sexually, and can cause other health complications. Some of these issues are to include, but not limited to, headaches, chronic pain, gastrointestinal disorders, unintended pregnancies, abortions, STIs, miscarriages, stillbirths, depression, post-traumatic stress disorder, anxiety, addiction to drugs or alcohol, suicide, and possibly homicide. In fact, 38% of women involved in IPV will end up murdered by their partners (WHO, 2024).

So, what is the *solution*? We take a stand together. We join the cause for awareness and prevention. We bring sexual assault and intimate partner violence to light! ***Don't be afraid to talk about it***! Understand that it is the victim's choice to report or not to report the abuse. There is no *shame* either way!! The resources and examinations are still available, should a patient choose *not* to report. The most important thing is that a victim is provided with the necessary resources to promote their healing and well-being.

Keep your heart and mind open to knowing and believing that you are worthy, and that you are not alone. You have the strength to make it through any situation. All the courage you will ever need, want, or desire, has been within you all along.

Action Steps: Victims of Trauma:
- Take a stand for yourself!
- Seek out resources or victim advocacy in your local area.
- Search for mental health counseling.
- Find Spiritual and Moral Support.

Lorina Sanchez, MSN, RN
Forensic Nurse
www.thesanenurse.com
lorinasanchez@gmail.com

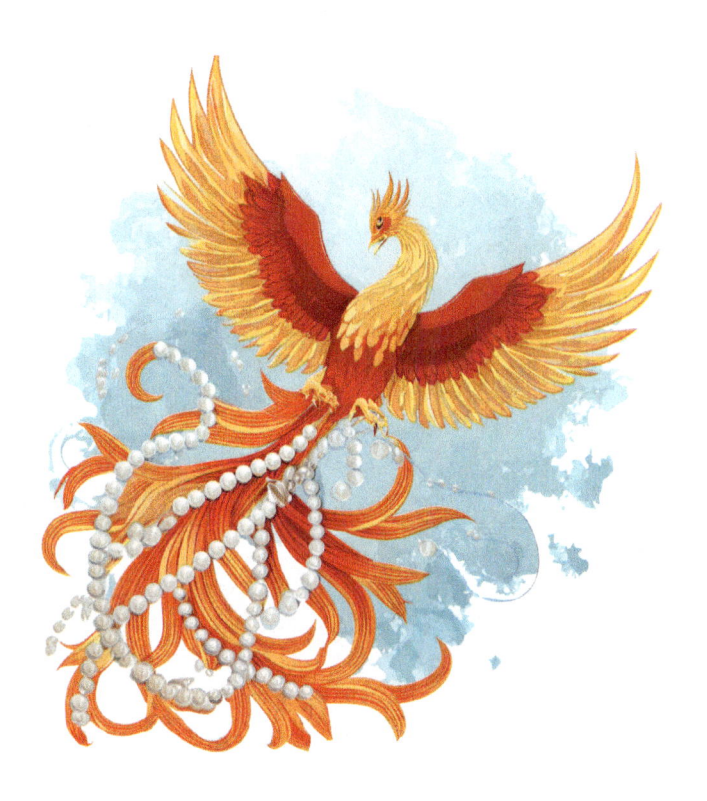

Lorina K. Sanchez, MSN, RN | 109

Anne Borow-Lawrence, MEd

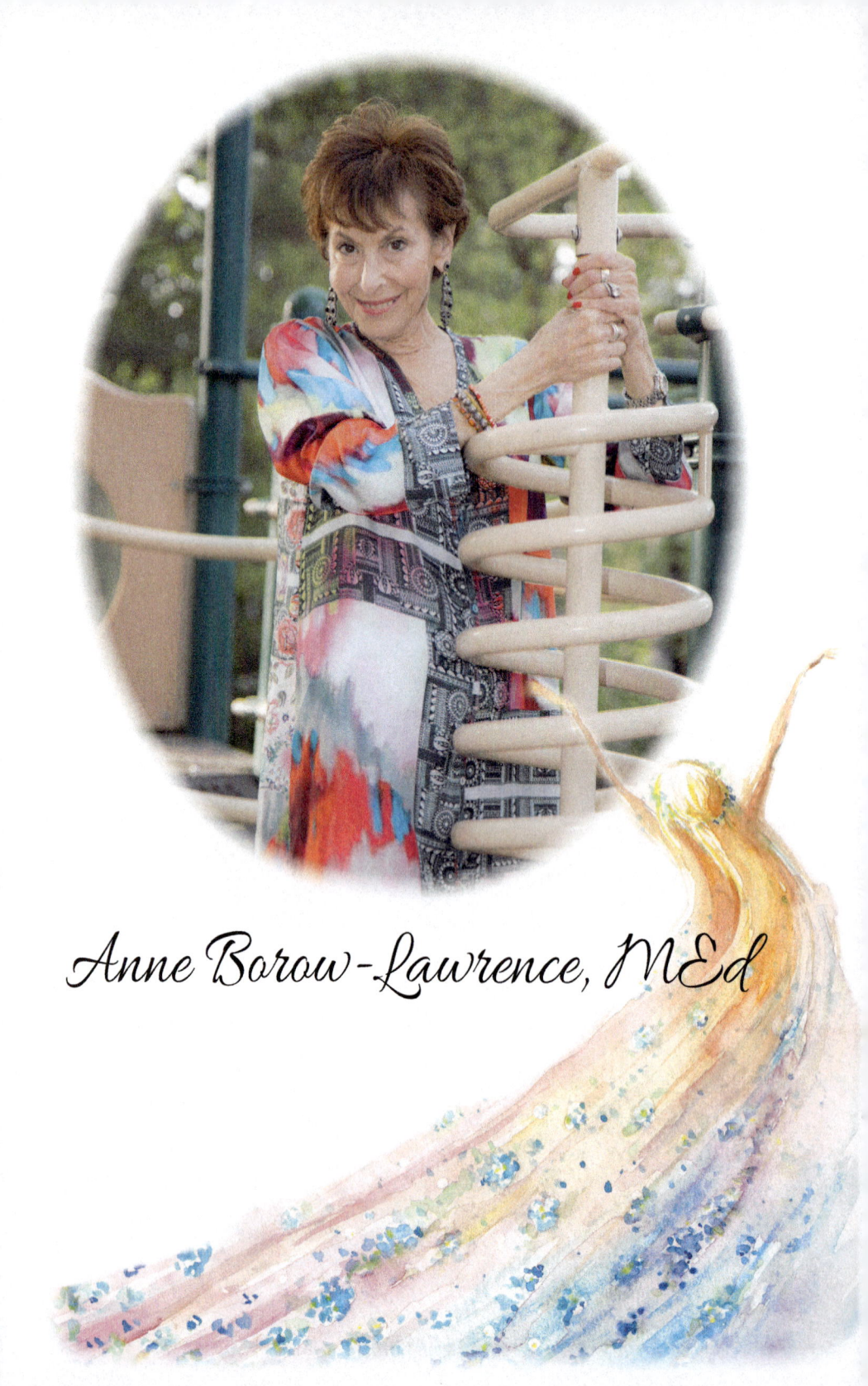

Discover Your Fountain of Youth: Myth to Mindset

"Age is merely the number of years the world has been enjoying you."

Intention:

Amidst the noise of modern life, a profound truth remains obscured—the real Fountain of Youth is not found in external remedies but within ourselves. May you feel a paradigm shift within these pages, hearing the message of mindset and heartfelt practices you can use. Experience the lightness of being touched by the music of nature, painting a new canvas in your life—embracing life itself in a new, uplifting, and unique way.

Story:

Since the dawn of civilization, human beings have been obsessed with reversing the natural process of life called aging. From ancient myths to modern advertisements, we are bombarded with the message that youth is paramount, and aging is something to be feared and fought against. This perpetual pursuit of the Fountain of Youth—whether through magical elixirs, lotions, potions, medications, meditations, or surgical interventions—pervades our society. While these modalities may have long-term value, without a fundamental shift in our beliefs and emotional states, the benefits we hope to gain may elude us.

Let's explore how society's obsession with youth impacts women, often making them feel inadequate as they age. We will delve into false beliefs and myths about aging, the power of a positive mindset, redefining creativity as we progress in our lives, the profound value of tapping into our creative spirit, and self-acceptance.

These are tools for reclaiming our essence and inspiring future generations. Personal anecdotes, scientific research, and practical advice will guide women to rediscover the Fountain of Youth within themselves.

From the beginning of time, The Obsession with Youth and the Fountain of Youth have captured the human imagination. This mythical spring, purportedly offering eternal youth to those who drink or bathe in its waters, symbolizes humanity's deep-seated fear of aging and death. Today, this myth manifests itself in a multitude of products and practices promising to halt or reverse the aging process.

Turn on the television, browse social media, or walk through any store, and you will be inundated with advertisements for anti-aging creams, supplements, and treatments. The underlying message is clear: youth is beautiful and desirable while aging is something to be hidden or feared. This relentless focus on maintaining a youthful appearance fosters feelings of inadequacy and insecurity, particularly among women.

Women, in particular, face immense pressure to maintain their youthful looks and vitality. Society often values them for their appearance rather than their wisdom, experience, or inner qualities. This external obsession can lead to a disconnect from the true essence of who they are and what they can offer the world. The real tragedy is not the physical signs of aging but the loss of self-worth and confidence that can accompany it.

I discovered my Inner Creative Spirit and life's passion when I was merely ten years old. A conversation that shaped my creative spirit for the rest of my life was one of intimacy and enlightenment with my father. As an aspiring professional ballerina, I had just spent the entire day in the Synagogue celebrating the Jewish High Holidays with my mother and my two older brothers.

There was a missing piece to this family worship. Someone was missing: my Dad, an internationally renowned muralist. He created worlds on walls like Michelangelo in the Sistine Chapel. I was bored to tears—which even flowed through my Jewish Holiday hat. I could not wait to escape. I knew my Dad was probably at home, as he usually was, reading or resting, maybe painting or drawing. It's hard to know because I wasn't there. As soon as we pulled into the driveway, eager to see him, I flew out of the car, ran up the stairs, and found him as I expected, sitting on my parents' bed reading the very same prayer book that I had been studying all day. I unceremoniously plopped myself down on the bed and bellowed, "Daddy, it's not fair. How come I have to go to Synagogue, and you don't? Don't you believe in G-d?"

He looked at me very endearingly and laughed. He then said, "Honey, of course, I do. I just don't believe that in the Bible when it says 'God created Man in His Own Image,' he meant some long-haired, bearded person on high. We are all created in the image of God. All of us have that Divine spark of creation contained within each and every one of us." He then asked me, "So who will you be? What will you be in your life, and what do you want to create?"

I said, "Oh Daddy! That's so easy. I'm a ballerina," and with an expressive response, I pirouetted out of the bedroom.

Then as a mature woman, at sixty, while caring for my 92-year-old mother, I witnessed firsthand the strength and resilience that came with a positive outlook on life. When I started caring for my Mom, we created a very special and unique environment. To me, with all I knew and experienced, it was so important to create a loving, nurturing, stimulating world so that my mom would make her transition peacefully, joyfully, and beautifully. I knew this was my gift to give to her. G-d used me to be this light in her life. This further reinforced my connection between longevity and mindset.

Mindset became paramount in my life. While still processing and grieving the loss of my mother, three months after her passing, through a somewhat "late" routine mammogram, I was diagnosed with a malignant breast tumor. I had no symptoms or awareness that anything had changed in my body. This sudden shift from caregiver to patient was a profound challenge. I had unknowingly overspent myself as a caregiver. I lost focus on my own self-care. Conversely, it also provided a powerful lesson in the importance of mindset, especially that caring for another also included caring for oneself.

During my early treatment, I was fortunate to have participated in a cancer support group session led by a pastor at the world-renowned Dana Farber Cancer Institute in Boston. As I compassionately listened to others share their journeys, I shared mine. At the end of speaking the Pastor said, "Anne, you must have been in shock when you received the phone call telling you that what was assumed to be a benign cyst was actually a lesion that could impact your "longevity," and especially after the loss of your Mom."

It was then I connected the dots. The feelings of fear and uncertainty. How did I want to handle this process? How would I navigate beyond the automatic survival response—Total Mental Shock!

Inadvertently, in an unconsciously competent way, I chose to again reject the common fears and negativity associated with cancer. Instead, I focused on maintaining a positive attitude, staying informed, and actively participating in my treatment options and decisions. Engaging in creative activities, practicing mindfulness, and surrounding myself with supportive people helped me navigate the physical, mental, and emotional challenges of treatment. Seven years later, I thrive with renewed vigor and purpose, embodying the message that the true Fountain of Youth lies within each of us and is by choice a matter of mindset. Dis-eases, and chronological aging, do occur, However; despair, depression, hopelessness, isolation, and being a victim—too are all choices we make.

At the heart of a woman's essence, all creeds, backgrounds, and ethnicities are the embodiment that women are creators and givers of life. This role extends beyond the physical act of giving birth to encompass the many ways women nurture, inspire, and transform the world around them.

Ruth Richard defines creativity as an Art Form. Creativity emerges in everyday occurrences—in the ordinary things—whether it's being a parent or a grandparent. For example, trying a new recipe, gardening, leading communities, or fostering innovation in one's chosen career. Women embody the spirit to bring into existence that which has not manifested before and with it, unique strengths and gifts.

This creative essence is not confined to traditional definitions of art but is found in everyday acts of innovation and care in life's relationships: the profound impact of mentoring and leadership of women as we continuously shape and enrich our environment. Embracing this role can serve as a powerful source of vitality and inspiration, helping women to feel empowered rather than diminished by the aging process.

So, what does creativity have to do with longevity? EVERYTHING! Forget everything you thought you knew about getting older. Integrate a positive mindset into daily life and triumph over it: Period!

Cultivating a rejuvenating mindset begins with daily practices that reinforce positivity and resilience. Mindfulness meditation, journaling, and engaging in new pursuits enrich our lives and fortify our mental health. Embracing lifelong learning and staying socially engaged also keeps our minds sharp and spirits high.

Professional research supports the idea that our mental state significantly influences our health and longevity. Positive thinking and emotional resilience are linked to better health outcomes, reduced stress, and longevity.

Neuroscientific studies show that a positive mindset can lower levels of stress hormones, improve immune function, and enhance overall well-being.

By fostering a mindset that embraces positivity and aliveness, we create chronicles within an internal environment that supports the energy of health and vitality. This concept aligns with the broader themes of *The Essence of a Woman*, highlighting our creative superpower and the importance of mental and emotional health in the overall well-being of women.

My most poignant and tender real-life example illustrates the very nature of our creative souls and spirits emanating from my father. His influence extended beyond personal conversations. Four days before he transitioned into the next realm of his body's existence, he lay in bed at home still drawing and sketching. His life was a testament to the idea that creativity and mindset are crucial to longevity and fulfillment. Even in his later years, he continued to paint his art which was still evolving within him. This relentless pursuit of creativity kept his mind sharp and his spirit vibrant, embodying the very essence of the Fountain of Youth. Despite his physical body breaking down, he was an artist, ever and always….He was on his—*life bed*—still creating.

Regular participation in creative activities, like my Dad until his final breath, enhances brain plasticity, reduces symptoms of depression, and anxiety, and improves social connectivity—an actual key to the longevity of health.

If you find yourself without a green thumb, a voice to tell stories, or even the ability to hold an artist's brush in daily activities, this practical advice will help you foster a mindset that supports a life full of vitality, vibrancy, relevance, joy, and health.

Engage in simple creative activities, such as sketching, writing poetry, or playing an instrument, to anchor your day and provide a sense of purpose and joy.

Practice mindful meditation to stay present and reduce stress. Techniques like deep breathing and body scans cultivate a calm and focused mind.

Engage in lifelong learning to stimulate the brain and foster a sense of achievement. Take up a new hobby, learn a new foreign language, or attend workshops to keep your mind active.

Participate in social engagement within a community. Joining clubs enhances social connections and provides emotional support, crucial for mental health in later life.

Adapt creative activities to suit your physical abilities. If mobility is an issue, consider digital art or crafts that can be done while seated. The key is to find joy and fulfillment in the creative process, regardless of the medium.

Harnessing mindset during health challenges requires a whole expanded skill set. A pivotal aspect of my journey was maintaining a positive mindset during my breast cancer treatment. This subsection highlights how mindset influenced my treatment choices and outcomes, providing a powerful testament to the role of beliefs and self-awareness as we face unexpected changes within our bodies. This sudden shift from caregiver to self-caregiver, with my breast cancer challenge, was a profound challenge, but I approached it with a steadfast belief in the power of a positive mindset. The Law of Attraction brought me to the program and methodology *"Prepare for Surgery, Heal Faster."* Now I am a practitioner in the methods that supported me.

I chose a combination and blended approach of Eastern and Western Medicine. My creativity and mindset-conscious decisions were based on my intuitive understanding of the dis-ease and the potential benefits of these treatments, balanced with my commitment to maintaining a positive outlook.

Throughout my treatment, I encompassed an indomitable spirit of wellness and wholeness. I was THE poster child! I engaged in creative activities, practiced mindfulness, and surrounded myself with positivity. This approach helped me navigate the physical and emotional challenges of treatment with grace and ease.

Today, I am over seven years cancer-free. My experience reinforced the importance that mental mindset overcomes any physical challenge. I share my inspirational message of healing and hope with others facing similar challenges.

This underscores the central message that a positive, resilient mindset is true power. It serves as a reminder that we have the capacity to influence our health outcomes through our thoughts, attitudes, and actions.

Start today by incorporating one new creative activity into your routine, one step and activity at a time. Remember, the true Fountain of Youth is within you—so drink up and enjoy the healthy cocktail so you can tap into this eternal source of personal power at any time you choose. You are the Creator of your life. Envision your superpower daily.

The Fountain of Youth we seek resides not in mythical waters or modern potions but brews within our being—through our thoughts, attitudes, beliefs, and daily practices. Embrace this empowering perspective, to craft a narrative of aging that is filled with fulfillment, happiness, joy, and vitality. Unlock your own Fountain of Youth, where mindset is the path to a life well lived, not just a life. As Mark Twain said, "AGE is just a number—it's mind over matter. If you don't mind, it doesn't matter."

Belief:

The real Fountain of Youth is a mindset. It is a place to think from, to create from. It's a context to abundance. Now is the time to rewire your brain, rewrite the rules, and redefine your pathway. Creativity is the access into your Inner Spirit.

Action Steps for the Fountain of Youth:

- **Never stop dreaming**: Now is the time. There is no time when we should stop.
- **Dream daily**: Make dreaming a daily ritual.
- **Create and explore new vistas daily**: Step out of your comfort zone and try new things.
- **Live a pirouette**: Pivot and keep on dancing, no matter your age.

Anne Borow-Lawrence, MEd
The Science of Being-Well
EnVisionCCS
www.envisionccs.com
anneblawrence@gmail.com

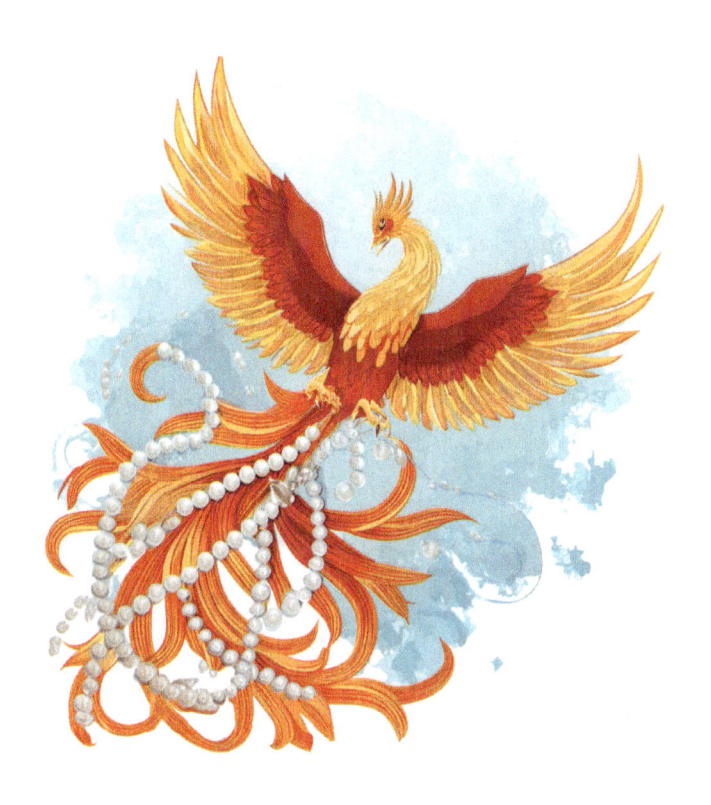

Betty (Elizabeth) A. Norlin

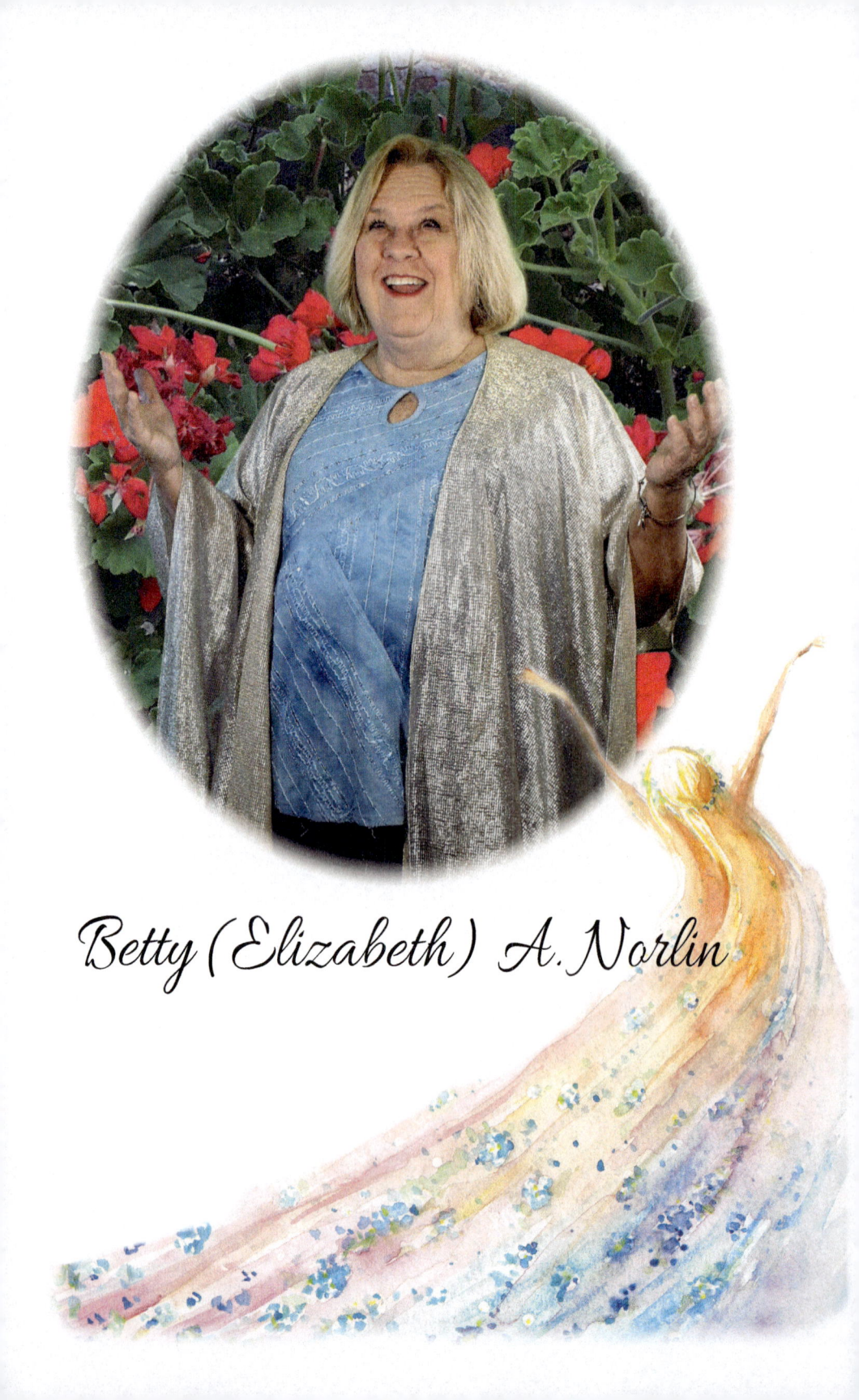

Our Bodies: The Optimal Design

"Dare to think differently. Discover unnoticed patterns to ask: What else is possible?"

Intention:

There is perfect order in the body. Your body and spirit speak to you and teach lessons you can apply in business, health, and life. Challenges can be stepping-stones, sages, and guides—if you allow it. My goal is to teach individuals and businesses how to discover these lessons.

Story:

My quest for life, for learning how to heal, began in my late twenties when doctors did not have the answers. I found myself exhausted—and figured "I was just getting old." The fatigue intensified until I was in bed 20 hours a day, too weak to move. After eight months, gradually I mustered enough energy to walk from my driveway to my next-door neighbors—and then sit down and rest until I had enough energy to walk back. Doctors told me I had a virus, and they did not have a way to "cure" a virus. My doctor said, "Go home. Rest. Let your body take care of itself."

I learned that 1/3 of the people never got better, 1/3 of the people had this recycling throughout their life, and 1/3 of the people got better—and stayed better. I knew deep within my heart I would be in the third that got better—and stayed better—I just didn't know how. Something deep inside of me told me, "Work on rebuilding your immune system naturally—and then teach others how to do it."

We do not grow unless given the opportunity—whether we create the opportunity, or are responding to a challenge.

Another growth spurt happened when I got *the shocking news* from my doctor, over the phone: *"They fully, fully, fully expect it to be malignant."* Imagine trying to tell your loved ones the news, and the word "malignant" was missing from your vocabulary. I would share, *"They fully, fully, fully expect it to be magnificent."* *(I would shake my head and think to myself, "No, that's not what they said.")* I would try again. The word malignant was gone. Gratefully. Graciously. Gone.

We cannot always control what happens to us, but we can control how we react to it. I thought to myself, "Cancer is just like malware on a computer. Malware can be fixed, so this can too." I came to understand that cancer was just cells gone astray. Misbehaving. Not doing what they were designed to do, the way they were designed.

I did a 21-day prayer and fast, with six friends. Every day, a new person, a new approach, and a new information download came into my awareness. I was learning more about "how to rebuild my immune system naturally, so I could teach others." I did not expect the lesson the way it arrived in my life, but I recognized and embraced it when it came.

I learned to talk to my body, talk to my disease. Make peace with both. I had several conversations with the diseased cells called cancer. The main question I asked was: "What are you here to teach me and how will you know when I have the lesson, so you are comfortable leaving?"

Ironically, this happened during the 2016 Presidential elections. President Trump became known for "Make America Great Again." My boyfriend, Frankie, looked at me and said, "Make your Boobs Great Again." I laughed. This is how I framed it when I told my family about my breast cancer…not in one breast, but in both.

I created a little "brochure" to share the news. Some of the points, that can be used as examples for any health crisis, are:

What are my boundaries and how can you best help me?
- *Laughter, Joy, Bring It On! It is healing!*
- *Questions, Discussions, Absolutely. Open to it. Might not always agree but want open communication.*
- *Be careful not to project your own fears or ideas onto me. It's my life. Own your own fears. Share your ideas.*
- *There will be rough times. I will let you know when I need to "go there."*
- *Positive, energetic people are welcome in my world! Positivity needed. Yet, you do not need to hide your fear. Just own it.*
- *Trust my decisions and my approach, yet feel free to voice your own when different.*
- *Feel free to ask any questions. Seek to understand, not judge. Watch critical spirit. It doesn't feel good.*

Later, after working with a life coach, I came up with my "life scripture verse:"

> *"The Father of compassion and the God of all comfort,*
> *who comforts us in all our troubles, so that we can comfort those in any trouble with*
> *the comfort we ourselves receive from God."*
>
> —1 Corinthians 1:3-4 (NIV).

As I went through these initial days of shock with a cancer diagnosis, and not knowing what the future would bring, I didn't feel scared. Fear lost its sting because I chose to share this message: I know who I am, who I belong to, and where I am ultimately going. This attitude didn't come from me, it came from deep within my spirit, not because of anything I did. I just believe I was fortunate enough to be chosen to share this message. I had to go through it in this way so that I could share with others that it doesn't have to be scary. I was given the gift to write: *The First 31 Days of a Cancer Diagnosis: Fear or Faith.* You can download it for free at my website: www.bettynorlin.com/31Days.

As I prepared for this book project, I started with prayer. I would suggest that anyone writing, preparing to speak or to create, get into "that place" through prayer, meditation, deep breathing, and nature. Listen to your spirit. Embrace your inner knowing. Here is what came to me:

- *I am the God of Perfection.*
- *Things can get out of order, but I can set them straight. I can help you use them for My purpose.*
- *It isn't about the human concept of perfection. It is about My concept, My plan, My order.*
- *I can reorder, restructure anything.*
- *Get right with Me to be right with yourself.*
- *If I am the Ultimate Creator, is it possible I planted a seed in you to manifest greatness through you?*

Now, relate that to you and your story.

Is the power in your challenge? Is the power in how you overcame? Or is the power in the people connecting to you, seeing themselves in your story, feeling your pain and joy, your fear and release, your power in surrender?

What is the message you are here to share?

What is your silver thread?

Dr. Jo Dee guides you to consider, "What is your 'Silver Thread?'" I wanted to understand this concept better, so I researched it. I came up with three meanings:

- A "silver cord" is the emotional tie between mom (Creator) and child (offspring).
- A "spiritual silver thread" is a silver cord that links our spiritual body to our physical foundation, so we will not be lost.
- "Silver" from ancient "Egyptian" beliefs is used to protect from evil spirits, ward off negative energies, and provide a life-giving linkage to purity and protection.

The better you know your 'Silver Thread' the more impact you will have. What idea comes from deep in your soul? How can you best use this to bless, impact, and help others? Each of us has a story.

Women are a creative source…so are men…all humans…all life. What is your creative genius? What was infused into you that you can infuse into others to help them grow and impact others?

As a result of continuing to follow my life path, MY BOOK emerged: *Our Bodies: The Optimal Design—A New Understanding of Our Miraculous Body*. In this book, I share the perfect order in our body in 10 different places.

From there came the online course: *Optimal Order: How to Revitalize Your Health*. The purpose is to bridge the understanding between Eastern and Western approaches from the patient's perspective, based on all I have learned over the years. The goal is to learn how to apply ancient wisdom in the modern world.

I have also been blessed to be an Ambassador of Health on our podcast: *Be Healthy in a Hurry*. It is a weekly show now in its 5th year. I speak on mindset, Dr. Wayne "The Mango Man" Pickering speaks on Nutrition and Food Combining, and Buddy Lee, The World Jump Rope Expert and two-time Olympian has spoken on Fitness. Our philosophy is that if we tap into our internal environment, and take care of that, we have the best chance to avoid, or address, the health issues we have. We believe you must be part of your own healing team, ask questions, and find the practitioners and approaches that work best for you and your loved ones. The podcast can be found on most podcast platforms or at www.behealthyinahurry.com.

In addition, through my own writing process, I now teach others to write and share their stories through book coaching, editing, and publishing. I strongly believe each of us has a story (or two) and we can use it to reach, teach, and bless others.

Philosophy:

I "heard" spiritually, early on, that I would be healed. I also knew that my definition of "healed" and my Creator's definition of "healed" may not be the same. It didn't scare me. It prepared me for whatever was next.

I am one who believes in natural approaches whenever possible. I will use Western Medicine if I feel that is where my spirit is leading me. I opted however, for the Eastern Approach, the more natural approach, first.

For me, through my prayer, my fasting, and speaking to both traditional and more holistic practitioners, my approach became the "blended" approach. That is a large part of what I teach audiences today. That, and how to listen to your body—in life, in business, and in health.

In creating this chapter, I thought about the creative power women have. A woman has the ability to birth a baby physically, A woman also has the ability to birth an idea globally, The fertilized egg grows within you. It is fed and nurtured by you. You have support from dad and others.

Let's take this to the idea level. When an idea, an inner knowing, comes to you, it is your opportunity and responsibility to pay attention to it, fertilize it, feed it, share it, birth it, and grow it.

How do you bring this back to your ideas, your purpose, and how you can influence and impact the world? I believe you:

- Listen with your heart. Listen to your soul. Be purposeful. Be intentional.

- Welcome the support, the love, and the ideas of others, and be open to what God and the universe bring your way.
- Create, guide, and let go. Honor the creation, the idea, and the gift of blessing others with your creation. It is in some ways only yours for a while, yet was begun in you, and will be nurtured by others. Work together and realize your creations belong to all of us, not just you.

One of my favorite Renaissance men is Leonardo da Vinci because he taught each of us the power of observation. A young lad, born out of wedlock, to a peasant mom and a landlord dad, grew up to bless the world with his creations, his observations, and his artwork. He made the Divine Ratio famous through *The Vitruvian Man*. The Divine or Golden Ratio, roughly 5 to 3, can be found in nature, art, your body, and financial markets. As a math teacher of many years like Leonardo, I was able to connect and teach this health and body connection. That, and how to listen to your body and learn the artful lessons that are built into each of us at a cellular and design level.

When you learn how to take those lessons and apply them in your own lives, in your own business, and in your own health, you begin to get a glimpse of the power within you. The power that can transform the world and those around you.

This is the Essence of Women, The Essence of Life, The Essence of Creation.

You can find more about my book: *Our Bodies: The Optimal Design*, my online class, my Zoom Classes, and my Speaking at www.bettynorlin.com.

"The discovery of unnoticed patterns will dare people to think differently…to ask what else is possible? … And isn't it about time?!"

—Betty Norlin

I believe my mission in life is to bridge and design the gap between the Eastern and Western Approaches to health. There is a beauty, science, and optimal plan in both. I am grateful for people who embody ancient wisdom and apply it to today's issues, challenges, and successes. You elevate and increase from others—from history, from different design approaches and beliefs, from varied cultures. Be willing to be open-minded, and curious, and listen with sensitivity in your heart.

Action Steps:

Ways to create balance internally, which impacts your health.

- Stimulate the Vagus Nerve: Turn head to right for 30 seconds, center for 30 seconds, left for 30 seconds, center for 30 seconds, repeat.
- Stimulate the Vagus Nerve: Massage and rub the side of your neck up behind your ears gently and back down seven times.
- Balance protons and neutrons in your body: Put your bare skin on the ground 10–30 minutes a day.
- Vitamin D: spend 10 minutes in the morning sun daily.
- Listen to Positive Prime 3 minutes a day—neuroscientifically changes mood (see podcast episode from 10-8-19 with Kim Serafini).
- Remember your internal words and focus: Are you Overwhelmed, or Overwhelmed by grace? Thanksgiving or Thanks-taking? Giving or Getting Mindset? Hopeless—or remembering sometimes less is more—so drop the "less" to have more—Hope!
- Music: Rife Frequencies or for Binaural Beats—(Melody Clouds—See 11-1-22 Podcast).
- Ask questions, learn, grow, and listen to your heart and the hearts of others.

Betty (Elizabeth) A. Norlin
Owner
What is Holistic Health, LLC
www.bettynorlin.com
whatisholistichealth@gmail.com

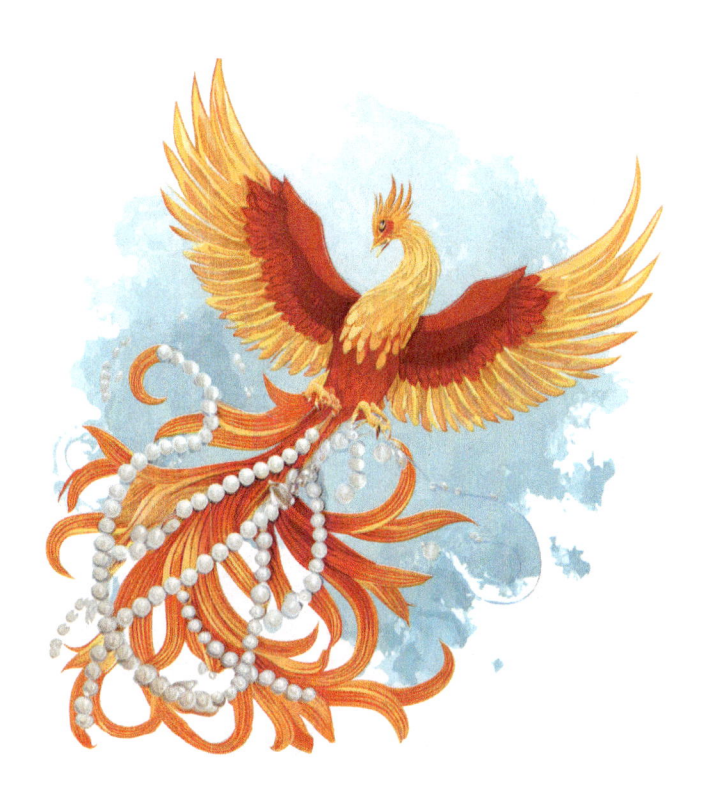

Renée Brown

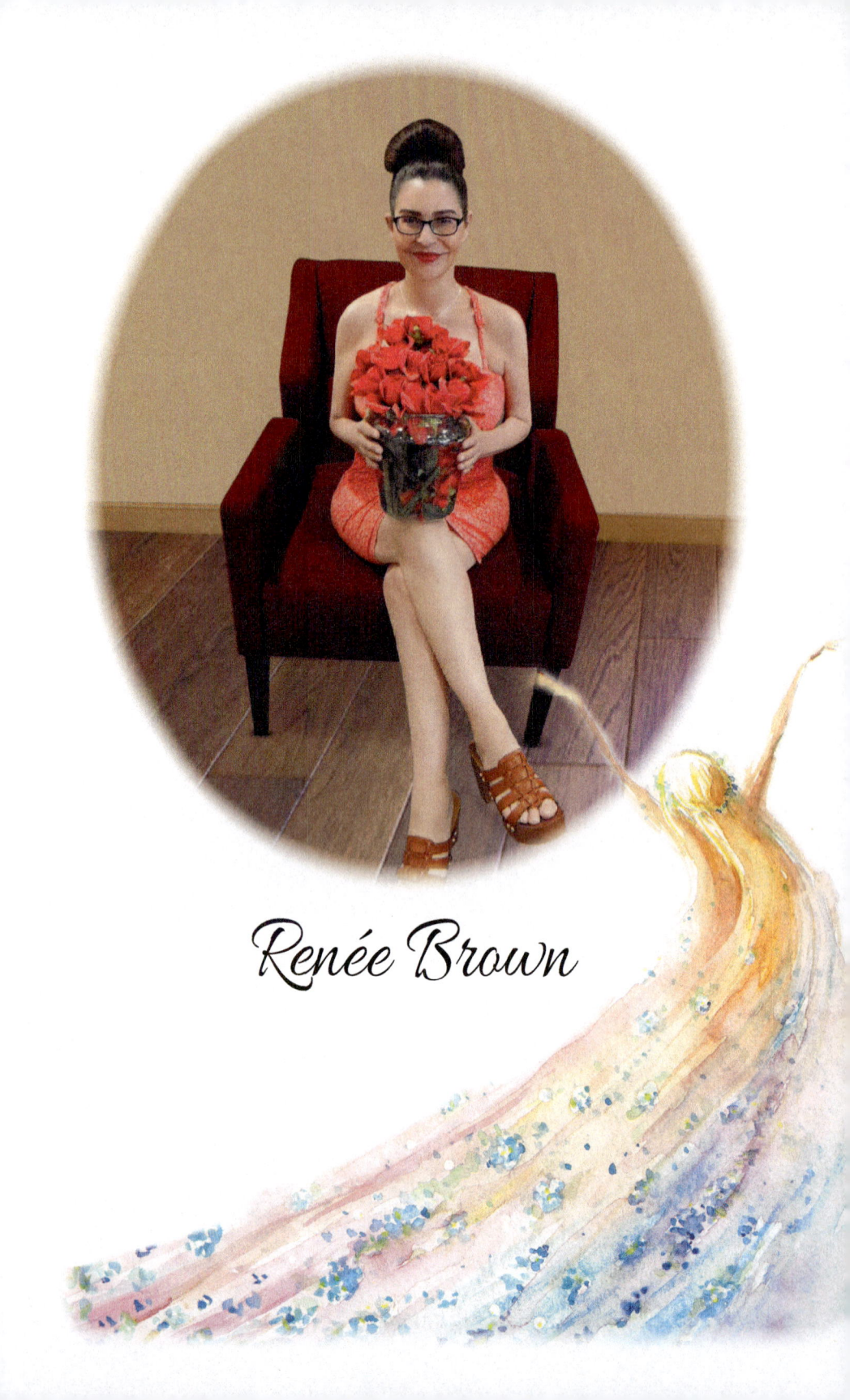

Unbreakable: From Trenches to Triumph!

"Receive, Overcome, Serve, and Inspire!" (ROSI) for Resilience and Optimism."

Intention:

This is a story from my heart, to inspire others to disrupt what isn't working or to create something new and novel for humanity to flourish.

Story:

Over the past 20 years, my husband, Mike, and I have partnered with thousands of patients to help build a new world of wellness! When I reflect upon the common missions of the companies that we have created, my personal experience and passion have motivated me to offer healing to those with trauma on a multidimensional level. In therapeutic settings, clients want to speak with someone who has "been there." There is an undeniable energy that is ameliorating when we feel understood. When we feel heard, we also feel loved.

We are very proud to stand behind many causes together with several successful businesses: Next Level Recovery (Treatment Center), Sober Living Properties (Recovery Housing), and Medical Mindshare (Integrative Medical Care). Our programs have been lifesaving and life-giving.

After many years of helping such an array of clients, we discovered something very alarming. Mike and I noticed that many of our clients, who were thrust in and out of foster care, usually had lives that continued to be riddled with abuse from correctional facilities well into adulthood. These patterns were similar to our clients who had survived intergenerational poverty and who typically experienced institutional style housing at a young age.

Some shocking statistics about children in foster care and correctional facilities include:

- PTSD: Children in foster care are diagnosed with PTSD at twice the rate of U.S. war veterans
- Incarceration: 20% of former foster care youth are incarcerated by age 21
- Homelessness: 30% of former foster care youth are homeless by age 21

- Substance abuse: 50% of former foster youth develop substance abuse by age 24
- Death Row: Up to 80% of death row inmates are former foster care youth

Life is sometimes composed of circles and semicircles that itch to be completed. One of the most ardent desires of my heart is to make a change or a dent in the current foster care system. It was a system that I wrestled with as a child along with my brothers.

It's unfathomable to know where to begin. In what seems like a lifetime ago, I was in the Los Angeles Foster Care System along with my brothers, Kevin and Eddie, in the late 70's and 80's. This was a time in Los Angeles County when institutional style care, Group Homes, Foster Homes, and other facilities were largely unchecked and unaccountable for the treatment of at-risk children.

Most institutional centers and group homes congregated kids who were considered "Emotionally Disturbed." This label was used for children who had experienced a multiplicity of traumatic events. This alienating label was supposed to commission the coordination of enriched professional services to take place. Traditionally, these children had been put in the most abusive environments. They were commonly discarded into specialized institutions where heinous acts were committed against them. These places had been rife with felonious acts in the most widespread and offensive abuses in the foster care system, which still happens to this day.

At the brink of turning ten years old, I was arrested for escaping a foster home. This shivering trauma began with a long chain of nefarious events. Sequestered in a locked room, I was forbidden to leave short of going to school. Another boy and girl, Danny and Anna, chose to run away with me and flee from contemptible circumstances. Emotionally weak from abuse but with an overarching feeling of nothing to lose, we ran away after school. I leaned on Danny for confidence since he claimed to know how we all could survive. Danny, who fully embraced his American Indian heritage like a magic wand, mistakenly thought he could assist us to live off the land. Naively I believed that he really did understand how we could sustain ourselves in the city.

The three of us began to slowly and aimlessly meander into a heavily populated city center location. On the walk, strong emotions welled up inside of me. As I looked down at the sidewalk and studied the lines in contrast to my strides. I felt isolated and alone, like no one cared. I was angry to be alive! I had never felt such despair until that day.

Eventually, we all began to tire. It had been a very long and arduous day. In the evening, Anna began to become nauseous. It was past midnight when her illness began to become more pronounced. Being kids, we all thought it would be fun to swim in the swill water under the sub-walk earlier that night. No one knew that we were making one of the worst choices possible. It was notoriously dangerous to hang out in that particular spot. The heavy rain that day filled the sub-walk up with at least three feet of water. That's what made it fun to explore and swim inside at the time. Miraculously, the heavy rain in the sub-walk most likely kept us alive and safe that night.

I had everyone wait for about an hour, hoping that Anna would improve and that we could continue our escape from the home. Starving, we hadn't eaten anything since our school lunch. I was wearing a summer crop top and shorts that day despite that it was December. Dressing for the weather didn't occur to any of us. Danny was nine years old and was about six months younger than I was. Anna was only eight years old but claimed to be almost nine.

Danny and I began to notice that Anna was declining fairly fast. It was time to make some quick decisions. Someone needed to stay with Anna, and someone also needed to run back to the home to get some help. Sizing up the situation the best that I could, I knew that I would have to be the person who could make it back to the home.

When we left the foster home, we had an understanding that we would never return. Dark and foreboding neighborhoods lay ahead of me, and I didn't consciously know where I was. My personality has always been detail oriented, and because of this, I felt like I was the natural candidate to make it back to the foster home. Confidence in my intuition would have to carry me through a five-mile run. I ran because Anna needed me to be quick, and it felt safer to run. There were menacing gang members, violent weapons, homeless people, and other dangers all around me. Everyone was clearly awake on the sidewalks. I decided that I would run in the middle of the street to keep as far away as possible from the apparent threats.

Raw instinct was triggered inside of me, and I decided to run head-on into where cars would come toward me. I was counting on perhaps one car rescuing me if I were to be attacked by someone. Running also kept me warm. Vague memories allowed me to make the right twists and turns through the unlit residential areas. I prayed throughout the run that I would be safe along with Danny and Anna. It was the most frightening and perilous run of my life!

Still in the ghetto, there were young men who made me feel vulnerable. My situation escalated when I saw them standing up from the porch where they had been sitting. They saw me, and it looked like they were deciding whether or not to run after me. At this point, I ran even harder and chose not to look at or make any eye contact with the young men. The landmarks were becoming familiar as I had just passed our elementary school. Thankfully, the first glimpse of dawn was on the horizon when I saw the first sliver of light. It gave me more hope and encouraged me to run the distance.

The police were called to arrest me as soon as I came to the house. They didn't ask any questions when they ordered me to take them to find the other kids. When we got back to the home, Danny was asked to settle in, and Anna was taken to the hospital. They both had prior arrests, but this would be my first one. I was about to be booked and incarcerated. Sadly, I knew that I would never see Danny and Anna again.

Behind bars, I wasn't aware that anyone would ever come for me. I was familiar with an adult jail as I had been dropped off there before when there wasn't any other place for me to stay. What few people know is that criminalization rates amongst abandoned children are very high.

Cruelly, the police teased me that I was there to stay! My biological mother finally arrived after receiving a phone call that I had been found. It was a miracle because statistically children were not known to survive a night on the streets of East Los Angeles. My mother was traumatized herself. She had panicked fearing that she might not ever see me again. No one asked me why I left the foster home or why I wanted to run away. That day was pivotal. I was about to permanently lose my voice as a ward of the state and become a child with a record. The truth was I was joining thousands of other kids who had lost their voices the same way. Adding insult to injury, it was then that I was labeled an "Emotionally Disturbed" child.

The greatest pain and trauma in my life was losing my younger brother, Kevin, to adoption. He was seven years younger than me and always felt more like my own first-born child than my brother. To this day I still have an indescribable pain in my soul from all the years Kevin was missing in my life. This type of grief is known as "Ambiguous Loss." It is defined as a loss without an intuitive path for emotional closure.

Against all odds, I reunited with Kevin after years of rigorous research from both of our sides. Faith and prayer have always filled my life with miracles. I couldn't feel more blessed, grateful, and complete that he is in my life again. Presently, Kevin has a beautiful family. He is a loving husband and father with a fulfilling career as a film writer and producer.

When my brother, William, and I were twelve, we shared our life stories. Technically, he is my step-brother but spiritually we are connected as brother and sister. Because of our unstable family situation, I felt troubled for him. I didn't know if he was going to be able to make it through the system again or life in general. By the time we had reached sixth grade, we both had attended twenty elementary schools and shared a lot of trauma. I found myself feeling very protective of him. I went on to experience adoptions that didn't quite work out, and William was sent to one of the most brutal institutions in the area.

There, his abuse was barbarous, he was chained up for more than six months as a young teen and was even denied the privilege to use a toilet. Because of this abuse, he had to learn how to walk again. William represents a sizable demographic that transitions from foster care to incarceration. It's commonly called the "foster care to prison pipeline." He was incarcerated for so long that he nested into the prison system.

After nearly a lifetime in prison, William was released five years ago. We continue to share the ability to read each other without many words. He is enjoying a good marriage and has been able to bond with his wife's family as his own. He is currently an author and is working on becoming a speaker.

Philosophy:

Years ago, I spoke with Les Brown, who was also a foster child. He asked me to visualize moments that have defined my life. Trying circumstances emerged like a cauldron in my mind. Les Brown's answer was in that mix.

What has defined my life has rested between the spaces of those difficult moments. I have always felt a reaffirming love from heaven, that has empowered me with fortitude. It has allowed me to receive love from other people as well as from nature. Receiving love into the inner core of who you are, can be a profound experience. This ability has often ignited a renewal of spirit inside of me and has sometimes enlightened me with an extraordinary sense of gratitude and compassion. Letting love in has even affected who I am on a physical level. Restorative wellness has come from the regular practice of prayer from the earliest memories of my childhood.

Allowing love in can become a spiritual practice that lets us nurture our state of being as well as a way to replenish ourselves on a cellular level. When energy vibrates at the frequency of love (528 Hz), our thoughts as well as the entirety of our senses become affected by "love hormones." It is then that we can find the connection to ourselves and others much easier. It's in this state that our rate of healing is also increased. I have been happy to hear of this broad concept utilized and researched in Quantum Biology, using the combination of intention and love.

ROSI (Receive, Overcome, Serve, Inspire) has allowed me to overcome many obstacles and has primed me to become more aware of serving others. When we merge the simplicity of faith, love, and intention into who we are on a soul level, every possibility can become possible!

Using my life experiences, I have come up with three concepts that a person can use as a foundation for starting a new nonprofit.

- **Discontent creates change:** There are many problems that make us feel disquieted, but there are some experiences that viscerally and spiritually move us. Evaluate if you would like to create the change in the world that you would like to see.
- **Vision:** Visualize your service or product as well as all the working parts. Work with other people to assist you with a top-down and bottom-up analysis. This should reveal a larger and more concrete picture.
- **Believe:** If you have the willingness to believe that your cause is really possible and achievable, everyone around you will want to embrace your vision. It is in this capacity that any obstacle can be overcome!

Action Steps for Optimism and Resilience:

- **R) Receive:** Let love land in your being to remind you of the very essence of who you are. A gush of gratitude might overwhelm you, let it resonate throughout your whole body!
- **O) Overcome:** Leverage your intentions with love and connection to overcome your obstacles.
- **S) Serve:** This action can transcend our entire body with positive context and healing. This act enhances our physiology immediately. A happiness trifecta of Dopamine, Serotonin, and Oxytocin will be released as you serve.
- **I) Inspire:** "Know what you know, Know how you know, and Know how to teach or tell what you know!" Renée Brown

Approximately six percent of the children in our country are in Foster Care, and 48,000 of them live in institutions.

I encourage you to make a change for foster care children by visiting this website: www.ImproveFosterCare.org.

Renée Brown
President and Co-Founder of
Sober Living Properties, Next Level Recovery
www.soberlivingproperties.com
www.nextlevelrecovery.org
www.medicalmindshare.org

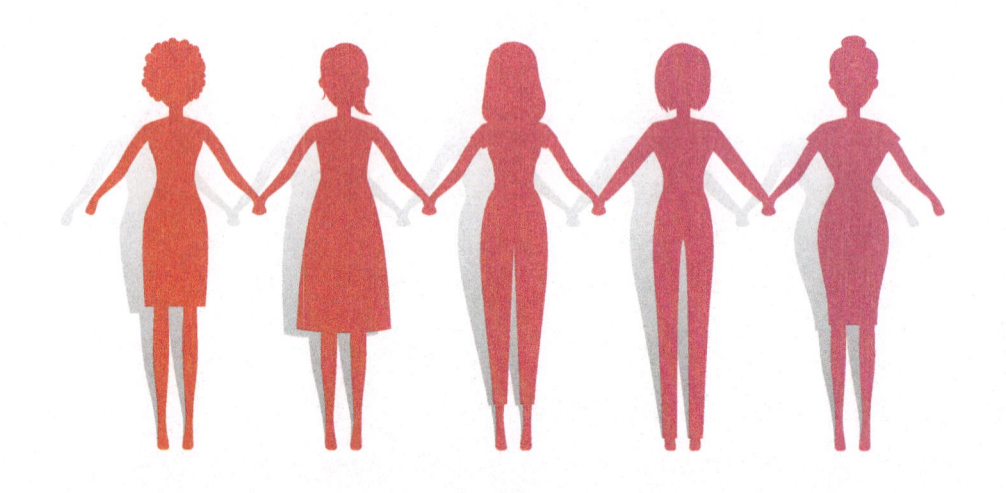

CHAPTER THREE

Emotional Pillar

"True beauty in a woman is reflected in her soul. It is the caring that she lovingly gives, the passion that she shows."
—Audrey Hepburn

"A woman whose smile is open and whose expression is glad has a kind of beauty no matter what she wears."
—Anne Roiphe

"Her own thoughts and reflections were habitually her best companions."
—Jane Austen

"We may encounter many defeats but we must not be defeated."
—Maya Angelou

"Do not dissect a rainbow. In other words, do not destroy a beautiful phenomenon by overanalyzing it."
—Denise LaFrance

"She walks in beauty, like the night. Of cloudless climes and starry skies."
—Lord Byron

"And in her smile I see something more beautiful than the stars."
—Beth Revis

"No matter how plain a woman may be, if truth and honesty are written across her face, she will be beautiful."
—Eleanor Roosevelt

Dr. Jacqueline Mohair, PhD

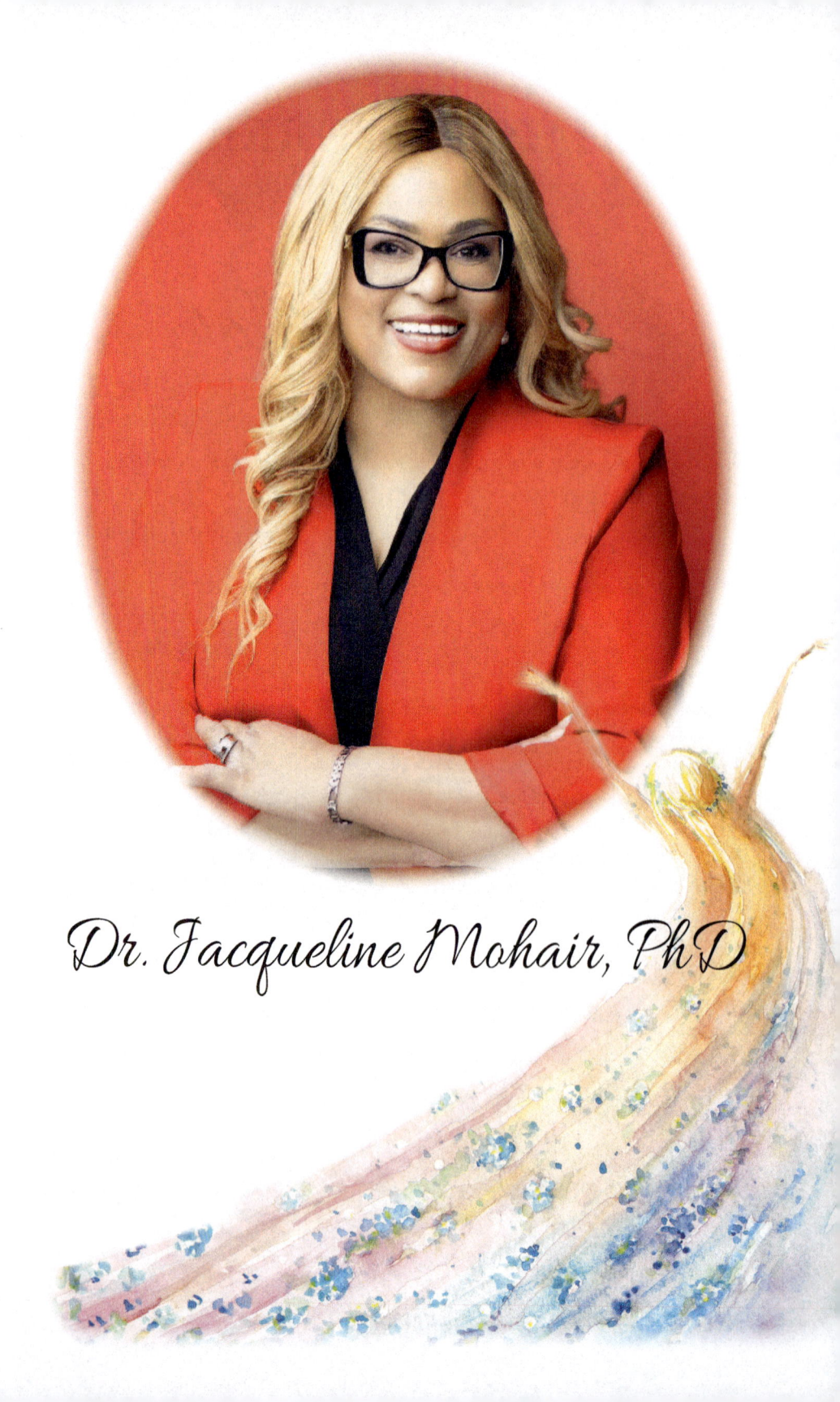

The Journey of Healing, Trust, and Transformation

"Bouncing Back: Embracing Resilience and Purpose."

Intention:

The Power of Emotional Intelligence

Emotional Intelligence (EI) encompasses the ability to understand, manage, and effectively express emotions. It's not merely about recognizing how we feel but about leveraging that awareness to navigate life's challenges, heal from trauma, and build profound, meaningful relationships. As Proverbs 4:23 (NIV) beautifully illustrates:

"Above all else, guard your heart, for everything you do flows from it."

This verse emphasizes the significance of emotional intelligence in our lives, urging us to protect and nurture our emotional well-being to fully embrace my quote: *"Bouncing Back: Embracing Resilience and Purpose."*

Life's challenges often come uninvited, shaking our sense of security and testing our resolve. For me, the journey from professional setbacks to entrepreneurial success has been a transformative experience, one fueled by resilience, faith, and the inner strength I discovered during the most trying times.

May you experience and appreciate the transformative power of emotional intelligence's power. It goes beyond managing emotions to enhancing self-awareness, empathy, and resilience. By offering practical strategies and biblical wisdom, may you be guided towards healing and growth. Together, may you also be inspired to use emotional intelligence to enrich both your personal and professional relationships.

Story:

The journey began during a tumultuous period marked by unexpected layoffs and professional uncertainty. I was challenged to confront layoffs and setbacks—Head On! The emotional impact of these setbacks was profound, leaving me challenged, grappling with self-doubt, and questioning my future. The stability I once took for granted was suddenly gone, and I was faced with the daunting task of redefining my path.

It was in this moment of uncertainty that I turned to my faith for solace and guidance. The scriptures became a source of strength, offering reassurance and a new perspective. Isaiah 40:31 (NIV) promises:

"Those who hope in the Lord will renew their strength."

This verse became a powerful reminder that my trials were not the end, but a part of a greater journey.

As I faced these challenges, my faith became an anchor, providing me with the courage to persevere. Immersing myself in prayer and reflection helped me to see my setbacks not as insurmountable obstacles, but as opportunities for growth and strength in all areas of my life. The spiritual guidance I received during this period reinforced my belief that these trials were shaping me for something greater. These challenges became an emotional anchor in my 'essence of a woman.'

Scriptures like 2 Timothy 1:7 (ESV), which states,

"God gave us a spirit not of fear but of power and love and self-control."

These affirmations were a source of my strength and capability. These verses helped me to confront my fears and uncertainties, turning them into a powerful force for change and resilience.

During this period of introspection, I discovered a newfound passion for entrepreneurship. What initially felt like a setback was, in reality, a powerful catalyst for transformation. I began to see these challenges as an invitation to step into a new realm of possibility, driven by a desire to fulfill my true potential as a woman. The Lioness of unleashing my feminine soul was born again.

Embracing this new path required me to channel this inner lioness—a symbol of courage, strength, and resilience. Rather than being deterred by obstacles, I saw them as opportunities to innovate and grow. The challenges became a source of inspiration, driving me to build a business that aligned with my purpose and values.

The Impact of Trauma on Emotional Intelligence

Trauma, especially from abuse, can significantly impair emotional intelligence. It affects one's ability to trust, connect with others, and even understand one's own emotions. Survivors of trauma often deal with long-lasting effects that complicate emotional awareness and management.

Unveiling these challenges to break through and reach into the soul of this trauma triggers a profound and emotionally healing experience. The following Four Steps to 'Understanding these Challenges' with Trauma are key:

1. **Hypervigilance and Anxiety:** Survivors of trauma frequently experience hypervigilance—a state of constant alertness and anxiety. This perpetual state can make it difficult to form meaningful connections and trust one's own emotions. Philippians 4:6–7 (NIV) offers solace:

   "Do not be anxious about anything, but in every situation, by prayer and petition, with thanksgiving, present your requests to God. And the peace of God, which transcends all understanding, will guard your hearts and your minds in Christ Jesus."

2. **Dissociation and Emotional Numbness:** To cope with overwhelming emotions, individuals might dissociate, distancing themselves from their feelings. This can lead to emotional numbness, where they feel disconnected from both positive and negative emotions. Psalm 34:18 (NIV) reminds us,

   "The Lord is close to the brokenhearted and saves those who are crushed in spirit."

   offering hope that even in emotional numbness, God's presence is a source of comfort and healing.

3. **Difficulty in Trusting Others:** Trauma can severely damage one's ability to trust, creating barriers in relationships with family, friends, and even oneself. Proverbs 3:5–6 (NIV) encourages us to:

   "Trust in the Lord with all your heart and lean not on your own understanding; in all your ways submit to him, and he will make your paths straight."

   underscoring the importance of trusting in God as we work to rebuild trust in ourselves and others.

4. **Negative Self-Perception:** Survivors often internalize trauma, leading to negative self-perceptions and feelings of unworthiness.

This can perpetuate a cycle of self-sabotage and emotional withdrawal. Psalm 139:14 (NIV) offers reassurance:

> *"I praise you because I am fearfully and wonderfully made; your works are wonderful, I know that full well."*

This verse reminds us of our inherent worth, regardless of past experiences.

Emotional Intelligence Tools are the first steps for reframing and rebuilding. Trust is a cornerstone of healthy relationships but is often the first casualty in the aftermath of trauma. Rebuilding trust involves:

1. **Self-Trust:** Emotional intelligence starts with self-trust. It involves acknowledging and honoring one's feelings, setting healthy boundaries, and making decisions aligned with personal values. Psalm 37:3 (NIV) advises,

    > *"Trust in the Lord and do good; dwell in the land and enjoy safe pasture."*

2. **Establishing Safe Relationships:** Surround yourself with supportive, trustworthy individuals. Emotional intelligence helps identify safe relationships and recognize red flags. Proverbs 27:17 (NIV) highlights the importance of healthy relationships:

    > *"As iron sharpens iron, so one person sharpens another."*

3. **Practicing Transparency:** Being open about emotions and experiences fosters trust. Emotional intelligence involves clear communication and honesty in expressing feelings. Ephesians 4:25 (NIV) encourages,

    > *"Therefore each of you must put off falsehood and speak truthfully to your neighbor, for we are all members of one body."*

4. **Forgiveness and Boundaries:** Forgiveness is crucial but must be accompanied by clear boundaries. Emotional intelligence helps navigate the complexities of forgiveness, ensuring it doesn't lead to re-exposure to harmful behaviors. Colossians 3:13 (NIV) states,

    > *"Bear with each other and forgive one another if any of you has a grievance against someone. Forgive as the Lord forgave you."*

Cultivating Emotional Resilience in Families becomes the next cornerstone to emotionally rebuild. Families play a critical role in supporting each other's emotional intelligence. To foster resilience within a family:

1. **Create a Supportive Environment:** Ensure that every family member feels safe, heard, and valued. Emotional intelligence promotes open communication and mutual respect.

   Galatians 6:2 (NIV) instructs,

   > *"Carry each other's burdens, and in this way you will fulfill the law of Christ."*

2. **Encourage Emotional Expression:** Allow family members to express their emotions freely and healthily. This includes regular family meetings where everyone can share their feelings without fear of judgment. Ephesians 4:29 (NIV) advises,

   > *"Do not let any unwholesome talk come out of your mouths, but only what is helpful for building others up according to their needs, that it may benefit those who listen."*

3. **Develop Coping Strategies Together:** Work as a family to develop coping strategies for dealing with stress and adversity. This could involve mindfulness practices, relaxation techniques, or shared hobbies. 1 Thessalonians 5:11 (NIV) says,

   > *"Therefore encourage one another and build each other up, just as in fact you are doing."*

4. **Focus on Collective Healing:** Healing from trauma is often seen as an individual journey, but families can—and should—heal together. Emotional intelligence helps families recognize that collective healing strengthens bonds and ensures that no one feels isolated in their pain. 1 Corinthians 12:26 (NIV) teaches,

   > *"If one part suffers, every part suffers with it; if one part is honored, every part rejoices with it."*

Empathy is essential for healing and strengthening relationships. Empathy is the ultimate healing tool. Developing empathy involves:

1. **Self-Empathy:** Treat yourself with the same kindness and understanding you would offer a loved one. Emotional intelligence fosters self-compassion, helping you forgive yourself and acknowledge your pain. Matthew 22:39 (NIV) reminds us,

   "Love your neighbor as yourself,"

   highlighting the importance of self-love.

2. **Empathy Towards Others:** Developing empathy for others helps build deeper, more meaningful connections. Emotional intelligence enables understanding others' emotions and experiences, aiding in the rebuilding of trust. Romans 12:15 (NIV) advises,

   "Rejoice with those who rejoice; mourn with those who mourn."

3. **Empathy in Action:** Empathy involves action. This may mean offering support, volunteering, or being present for someone in need. James 2:15–16 (NIV) states,

   "Suppose a brother or a sister is without clothes and daily food. If one of you says to them, 'Go in peace; keep warm and well fed,' but does nothing about their physical needs, what good is it?"

Philosophy:

'Transforming Pain into Purpose' is a powerful aspect of emotional intelligence. This key component creates constant forward momentum. To achieve this transformation:

1. **Identify Your Passion:** Emotional intelligence helps you connect with your passions, activities, or causes that bring you joy and fulfillment. Romans 8:28 (NIV) offers reassurance:

   "And we know that in all things God works for the good of those who love him, who have been called according to his purpose."

2. **Share Your Story:** Sharing your story can be empowering for both you and those who hear it. Emotional intelligence encourages you to find the courage to share your experiences, providing hope to others. Revelation 12:11 (NIV) says,

> *"They triumphed over him by the blood of the Lamb and by the word of their testimony."*

3. **Advocate for Change:** Channel your experiences into advocacy. This might involve working with nonprofits, speaking out against abuse, or participating in legislative efforts. Micah 6:8 (NIV) teaches us:

   > *"To act justly and to love mercy and to walk humbly with your God."*

4. **Mentor Others:** Mentoring allows you to guide others who are going through similar struggles, offering support and hope. 2 Corinthians 1:4 (NIV) encourages,

   > *"Who comforts us in all our troubles, so that we can comfort those in any trouble, with the comfort we ourselves receive from God."*

Navigating Emotional Intelligence in Family Dynamics becomes the next level for all within the Psychological Hierarchy of Emotional Health. Several key components for the core of the emotional health of the family are gained through support. Families play a crucial role in emotional intelligence and healing. Understanding how family dynamics support or hinder emotional growth is essential. To emotionally succeed, especially women need to embrace the following:

Creating a Safe Space:

1. **Active Listening:** Foster an environment where family members listen actively and empathetically. James 1:19 (NIV) says,

   > *"Everyone should be quick to listen, slow to speak and slow to become angry."*

2. **Non-Judgmental Responses:** Ensure emotions are expressed without fear of judgment. Romans 14:13 (NIV) advises,

   > *"Therefore let us stop passing judgment on one another."*

3. **Regular Check-Ins:** Implement regular family check-ins to address emotions and prevent misunderstandings. Proverbs 15:1 (NIV) highlights,

"A gentle answer turns away wrath, but a harsh word stirs up anger."

Building Resilience Together:

1. **Modeling Resilience:** Demonstrate resilience by handling adversity with grace. 2 Corinthians 12:9 (NIV) states,

   "My grace is sufficient for you, for my power is made perfect in weakness."

2. **Encouraging Problem-Solving:** Work together to solve problems and find solutions. Ecclesiastes 4:9 (NIV) notes,

   "Two are better than one, because they have a good return for their labor."

3. **Celebrating Successes:** Acknowledge and celebrate achievements to build confidence and motivation. Psalm 126:3 (NIV) says,

   "The Lord has done great things for us, and we are filled with joy."

Healing from Trauma:

1. **Family Therapy:** Engage in family therapy to address relational issues and develop healthier communication patterns. 1 Peter 5:10 (NIV) offers hope:

   "And the God of all grace, who called you to his eternal glory in Christ, after you have suffered a little while, will himself restore you and make you strong, firm and steadfast."

2. **Shared Healing Practices:** Incorporate practices such as prayer or meditation into family routines. Psalm 46:10 (NIV) encourages,

   "Be still, and know that I am God."

3. **Forgiveness and Reconciliation:** Address forgiveness and reconciliation within the family. Matthew 18:21–22 (NIV) teaches about forgiveness:

   "Then Peter came to Jesus and asked, 'Lord, how many times shall I forgive my brother or sister who sins against me? Up to seven times?'"

   "Jesus answered, 'I tell you, not seven times, but seventy-seven times.'"

Embracing Emotional Intelligence for Healing and Growth as a strong, resilient, and powerful woman requires a heart arsenal of emotional intelligence tools. Emotional intelligence is a powerful tool for healing from trauma, rebuilding trust, and fostering deep, meaningful relationships. By embracing emotional intelligence, individuals and families can navigate the challenges of trauma, cultivate resilience, and transform their pain into a source of strength and purpose. This healing, especially with women, cultivates healing, fosters trust, and creates transformation on every emotional plane. Embracing these qualities fosters power in every Universe of life.

Action Steps: Transformative Practices for Families:

- **Gratitude Practices:** Cultivate gratitude within the family. 1 Thessalonians 5:18 (NIV) advises,

    "Give thanks in all circumstances."

- **Emotional Check-Ins:** Regularly check in with each other's emotional state. Proverbs 12:25 (NIV) states,

    "Anxiety weighs down the heart, but a kind word cheers it up."

- **Encouraging Independence:** Support each member's emotional independence while maintaining strong connections. Galatians 6:2 (NIV) advises,

    "Carry each other's burdens, and in this way you will fulfill the law of Christ."

Dr. Jacqueline Mohair, PhD
President: Trinity School of Business
www.trinityschoolofbusiness.org
themohairs@gmail.com

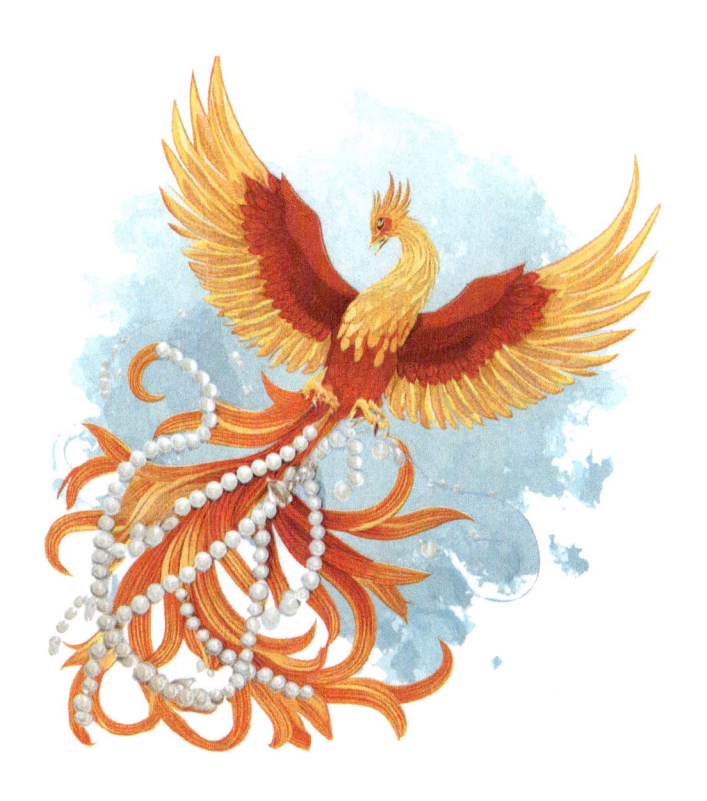

Sonja Rechnitzer

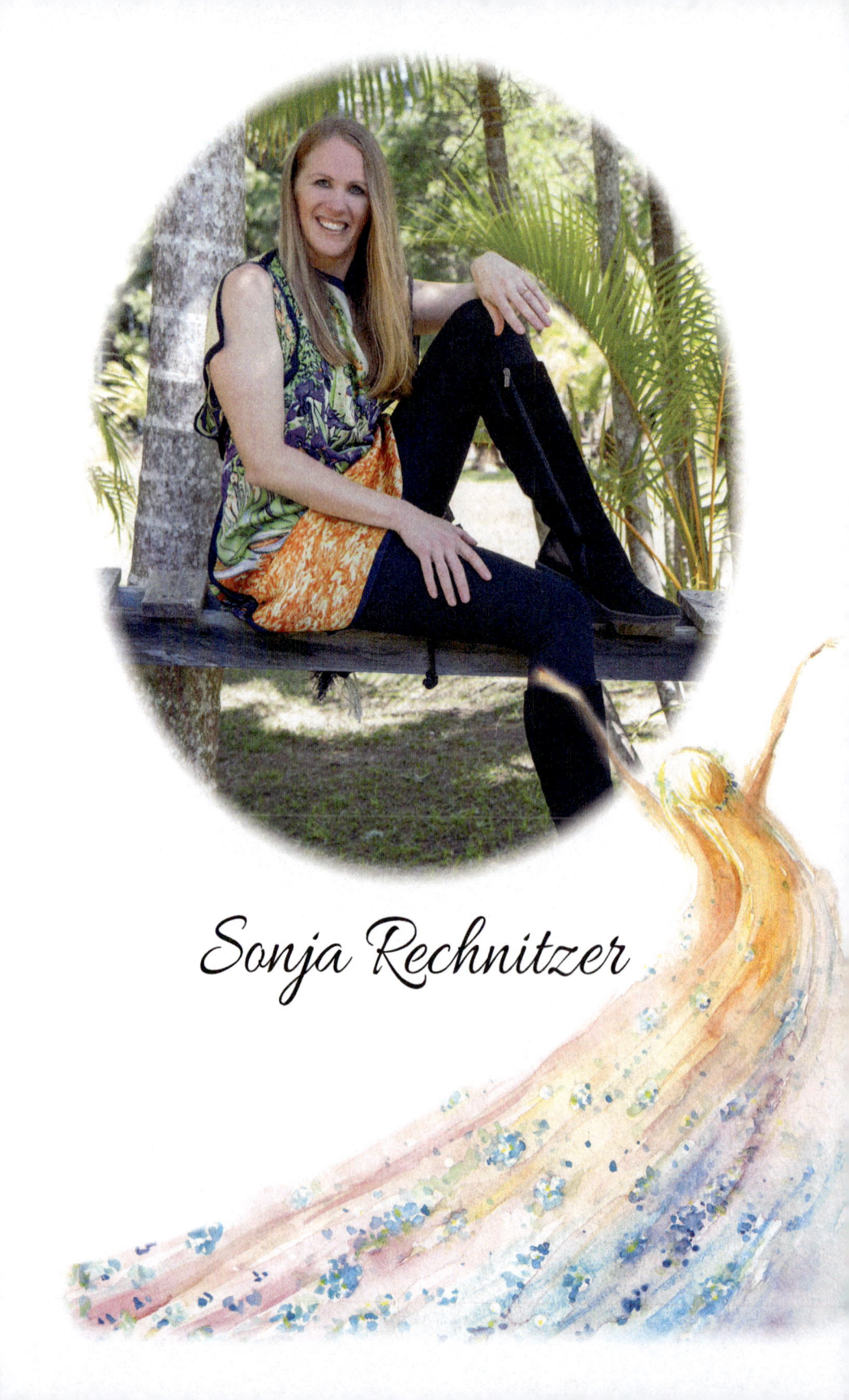

The Full Power of Intuition and Purposeful Living

"To live your life fully, be your empowered self and make a difference."

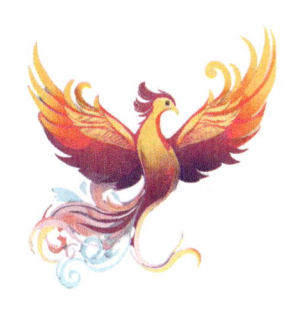

Intention:

Recognizing and living out your purpose is every woman's true life—a life lived fully—the life you were born to live, making the difference only you can make. From that space, you will experience all the love, joy, success, fulfillment, and abundance you have ever dreamed of—and you will be living your best life.

Every woman can find the strength to break societal norms and live her soul purpose—her reason for being.

To achieve this, we need the courage to always live our purpose, not just during designated hours or after fulfilling others' needs. Women often fall into the role of nurturer, prioritizing others over themselves.

True sustainability comes from acknowledging our divine purpose, embodying it, and sharing it—which often requires stepping into visibility and away from supporting someone else's dreams.

When we align with our life purpose, it supports and sustains us, allowing us to focus on what is real and bringing daily joy and fulfillment. Our purpose becomes monetized, shifting from sharing our skills with a few to offering our unique gifts to the world.

Enlightenment is not achieved in a brief meditation or journaling session; it is lived daily through our soul purpose. It is not about working for someone else's goals but fulfilling our own. If enlightenment is not your goal, substitute it with living an ***awesome life***—the result remains the same.

So let us embrace our truth, love, passion, and purpose—it is time to ROCK this world with our greatness!

Story:

I felt it again, 40 years after the first time…tha-thump, tha-thump, tha-thump. That familiar rhythm, that calm…when everything aligns perfectly, the focus is crystal clear, and all that is felt is pure happiness—a blend of love, joy, peace, fulfillment, and connectedness.

The rhythmic beat of my heart matched the clip-clop of my pony's hooves—I was ten years old, having questioned the meaning of life, wondering what life was all about. Why are we here? What does it all mean?

It all made sense for the first time in that moment as I breathed in deeply, a massive smile covering my entire face...and being. I am here for a reason. I am here to connect and make a difference. Making that difference brings me love, joy, peace, fulfillment, connectedness, and oneness.

Finding that purpose—the purpose of my life, the difference I am here to make—I felt close to it when riding my pony. It was like whispering the beat into my heart as we trotted along the creek, happily bouncing forward. I was one with him—we moved together, understood each other completely, and loved each other unconditionally.

Twenty-three years later, I understood why those years with horses were crucial. I was connected to my intuition, experiencing oneness, trusting my instincts, and living my best life—teaching, loving, and embodying joy. Whenever I faced a problem, I would seek solace with my horses, connecting to my true self and what was meaningful.

After disconnecting from horses due to a demanding corporate life, I lost touch with my intuition. I became a corporate robot, juggling work, fitness, and trying to become someone worth loving. Meanwhile, my pony loved me unconditionally—what was real always did. Nature and horses were my connection to myself and self-love.

At 33, I met Daniel Rechnitzer, who helped me reconnect with my intuition. Through this, I found my life's purpose: teaching women to connect fully with their intuition, discover their life purpose, and live their best lives—fulfilled, connected, and in awe of themselves.

But it was 40 years since that first moment on my pony, when I was ten years old, that I next rode and felt that feeling again...tha-thump, tha-thump, tha-thump. That perfect rhythm, that spectacular alignment, where everything is right with the world, where the focus is crystal clear, and all you can feel is truth, love, indescribable happiness and joy, and absolute peace of mind.

As I go on the journey toward the 2025 World Cup in Horseball, representing Australia for the first time at 51, learning to conquer a whole new set of fears stepping into courage once again, I am reminded of David R. Hawkins's Map of Consciousness Levels.

Wayne Dyer's concept on the journey from ego-driven ambition to a life of meaning is a great starting point for understanding how we can gracefully move in this ego-driven world. I first learned about this concept from a dear friend and psychology expert, Joe Pane, who wrote an excellent book: *The Courage To Be You*. Joe also introduced me to the Map of Consciousness Levels, which shows as we expand our energy through practicing courage and ascending the scale out of fear, desire, anger, and pride and into willingness, acceptance, reason, love, joy, and peace—we can achieve everything we ever dreamed about.

Moving from the ambition and ego-driven part of the scale into the meaning-driven section, we can move through life without all the emotions that drive us to 'need' and 'want' and 'have to have.' Happiness is easily achieved through fulfillment and purpose rather than 'stuff.' When you are fulfilled, you no longer 'want' things—you are just…happy.

As I have taught millions of people how to connect to their full power of intuition, I have noticed that the life we experience is simply a reflection of our overall energy and consciousness. When we spend some time and energy aligning our consciousness, climbing the energetic ladder to true power, which lies in the feminine, intuitive energy, we are paving the way for truly great experiences to unfold in our lives…effortlessly.

The emotions we experience at this level charge our true creative power of manifestation—fulfillment, love, abundance, joy, and peace.

A friend recently noted that everything we own will be gone in 100 years. Who remembers their great-grandparents' names? The car we drive will become scrap metal. As we packed up my parents' house, I saw how much 'stuff' was no longer meaningful. Choose things that hold long-term value.

That brings me to two things:

Be Mindful of Your Creations: Reflect on what you are creating. Will it have meaning in 50 years? Is it worth the expense, not just financially but energetically? Ensure your energy is directed purposefully.

Discover Your Legacy: Consider what will remain after you are gone. What difference will you make? This leads us to my ultimate philosophy:

Live your purpose in life, discover it, live it, embody it, and monetize it so that you can live it **fully** and contribute **all** of your purpose to this beautiful planet and the incredible beings on it. You can dedicate your life to something so meaningful that it makes your entire being smile from ear to ear, from top to toe. You can live feeling the tha-thump, tha-thump, tha-thump, clarity of vision, and unbound joy and happiness that come from purposeful living, guided intuitively by every step.

Live each day as if it is your last: Embrace it, enjoy time with loved ones, connect meaningfully, do what you love, and express gratitude. I remember being frustrated with my son's eating habits until I heard about a friend's stillbirth. That perspective shift made me grateful for my healthy child. Now, with two healthy children, I cherish this blessing every day.

It takes discipline to live life fully, to move away from what is 'normal,' and to create **your best** life. People think it just happens to you that those of us with incredible fortune and love just got lucky. I used to think that about people like that. Until I went on my journey from being a corporate robot to discovering my true self, purpose, and contribution. Let me tell you, it is the most incredible journey, and if there is anything worth spending time and effort on, this is it. The best thing is, when you put a few things in place, it becomes effortless—which is strange to say, I know. When focused on what is **real and true** for you, your effort is joyful, fun, and loving. So, make a start, take action, and be disciplined and focused on those actions. You will be grateful for the rest of your life for taking that first step and then continuing to take one step at a time on your life-purpose path.

Belief:

When we focus on needing something, we are in the energy of desire—a contractive, destructive force. Instead, focus on a powerful way of being.

Consider who you will BE when you have what you want. How will you feel? What emotions will you experience? Write them down. Can you already embody these feelings? Finding more straightforward ways to feel accomplished and happy creates the energy for the next step and fast-tracks achieving what you desire.

Action without purpose is a significantly diluted energy. As a result, we often spend our days doing, doing, doing, doing, doing a million things and not seeing much result. Focused and disciplined action is the ultimate way to live in abundance.

On the other hand, purposeful action comes from deep inside, focused on a powerful way of being that drives inspired action.

I saw in my tune-ins that the best way to make the money needed for a deposit on a family home was to inspire people to live their purpose in life and make a difference to people. I wanted to make a difference to as many people as possible, so I decided to exhibit and speak at the next Mind-Body-Soul Expo.

To keep a long story short—let me share my realization. I went to the expo with just one goal in mind, and yes, it was NOT the goal of how much money I would make. I went to change lives, show people their purpose in life, tune into their energy, show them their unique gift to this world, and inspire them to create their passion project to help people in the way that only they can. I did two speeches and four days of back-to-back 15-minute sessions, bringing to light over 150 people's purpose in life and how they can take the first steps toward monetizing and living that purpose.

I did it for free—to contribute and make a difference. I felt terrific—fulfilled, full of love and gratitude for my abilities, accomplished, successful, focused, relaxed, and in awe of myself. To say people were inspired is an understatement, and to say the results from that expo funded my house deposit would also be an understatement.

In contrast, I saw other booths scrambling for clients, fearful of not making their money back (expos in Australia can be pretty expensive), and putting on the hard sell. They went in afraid of failure, and that is precisely what they experienced: a failure to inspire, a failure to make it worth their while, and indeed a failure to have fun.

Success comes easily when you work with inspired action, but watch out for your fear of failure! People think failure is the opposite of success when it is integral to success. Each so-called failure brings you closer to the success you are reaching for and fuels your strength and courage to ensure you have become the person you need to be when success—as you define it—arrives.

The most important thing is to take steps—even if they are very small steps on days when action is hard for you. Finding the discipline to take even a tiny step each day—or each hour if you are able to operate on that level—will create results unlike any you have experienced so far.

When those steps are taken on your life purpose path, they are transformed into giant leaps, taken in the right direction (purposefully) and from the right being-ness. So rather than taking steps on a wiggly path in an awkward direction, even tiny steps in the right direction will get you there much faster and with much less effort.

Remember to enjoy the result and practice gratitude.

When practicing gratitude and living with a frequency of discipline and focus, creating a powerful, purposeful life will appear effortless.

Now this is very important—enjoy it!

That sounds tongue-in-cheek, but it is a crucial component to the success you are after.

I watch my friend's dog at the beach. Now he is getting old, but he is still excited every morning like a puppy. You can almost hear him say, "It's daytime!!! Let's play!!! Let's go!!! Let's do something fun!!!" He is not thinking about what happened yesterday, he is not worried about tomorrow, and he is just excited right now. You take him to the beach, and he is excited, grateful, and happy. He is not concerned about whether he will get to go again or that you did not take him yesterday—he is just having a great time.

When you are enjoying your life, living each day with the enthusiasm of a puppy that lives just for **this moment**, you are in the vibrational frequency that creates more of the same. You are manifesting intentionally more of these experiences that bring you love, joy, happiness, fulfillment, abundance, success, creativity, laughter…enlightenment and an extraordinary life.

The gratitude and love you find in these moments (every moment from now on) are working hard in the background to keep creating for you.

Remind yourself daily that you were born with a unique purpose, and in every way, you were born with what it takes to fulfill that purpose. In remembering what is important in your life, abundance will overflow. So you are enough; you have what it takes; you just need to find your path.

Immerse yourself in your Soul Purpose. I see an image of the world—lush and vibrant, and its pores are open and ready to receive. Each pore is a connected being living its sole purpose in this lifetime, feeding the planet everything it needs to flourish. In return, the earth provides energy, comfort, and sustenance—everything a being needs to live. Give yourself the gift of being part of an ecosystem where nothing is taken from you because what you give and need is readily available.

Be your true self—unapologetically shine the **true you** out in the world. Imagine an entire planet filled with people who are their true selves instead of the limited, damaged ego selves they have been living as. That is how you change the world!!

Action Steps:
- Create a Powerful Way of Being
- Take Inspired Action, Focused and Disciplined
- Enjoy the Result and Practice Gratitude
- Remind Yourself of What is Important

Sonja Rechnitzer
CEO, Global Trainer
Intuition Wisdom Institute
www.IntuitionWisdom.com
1@intuitionwisdom.com

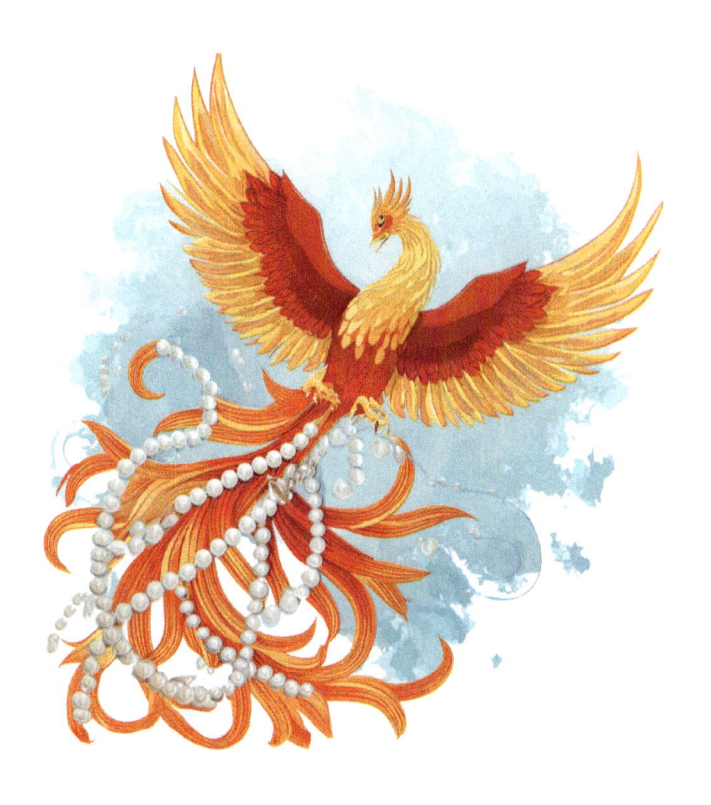

Sonja Rechnitzer | 163

Karen Rudolf

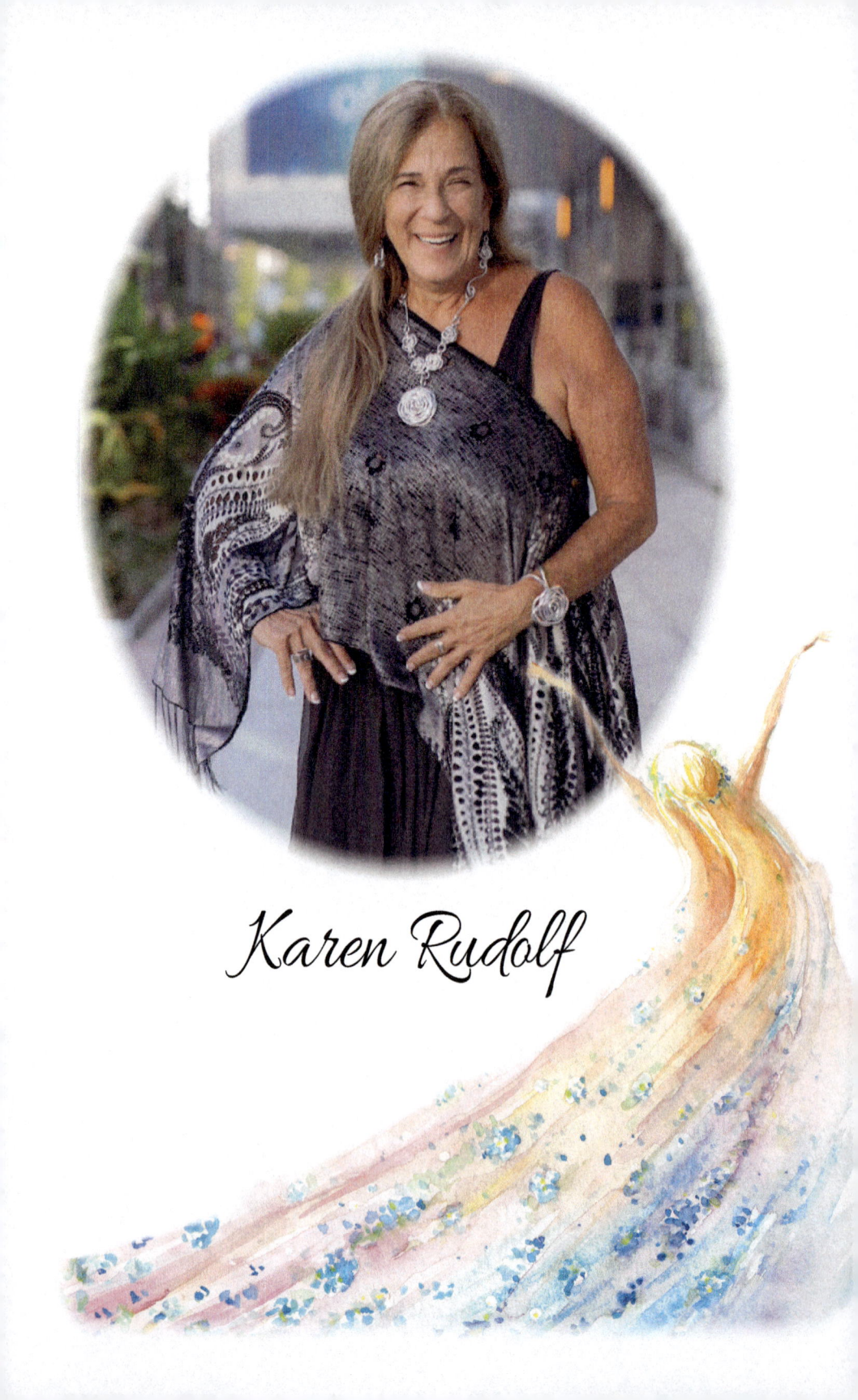

Dancing with The Divine: A Graceful Journey Within

"Embrace the beauty of the journey starting with your own."

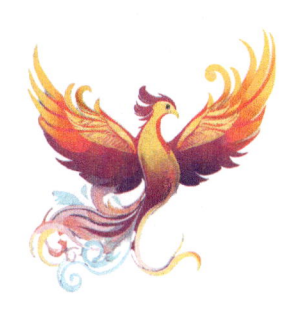

Intention:

Step into the transformative journey of a butterfly within these pages, where each word encourages you to unfold the wings of your true self. Beginning with affirmation and personal perceptions, I invite you to explore the delicate balance of strength and vulnerability, like a butterfly emerging from its cocoon. Engage your tales and introspective insights that call you to delve into the depths of solitude and the richness of connections, discovering the unique melody of your own life's story.

More than a narrative; it's a call to action to live authentically, resonating with your deepest values and aspirations. Embrace this guide to vibrant authenticity and elegant transformation, and find encouragement in pursuing self-discovery, recognizing the power of your authentic voice through the beauty of your metamorphosis.

Story:

"How do you do what you do?" This question, posed by a friend who saw in me a strength I had never acknowledged, shook the foundations of my self-perception. It was a moment that blurred the lines between perceived weakness and hidden resilience, revealing the intricate dance of strength and vulnerability of the delicate butterfly within me. This moment of unexpected recognition sparked a profound journey of self-reflection.

Imagine a divine soul as a vast stage where the motion of 'The Dance Within' takes place—a dynamic performance of contrasting emotions, experiences, and aspirations. This dance represents the eternal interplay between our exposed and hidden facets, where every step, twist, and turn reflects the continual negotiation between the person we present to the world and the essence we hold within. Pursuing this dance not just as a metaphor but as a lived experience—guiding us through the harmonious and sometimes challenging rhythms of self-discovery and transformation.

My first perception of my early childhood was a complex tapestry woven with threads of vulnerability and resilience. Diagnosed with asthma, I was frequently labeled as 'sickly' by my mother, a tag that enveloped me in a shroud of limitations. This medical label not only defined my physical activities but also cast a long shadow over my self-esteem. The familial atmosphere, strained with frequent conflicts, deepened my sense of being trapped in a role I didn't choose—perpetually the victim of circumstances beyond my control. These early experiences of health struggles and family dynamics instilled a narrative of helplessness and confinement within me. The asthma was a physical manifestation of my emotional suffocation.

Growing up, my voice seemed to dissolve in the cacophony of louder, more authoritative voices. Feeling isolated, my questions and curiosities were displayed with a dismissive wave of a hand, encapsulating the message that children were to be seen, not heard, pushing me further into a cocoon of isolation. This silence was not empty but filled with the vibrant, though often painful, explorations of my inner landscape.

My retreats into the nearby woods became my sanctuary, where the natural environment embraced me in a way people didn't. There, hidden under the protective canopy of trees and accompanied only by my thoughts and a handful of dolls, I found solace where my internal dialogues could breathe. These solitary moments amidst nature shaped my early understanding of myself—highlighting a stark contrast between who I was told to be and who I felt I could become. There in my little igloo, I "healed" my dolls with leaves. I was a Healer.

At a fragile time when a child is first experiencing the change from self to community, one April Fool's Day in first grade was not April Fools, but a turning point marking a pivotal moment that would quietly shape much of my early life. During a class exercise, my earnest attempt to participate was met with unexpected laughter—not with me, but at me.

The teacher had crafted a playful jest that everyone but I was in on. As laughter echoed around the room, confusion turned into humiliation; with a room full of faces blurred into a sea of mockery. I was left out. At that tender age, the classroom—a place that should have fostered learning and curiosity—became a theater of embarrassment and humiliation.

Like a rose ready to bloom—I shriveled up. It was then I made a silent vow to myself: to never open up again. This incident wasn't just a fleeting moment of childhood embarrassment; it symbolized the start of my imposed silence, a heavy cloak that I would wear for years to come.

This moment intensified an internal conflict and personal dissonance that had been simmering beneath the surface: the battle between my desire to be heard and a deep-seated feeling of unworthiness. This conflict did not stay confined to my childhood but stealthily followed me into adulthood.

Each opportunity to express myself or share my thoughts became a battleground where the desire to speak was met with the haunting echo and backlash of that initial classroom laughter, reminding me of my perceived inadequacy.

As I navigated through life's stages—adolescence, young adulthood, and beyond—this internal conflict often manifested in my relationships and professional endeavors, where I grappled with the dichotomy of wanting recognition yet feeling undeserving of it. This struggle between seeking a voice and shying away from the spotlight became a central theme of my journey toward self-discovery, empowerment, and dancing with the divine.

The awakening and turning point of my grace journey towards self-empowerment began with growing discontent with the labels and constraints imposed upon me from a young age. This awakening was not sudden, but rather a series of moments and insights that gradually illuminated the limitations I had unknowingly accepted.

One such moment occurred during a particularly reflective evening when I realized that the narrative of being 'sickly' and 'incapable' was not my own, but one I had inherited and internalized without question. This realization was both jarring and liberating. It propelled me to question other areas of my life where I had allowed superficial perceptions to dictate my self-view and concrete experience. Each question was a step towards dismantling the old beliefs and forging a path to self-empowerment.

As I peeled back the layers of my imposed identity, I plunged into the realms of Quantum Physics and Neuroscience. This self-discovery and exploration were driven by a deep desire to understand the fundamental principles of the universe and the complexities of the human brain. Studying these subjects, I started to recognize patterns and connections that transcended my previous understanding of life and my role within it.

Quantum Physics taught me about the potential for multiple realities and the power of observation in shaping outcomes. Neuroscience unlocked insights into the plasticity of the brain, revealing that change and growth are always possible. These disciplines not only expanded my intellectual horizons but also transformed my perception of Self. They provided a scientific foundation for the idea that I was not fixed by my past or my conditions; rather, I was a dynamic entity capable of profound transformation and growth—from cocoon to butterfly This insight became a cornerstone of my journey to self-empowerment, fueling my quest to redefine my narrative and embrace the possibilities of a new self-crafted identity.

My path to reclaiming my voice was embracing personal authenticity, evolving into a butterfly struggling to escape its cocoon. Initially, this process was fraught with personal and professional setbacks that tested my resolve. While painful, each setback served as a critical learning point, paving the way for a rebound, and pushing me to speak up and assert myself in situations where I had previously shrunk back.

My cocoon of silence had become a fortress, now breaking apart, as I began to voice my opinions and express my needs openly. My wings emerged in my metamorphosis, challenging but gratifying, as I confronted deep-seated fears and endured the discomfort of growth. As I persevered through these layers of resistance, much like the butterfly exerts effort to strengthen its wings, I discovered that with each attempt, my voice grew stronger, more confident, and unmistakably mine.

As I emerged from my metaphorical cocoon, transformed and vibrant, I began to embody the essence of the woman within and empowerment realized—that had been lying dormant within me. This newfound strength was not just a personal victory; it became a platform from which I could lead and mentor others. I leveraged my journey to guide those who were also struggling to find their voices and assert their authenticity in a world that often tries to impose silence.

My journey of transformation became a beacon for others, illustrating that it is possible to turn vulnerability into strength and authenticity into a powerful tool for leadership. Just as the butterfly emerges with wings ready to soar, I stepped into my role as a mentor with the grace and dance of confidence needed to uplift and inspire, showing others that embracing their true selves is the ultimate expression of empowerment.

My journey of transformation from a silenced observer, constrained by suffocating labels and self-doubt, to a vocal advocate for self-empowerment encapsulates a profound journey of growth and self-realization, navigating life's complexities. Like a butterfly finally freed from its cocoon, I have learned to embrace the entirety of my experiences—both the struggles and triumphs—that have shaped my path. A path that leads me to wholeness and wellness, *"W"Holistically*. This journey has taught me the power of resilience and the importance of finding one's voice in the chorus of life's challenges.

Pause and reflect on your own life's narrative. *Consider* the labels that have defined you and the moments that have silenced you. T*ake actionable steps today to start reclaiming your narrative. Assert your voice to echo your truest self. Remember, the journey of transformation begins with a single act of courage—a move into your divine dance of beauty toward understanding and embracing your authentic essence.*

Welcome the strength that lies in your story, for each challenge faced and every silence overcome adds a verse to the powerful song of excellence in your life. Stand tall in your journey, for you are the author of your own story, the sculptor of your destiny, and the only one who can grant yourself the power to live with boldness and purpose. Let your life be a testament to the fact that when we choose to lead with the voice of our authentic selves, we not only transform our own lives into beauty like none other, but also inspire those around us to embark on their paths of ease, empowerment, and grace.

In my 40 years of healing work, I've witnessed the transformative power of holistic approaches, which address the mental, emotional, physical, and spiritual health for lasting impact.

Effective communication helps guide individuals through their challenges and unlocks one's potential to live a healthy fulfilled life. Fostering resilience and self-leadership is crucial in supporting others to navigate their personal and professional lives. Just like a butterfly unfolding its wings, individuals will discover their inner strengths and harness them for personal growth.

Being a compassionate partner emphasizes the importance of empathy and genuine support within your personal journey. Continuous learning and adapting to new methods ensures better service to others. Comprehensive well-being elevates lives and nurtures growth, both personally and professionally. Collaboration and community impact and highlight the value of shared wisdom in driving positive change.

Belief:

To thyself be true; for in the depths of our understanding lies the unparalleled power to shape your destiny. It is through the unwavering embrace of our authentic essence that we harness the strength to navigate life's vast seas, not merely to weather the storms but rather to chart a course that resonates with the truth of our being. In knowing oneself, we unlock the door to boundless potential, forging paths illuminated by the light of our conviction and courage.

This chapter, akin to the transformative journey of a butterfly, invites you to unfold the wings of your true self. Here, amidst personal tales and introspective insights, you are encouraged to explore the delicate balance of strength and vulnerability. Just as a butterfly emerges from its cocoon, you are called to delve into the depths of solitude and connect deeply, discovering the unique melody of your own life's story. This narrative is more than words on a page; it is a vibrant call to action to live authentically, resonating with your deepest values and aspirations. Embrace this guide to elegant transformation, and find encouragement in the beauty of your metamorphosis, recognizing the power of your authentic voice as you chart your course.

Remember: Finding your true essence lies within finding the dance within. Find your wings and soar. The view is amazing from up there!

Action Steps for Your Metamorphosis:

- **Early Challenges**: Recall a label or expectation from your childhood. How did it shape your self-view? Reframe it to reflect your true strengths.

- **Turning Points**: Identify a pivotal life moment. What lesson did you learn, and how have you grown from it?

- **Journey to Self-Empowerment**: Reflect on a time you overcame a setback. What strategies helped you? How did this enhance your resilience?

- **Embracing Authenticity**: Define what authenticity means to you. Are there parts of your true self you hide? Why?

- **Empowerment**: Assess your life's current narrative. What would you change, and what steps can you take to start that transformation?

- **Be grateful for life's experiences:** Gratitude in all things serves you well. The road may be long and rocky, but find happiness in all situations.

Karen Rudolf
Empowerment Coach, Catalyst for Change
Tranquil SOULutions, LLC
www.tranquilSOULutions.com
karen@tranquilSOULutions.com

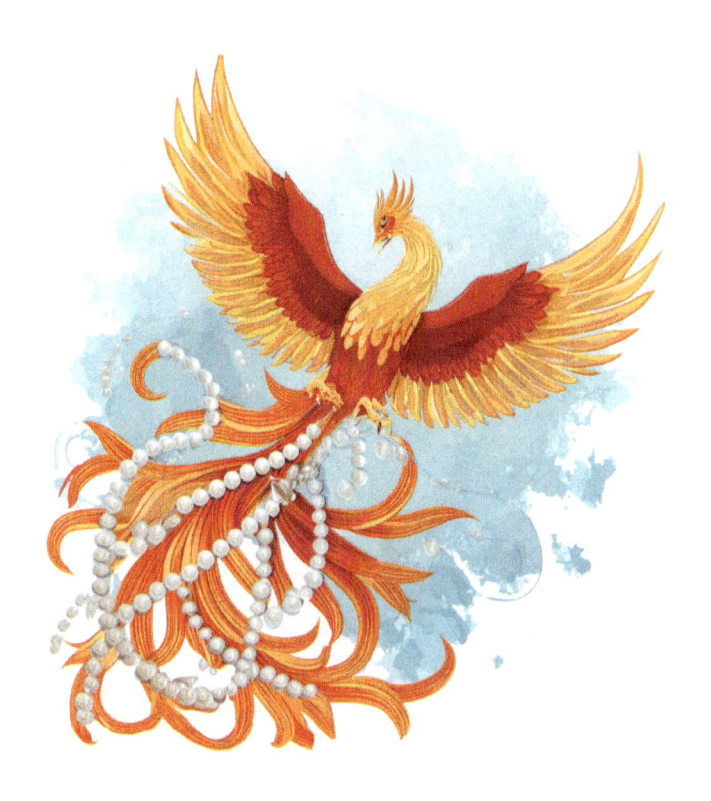

Cynthia Hammel-Knipe, CPE

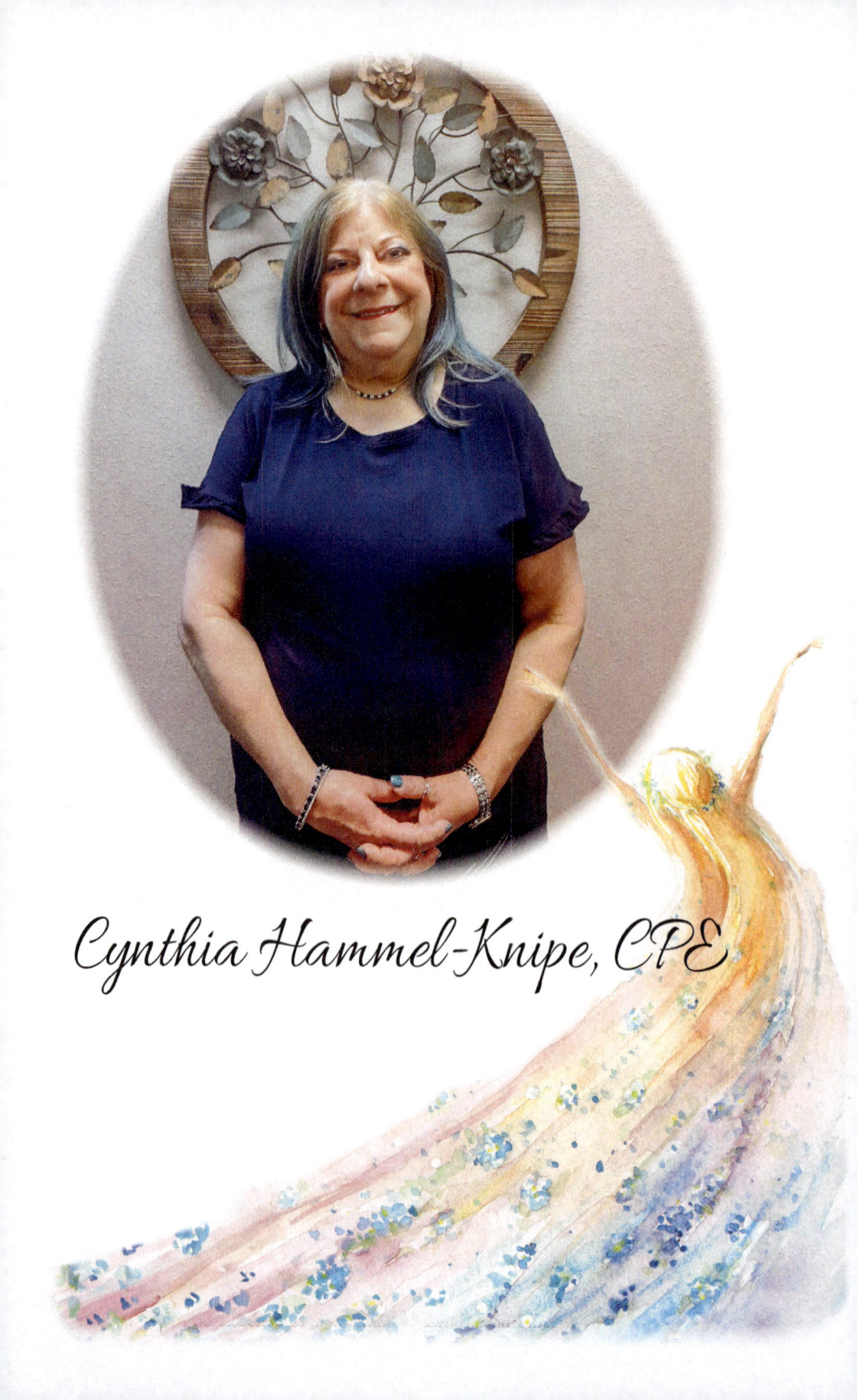

Self-Esteem:
The Road to Self-Empowerment

*"The beauty you feel on the inside
is the beauty you show to the world."*

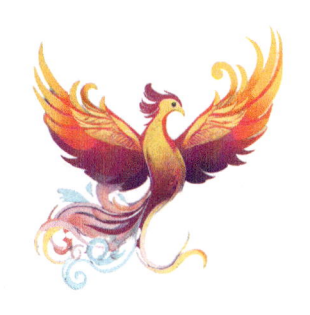

Intention:

Self-love is a journey. Women struggle more with this self-actualizing journey because of the world's expectations of women. May you unearth your own road to self-empowerment by discovering your unique footprint of beauty in your world.

Story:

Women struggle being the sole provider. Not until the Suffragette Movement did women earn this right, yet missed integrating it into their lives. Fighting for this right is nothing new.

Throughout time, women have had to fight for their rights to be sovereign souls. Women have had to maintain households, bear children, raise children, care for ailing parents, and answer others' demands. Many have the right to vote, and it was just a start for change. Change, however, is slow. Today's true battle is to maintain control over their own bodies. Women have always been judged for their appearance. They have been held to beauty pageant standards. TV and movies portray women as sex objects. It's amazing we've come this far. It's a struggle to keep one's self-esteem intact. As an electrologist, esthetician, permanent makeup artist, master herbalist, and iridologist; I have worked with countless women to help them achieve better self-images.

I have experienced this lack of self esteem as a young performer on stage. I was very self-conscious of an underarm rash. Thus, my own electrolysis journey began when I was in my 20's. My Native American friend had a 5-year-old son. His son, with childlike curiosity, was examining his father's upper lip and then my upper lip. His father had almost no hair on his upper lip. I, on the other hand, had a very healthy dark brown mustache. With the true innocence of a child, he asked why I had a mustache and his dad didn't. I was mortified! I tried the best I could to explain the genetic differences between us. My self-esteem plummeted in that minute. I had always been a little embarrassed by the hair on my upper lip. This was my breaking point. Desperate to find a solution to my problem, I went on a frenetic search to do something about it. To top it all off, I was afflicted with issues found in my underarms. Every time I shaved, my skin became irritated and I broke out in a painful rash. When I applied the usual deodorant it became even more painful. Many costumes I wore on stage were sleeveless, exacerbating the situation. I had to shave to look like a girl. I would try to hide the redness and rash with make-up. That wasn't a great solution, but it was the best one I could think of at the time.

Enter my best friend and my saving grace. Sue had gone back east to study electrology with her aunt. She came back needing practice as her business was building. I was a more than willing recipient. We worked out an amiable deal and that started my journey of electrolysis.

I discovered that permanent hair removal is achieved with a series of treatments. After a while, my dark, thick upper lip hair began to get lighter and finer. As it began to disappear, we were able to tackle those armpits! The more progress we made, the better I felt physically and emotionally. I was no longer afraid to go sleeveless. I could wear any color of lipstick I desired. I was no longer afraid to attract attention to my lips. It was liberating!

I was still pursuing my music career, as I expanded upon in *Health-a-Pedia*. Music is a healer; listen with your heart. Life is filled with music; listen with your soul. After an audition with the San Francisco Opera Association, I was offered a position with their sister company in Cologne, Germany. As ecstatic as I was about this offer, I had to discuss it at length with my husband and parents. This was one of the hardest decisions I would ever have to make in my life. My dream was to sing opera. I often practiced five hours a day. However, the circumstances surrounding the offer weren't ideal. My husband and I would have to live in different countries for a year. He was willing to move to Germany, but he would have to find his own work. Also a musician, he was a fabulous drummer. We were both well established musicians and instructors in Colorado. After looking at the big picture, Germany was not going to be in my future.

I was a private voice instructor and sang professionally with a couple of different bands. To supplement our income, I was also a bar manager. I was still looking for another profession that would allow me to continue music and add to my repertoire.

Enter a lunch date with Sue, the electrologist, who was now the President of the Colorado Association of Electrologists. She had to stop by the treasurer's house to take care of some association business. I accompanied her to Helen's house. Helen was going to start an electrology school herself. She was looking for a couple of candidates to try her curriculum. The students would then be grandfathered into the licensed school upon state approval. By the time we left Helen's house that day, I had my book and first pair of tweezers in hand. My future calling had been born inside of me. Since my hair disappeared and my self-esteem rose, I was excited about this amazing opportunity to help others feel the same way I felt. I could help others become their best selves. The more I studied electrology and the more I practiced inserting the needle; the more confidence I had that this was the right choice. Helen was a great teacher. She was very encouraging and very detailed in her instruction. She pointed out that this would be a stable profession for a woman. You could be your own boss.

The more I delved into the causes of hair growth, the more assured I was that I was in the right place, at the right time. I began to understand the importance of hormones in relation to hair growth. I was understanding why a woman might present with a full beard and mustache. A syndrome can present with one or more symptoms and can be hard to diagnose. This condition is now known as polycystic ovarian syndrome. The acronym for this is PCOS. When I first became an electrologist, it was known as Stein-Levanthal or Cahn's Syndrome. As the years passed and research progressed, PCOS was found to be the most accurate diagnosis. Among the symptoms are excessive hair growth on the face and midline of the body, weight gain or difficulty maintaining a normal weight, acne, possible depression, and a precursor to Type-2 diabetes. The inability to have a child may also be a result of Polycycstic Ovarian Syndrome. Although this is one of the most common reasons for hair growth, there are others. Stress is a major cause of unwanted hair growth. Stress, both internal and physical, may cause the free ranging androgens to produce unwanted hair. Heredity is a common reason as well. Certain ethnicities are prone to the hereditary cause of hair growth. Less common is tumor-related hair growth from a glandular condition.

There is a difference in hair removal methods, as most aren't permanent solutions. Waxing, tweezing, sugaring, and threading are all temporary solutions for hair removal. The most common side effects of these are skin irritation and scarring. They can actually cause the hair to become thicker and deeper in the follicle over time. The follicle may also become distorted or ingrown under the skin and cause a major eruption. Shaving is also a temporary method of hair removal. In some cases, one has to shave more than once a day. A shadow and roughness may occur, along with bumps and ingrown hair. Laser is only approved for a permanent reduction in hair growth. It doesn't work well on hair that is anything but dark in pigment. Issues may also occur in darker pigmented skin such as hypopigmentation.

Electrolysis is the only FDA (Federal Drug Administration) approved method for hair removal. It has been around for over a hundred years. The equipment keeps improving and the process keeps getting better all the time.

I'm always satisfied when I see great progress as the hair disappears and the smiles that appear from the smooth feel of hairless skin. When my client's confidence blossoms, it gives me reassurance that I made the right decision in choosing this career path.

Another very rewarding aspect of electrology is working with the Androgen Insensitivity Syndrome community. I began working with the LGBTQIA the first year I came into the profession. There has been good progress in the acceptance of the community since I began over 35 years ago.

Early on, many transgender clients wanted an appointment when they wouldn't be in contact with anyone else. Usually, that meant the last appointment of the day. Now, most have found acceptance and are very comfortable coming in anytime.

I have taught many electrologists how to work on the transgender client. Not only are we removing unwanted facial hair, we are helping them prepare for sexual reassignment surgery. This is a very specific pattern of hair removal. It's imperative that the surgical area be free from hair. This is a very sensitive procedure for the client to endure. The decision to become the person one feels they are on the inside isn't a choice that is made without difficulty. One must live as though they are the gender they feel. They must dress in accordance with their perception of who they wish to present to the world. Most require hormone therapy and two years of counseling minimum in order to initiate the transition. The hair removal process alone involves hours of work. One doesn't ask to be androgen insensitive, it simply happens. Many of the people I have worked with have known since they were children, that they were in essence, in the wrong body. I was merely a conduit for their journey to self-empowerment.

Many tried for years to follow societal norms. They married, had children, and tried to be someone they weren't. Some have been able to salvage their relationships. Most have struggled to maintain any contact with their previous partners. They have sacrificed a lot of their lives, to live in their truth.

I have become empathetic to their plight. It has brought me fulfillment in knowing I have been a part of someone's healing soul journey to their person and unique beauty of self empowerment.

Who knew that a musician who spent most of her younger life in the healing frequencies of music; would find healing in the medical arts? The beauty I found within, is the beauty I have been blessed to help others find in themselves.

Philosophy:

Being an esthetician has given another avenue to help others with their skin and permanent make-up. Teaching people the importance of skin care has been my parallel mission. Living in Colorado, at a mile above sea level, has its own challenges. This is a very dry climate as a rule. The importance of a good skin care regime is key to aging gracefully, with minimal wrinkles.

Many who come to see me initially for electrolysis, become skin care clients. Once the hair is under control, it's time to take active care of your skin. Keeping a good self-image is key to eternal happiness. When we look in the mirror and like what we see, we feel good to the depths of our soul. We transfer that self-confidence and all is good with the world!

My dual approach is internal and external. An enhancement to health is Iridology and Herbology. Iridology is the study of the Iris of the eye—a reading for foundational health. The reading is then accompanied with personalized supplements. The external with the proper skin care for their skin type. When you look at the whole person you get remarkable results.

Once health is achieved, why not permanent make-up? It brings out my artistic nature. I love giving eyebrows to people who have lost them. The eyebrows are the windows to the face. The shape of your eyebrows says a lot about you. The beauty of permanence is that you always look your best. I have had liner and brows since I was in my twenties. I must state that over time they do fade with exfoliation. Every now and then you do have to touch them up. It's totally worth it!

Being blessed with a thirst for knowledge has kept me evolving and expanding my horizons. I feel I have been guided by God, the universe, and angels every moment of my life. First to have been blessed by a career in music that still inspires me. Then to have been given the opportunity to learn a vocation in allied medicine, that brings such joy. The addition of permanent make-up and esthetics that brings variety. The training in vitamins and herbs (that started at fifteen years old), has given me a sense of purpose beyond breathtaking. Helping clients develop better self esteem and watching them transform into better versions of themselves provides me the gift of seeing their joy—that comes with the improvement of one's self-image.

The wonderful relationships I have developed are priceless. Everyone has their own path. We can walk the path together in love and peace, empathy and understanding. Be willing to learn from one another, and we will create a beautiful and better world.

Action Steps: T-A-K-E

- **Take Care of yourself from an inner and an outer standpoint:** skin care, electrolysis, nutrition, supplementation, exercise, meditation, loving your whole self, unconditionally

- **Acidity to Alkalinity:** One go-to remedy to help alkalize your body is to start your morning with six ounces of lemon water, and a recipe of: apple cider vinegar, cranberry juice, cinnamon, and cardamom, upon rising.

- **Keep Track:** Use pH strips to measure your pH by urinating upon rising.

- **Energize:** Take a good organic multivitamin—make sure it is bioavailable and bio-soluble.

Cynthia Hammel-Knipe CPE
Certified Professional Electrologist
Integrated Wellness Services, Inc.
www.electrology.com
crhkiws@gmail.com

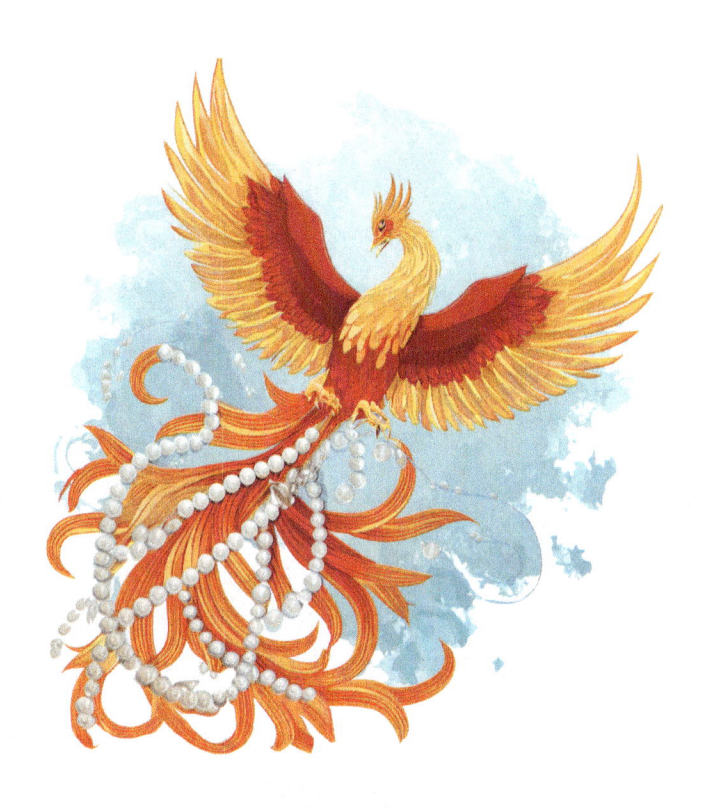

MarBeth Dunn

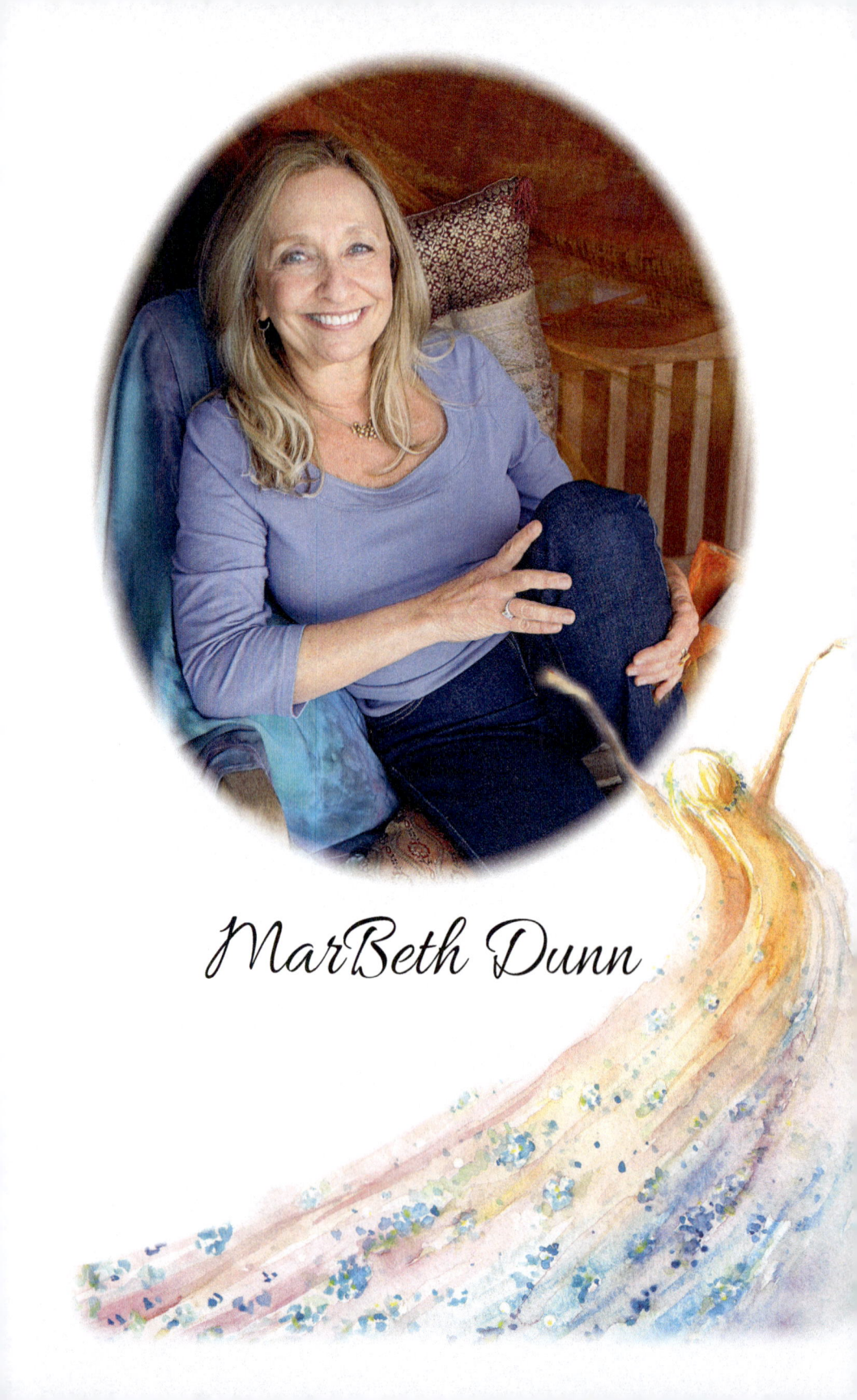

Your Body Loves You

"Your body heals from emotional and physical trauma: in an easy-to-learn language."

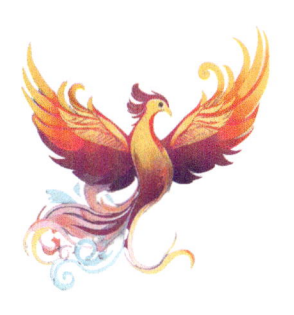

Intention:

Your body loves you and offers you a way to heal from emotional and physical trauma using its own easy-to-learn language of communication, through Somatic Healing. It stores the memories of past trauma, which is also the key to releasing them. As an empath and intuitive, may my journey of somatic healing be a blessing passed forward to you through my Intuitive Energy Management process.

Story:

I lay awake, checking the clock. It is only 4 a.m.

"Why am I up? Why is my throat sore? Am I coming down with something?"

I coughed and sneezed.

"Uh oh! There is a pain in my chest! I must be getting sick just before we leave Las Vegas! I don't want to travel sick!" I'm getting panicky, ready to unleash the immune-boosting brigade of elderberry, zinc, and hibiscus tea.

But wait! Better check in with my body first.

In the darkness, I sat up and muscle tested, joining my fingers together, and looping my thumbs with my forefingers. "I am physically sick," I said tentatively. My hands split apart. "No," responded my body.

"My symptoms are emotional." My fingers held together. "Yes."

"I'm feeling sad. I don't want to leave my family!" "Yes!" My body spoke again.

After a week-long vacation with my daughter and her family, I didn't want us to separate the next day and return to our respective homes across the country.

Gently, my awareness settled into the pain and heaviness in my chest and throat, and the knots in my gut. Holding the space, I quietly felt the physical feelings.

Sensations began to move through my body as I stayed with them. The physical symptoms finally left, and I, thankfully, was restored to my normal self and able to sleep. The next day, I expressed my sadness to my family. They felt it too. It brought us into a deeper connection as we traveled home.

My body had communicated in its special language. I released the sadness and accepted my feelings. In the past, I might have come down with a cold, but now I understand my body's signals to accept and release troubling emotions. Such is the power of the body-mind somatic connection.

My family was stoic as I was growing up and didn't express their emotions easily, so it's not surprising that I learned to disconnect from my feelings throughout a traumatic early childhood. Although I wasn't aware of my feelings and emotions, my body tried to help me access them with signals I didn't understand. I developed asthma, pains and aches, a slumped posture, and a feeling of being lost.

The body and mind are two integrative parts of a functioning whole. When they communicate poorly, stress, illness, and pain can result, thus we have DIS-ease. Thankfully, there are many ways to restore this connection, and I have learned them through my personal growth, training, and healing journey.

For years, I thought something was radically wrong with me. I had asthma attacks at parties, my energy was depleted around other people. I felt weak, subject to social anxiety, and toxic relationships.

After my divorce, in a vivid vision during a meditation, I saw myself inside a neighborhood new-age store. Intrigued, I visited the store in real life and signed up for their upcoming Friday night Reiki Circle.

At the Reiki Circle, practitioners channeled energy through their hands by candlelight, and we received this energetic gift. This powerful experience opened a doorway into a world of healing and consciousness-opening techniques. I lapped up the powerful, new intuitive knowledge and healing capabilities as I became a Reiki Master, Kundalini Yoga instructor, Matrix Energetics practitioner, Emotional Freedom Technique master, and practitioner of several other modalities with Somatic Healing techniques.

My practice originated in a physical location, and gradually transitioned to online coaching and mentoring. As a multi-faceted Energy Intuitive and Empath, I mentored and coached my clients to access their inner knowing and release their blocks to health, financial freedom, and happiness through their body wisdom.

One spring afternoon about twelve years ago, I sat at my desk on my glassed-in balcony-turned-office, surveying the dark cumulus clouds gathering over the lake. It was just about to storm when I reached out via Skype to a man in Germany I had never met to see whether we were a good fit to work together.

"Hello, Franz, what made you decide to contact me?"

"I've been feeling stuck, and I'm unsure which direction to go."

I noticed a deep pain and heaviness in my chest. Instinctively, I wrote on my notepad, "Deep sadness, heartbreak, grief."

"Tell me about the work you do."

"I have a business with my brother selling art reproductions."

The pain in my chest subsided, and I felt a stabbing pain under my left shoulder blade.

I wrote, "Betrayal."

"Are you happy in your business?"

"I'm feeling restless. I want to try something different, but I'm unsure what."

The pain left my back, and my solar plexus became a twisted mass of knots.

I jotted down, "Relationship issues. Difficulty maintaining power."

"Tell me about your relationship with your brother. Do you get along well?"

"We have our ups and downs. It's been rough since our mother died."

Instantly my pelvic floor was on fire.

I wrote, "Rage."

"Are you married? In a relationship?"

"My wife died a couple of years ago, and I've started seeing someone."

A golf ball lodged in my throat. It was sore.

I noted, "Unexpressed and trapped emotions."

My body returned to normal, leaving me astounded at how his body had communicated what it needed and how easily I had understood the messages from across the ocean.

"Franz, this is going to sound a bit weird. I'm an empath and I work with energy. As we've been talking, you've been communicating with me on a deeper level. Do I have your permission to send you healing energy?"

"Yes!"

Instantly, I knew what to do and where to send the energy. I felt his body release the trapped emotions, and his old traumas healed.

I sat back in my chair, astonished. Not only had I received a "computer printout" of Franz's emotional issues, but we had learned to communicate in a new language and were guided to the solution. My Intuitive Energy Management process was born!

Over the years, I have learned to appreciate my body's language of love and support, which correlates to ancient yogic traditions. The throat is the energy center for expression. It holds emotions that need to be expressed and acknowledged. Heaviness or pain in the chest, which is home of the Heart Center, can reflect grief or sadness. The solar plexus chakra is a center for personal power and complex relationships.

Let's look at the story of Georgia, a composite of several of my clients.

"My husband and I were in a traumatic car accident five years ago," said Georgia slowly, as she brushed her hair from her sad brown eyes. "He was so strong and vital before the accident, but he was injured so badly he can't work anymore. I am our only breadwinner."

"Were you hurt in the accident? How did it affect you?"

"No, not like Joe," Georgia replied, thoughtfully sipping her latte. "I've had chronic low back pain ever since, but it really affected me emotionally. I panic and freeze when I see a truck anywhere near me on the highway. My heart races so fast and beats so hard. Sometimes, I can't catch my breath. I have to pull over to the side of the road until I can get it together and feel safe. I avoid driving now. It stresses me out." And, she continued, "Our relationship has changed so much. He hates the way he is now, and I feel so lonely I can't sleep."

The car accident traumatized Georgia, as she continued to experience Post Traumatic Stress from the shock of the accident. She didn't feel safe in her body when she drove, and she would freeze, panic, and hyperventilate around large trucks. Her body, in its desire to protect her, had encapsulated the trauma of the accident as evidence she was not safe driving. Georgia recovered from both the physical pain and trauma responses with four sessions of Intuitive Energy Management. After Georgia's positive results, her husband also responded to treatment. Joe released his PTSD from the accident, along with much of the physical pain, anger, and resentment he was carrying. Their relationship improved significantly.

Philosophy:

In my practice, my clients are taught the simple and easy ways—the language to reconnect with your body.

- **Breathe:** Did you know that when you are stressed, your breath tends to be shallow in the upper part of the chest? This clavicular breathing doesn't allow a full oxygen flow, perpetuating stress. Below are two types of deep breathing that can help your body relax. They stimulate the vagus nerve, an integral part of the parasympathetic nervous system that signals your brain to exit its fight-or-flight mode after stress.
  - *Breathe deeply into your belly while sitting up or lying down.* This helps stimulate the vagus nerve, which can help calm you. Put one hand on your belly and the other on your chest. Your belly should rise on the inhale and move toward your spine on the exhale. Visualize the breath moving through your nose and down into the belly, and then up through your torso and out again through the nose.

- *Slow your breathing down.* Inhale for a count of four. Hold your breath for a count of six. Exhale for a count of eight. Practice for a minute. Notice how you feel. Repeat for another minute or two to release stress and feel calmer.

- **Love Yourself With Mindfulness:** The present is your Pivotal Point of Power. You have no power in the past, and it's impossible to change it. You have no power in the future because it doesn't exist. It is only in the present that you can create a different future. The following is an exercise to help you cultivate your awareness of the present moment.

  - *Tune Into Your Senses:* Sit straight, close your eyes, and breathe deeply. Notice where your body intersects with the chair and feel its weight. Feel your feet on the ground, your clothes on your skin. Notice any sounds you hear and try to identify them. Notice the breeze on your skin. Is it warm or cool? How does your skin feel? Are you smelling anything? Are you tasting anything? Are there any sensations on your tongue as you move it in your mouth? Are your muscles tense or relaxed? Bring your awareness to your breath as you breathe, and notice any corresponding body sensations. When you're finished, walk around your house or outside and notice what's happening in your body. Are you more peaceful and calm? What's different?

  - *Ground:* Experience the blades of grass between your toes! Walking barefoot in the grass, working in the garden, or hugging a tree can ground your energy. These activities are great ways to bring you into the present moment and calm stress. Here's another grounding method you can use wherever you are.

- **Root to the earth:** Sit quietly and visualize roots growing from the soles of your feet and/or the base of your spine deep into the earth. Imagine stress and negative emotions draining from your body and feeling them move into the earth. Then, see positive healing energy moving up from the earth, replacing them. Imagine this positive energy as a golden light moving up through your body. Notice how you feel.

- **Meditate Daily:** There are hundreds of ways to meditate. Breathing meditations focus on the breath. Mantra meditations focus on a word or a short phrase you repeat silently to yourself, such as "Om," "I am love," or "I am safe." Recorded guided meditations can take you to deep places and leave you feeling calm and expanded. You can practice the following simple meditation anytime to develop your awareness.

- *Heart Love Meditation:* Sit straight. Place your hands over your heart and bring your awareness to the warmth under your hands. Imagine golden light entering your heart as you inhale. See your entire being filling up with this light, but keep your focus on your heart. Repeat to yourself silently, "I am love," on the inhale and again on the exhale. Start with a few minutes, but extend the time as you become more comfortable. Notice how you feel when you've finished.

- *Soothe Yourself:* Love is the most powerful healer. When you are distressed, a simple way to soothe yourself with self-love is to place one hand on your heart and the other on your solar plexus, the space between your navel and your breasts.

   Gently stroke yourself with your hands and tell yourself, "I love you." "You are safe." Notice any feelings that show up. How are you responding to the love you're offering yourself? Notice any changes in your body.

- **Exercise:** An easy way to help you re-establish your body-mind connection is through exercise. Exercising your body, from walking to weight lifting, offers many health benefits. Regardless of your choice, tune your awareness into your body while you do it.
  - Yoga, Qi Gong, and Tai Chi are excellent ways to connect with and heal your body and mind using the life force energy, also known as Prana, Chi, or Qi, while getting into shape. They help rekindle the body-mind connection and can be considered somatic exercises.

We are all beings of light, created in the image of our Creator—Who is Love. I was guided by a sherpa, and now I am the sherpa—guiding souls to remove the blocks of distress to the awareness of Love's Presence, Remember that you are a powerful, unlimited being not defined by your past.

In the School of Life, we are each given a unique curriculum, and our lessons help us grow in the language of *strength, resilience, and love.*

Our bodies hold our unresolved emotions, stress, and trauma. Unfortunately, many people are disconnected from their physical selves and are unaware that their bodies are key to unlocking their emotional and physical health. Simple mindfulness, grounding, and breathwork are a few of the techniques that can help rebuild a somatic body-mind connection and foster better health. Being an Empath, I am grateful for the ability to use somatic healing to access people's emotions and body awareness, when they're not able to. Always love your body, your temple, it speaks to you in a simple easy language.

Action Steps to Love Your Body:
- **Breathe:** Breathe deeply and count your breath to stay in the moment!
- **Be Here Now:** Mindfulness returns you to the present moment.
- **Ground:** Experience the blades of grass between your toes.
- **Meditate:** Daily.
- **Soothe Yourself:** Love is the most powerful healer.
- **Exercise:** Move while you tune in to your body.

Marbeth Dunn
Somatic Healer
www.marbethdunn.com
marbethdunn@gmail.com

Barbie Layton

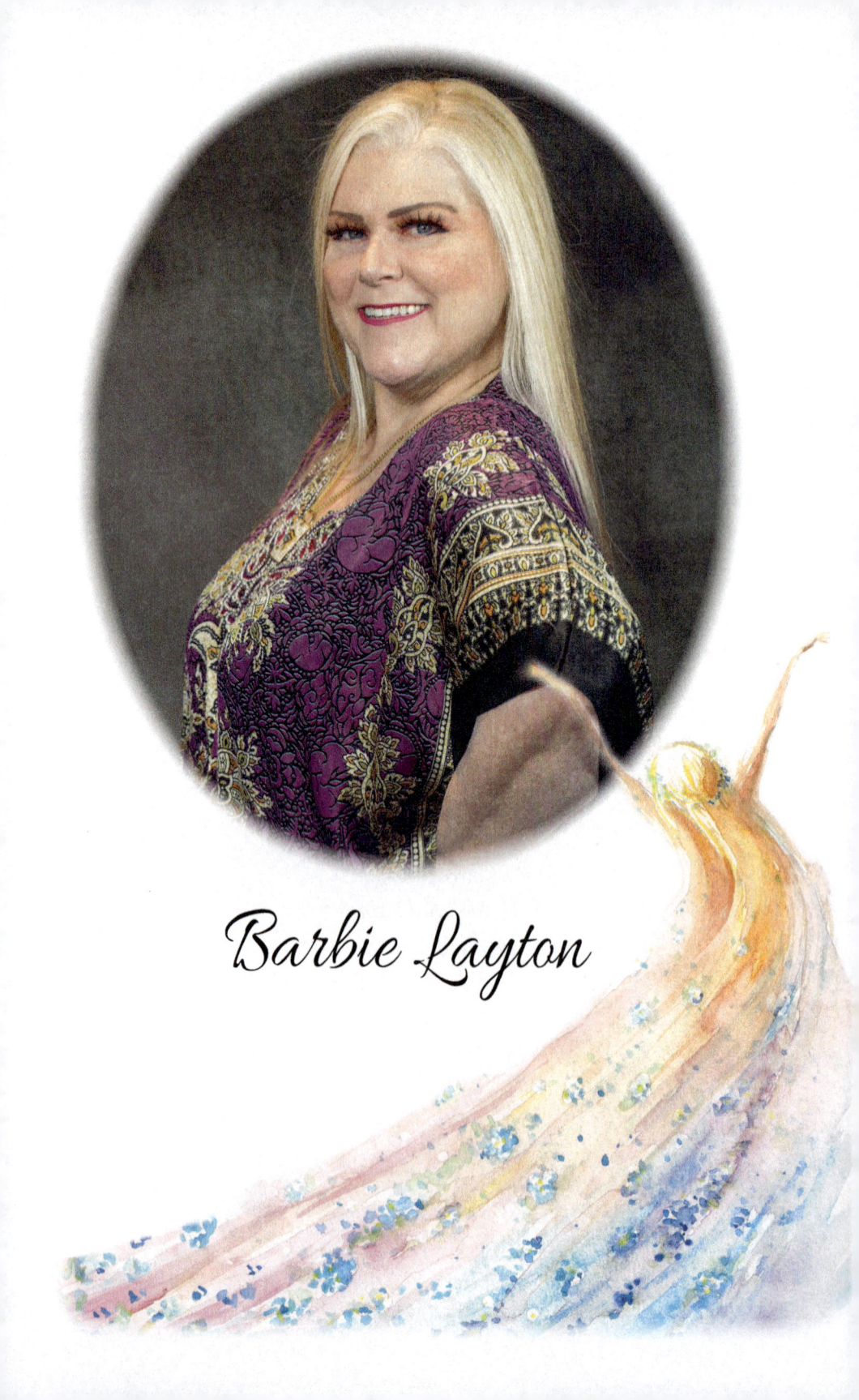

A Woman's Weight is Not Her Worth

"Rock what your mama gave you!"

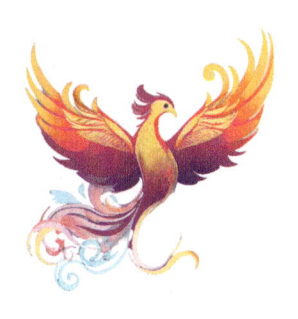

Intention:

How often have you felt your value as a woman is tied to your beauty or your weight? Throughout history we have had different beauty standards yet only one body. The Elephant in the Savannah does not look at a gazelle and wishes it had thinner legs. Beauty truly is in the eye of the beholder and comes in all shapes, colors, and sizes.

Story:

In the hustle of today's Global Society, the essence of being a woman unfolds in layers as complex and vibrant as the lives we lead. One struggle that is still a defining issue for women worldwide is the issue of weight. Standards of beauty change over time but we are only born with one body. Throughout history and across cultures, perceptions of women's weight and beauty have varied significantly, shaped by cultural norms, socioeconomic factors, and evolving ideals.

In many ancient cultures, such as Greece and Rome, plumpness was associated with wealth, fertility, and prosperity. A larger body size indicated access to plentiful food, which was a luxury not afforded to everyone. The Baroque painter Rubens from the Netherlands was famous for women who had ample curves and saw those as a status symbol. Similarly, in some African and Pacific Island cultures, larger body sizes have been traditionally revered as symbols of beauty, health, and fertility as well. Women with fuller figures were considered attractive and desirable mates. The Western World saw a significant shift towards thinner ideals of beauty starting from the late 19th and early 20th centuries. This was partly influenced by changing fashion trends, which favored slimmer silhouettes. You had the flappers of the 1920's who were thinner and then in the 1950's you had sex sirens like Marilyn Monroe and Jane Russell who had sexy hourglass figures. Hip to waist ratio is a biological phenomenon that our cavemen used as they saw an expanded waist and they didn't waste their resources as it was evident that the woman was already pregnant. The Golden Ratio that Leonardo da Vinci used for the aesthetic of beauty is also a way to show that symmetry is the most attractive quality of a woman. With the rise of mass media, particularly in the 20th century, images of thin models and celebrities became pervasive, shaping societal standards of beauty. This was further reinforced by the fashion and entertainment industries, which often promoted thinness as the ideal for women. There's also a persistent pressure on women to conform to unrealistic beauty standards. This can lead to unhealthy behaviors, such as extreme dieting or excessive exercise, in pursuit of an idealized body image. Many social media algorithms already start to transmit harmful ideas about eating disorders as early as age twelve.

As a girl growing up in the suburbs the worst crime was to be overweight. I was always a big-boned girl. At school, I was bullied. Calling a girl 'fat' weaponized the word. It's like throwing a hand grenade into a room. Certain words are explosive and incendiary. While growing up in the 80's in Malibu, California, one could even witness stickers saying: ***"no fat chicks"***! Spending so much time agonizing over calories and carbohydrates while jogging two miles a day, competitive ice skating every weekend with a National Gold Medalist Coach, and dancing ballet twice a week, I desperately needed the calories but had to focus on sheer willpower. I so thoroughly enjoyed the quick and brisk icy rush as I did powerful backward crossovers and spins on the smooth and elegant ice rink!

One fateful day, I was suited up to go jogging and I had treats for my beautiful dog, Chula, who was half Siberian husky and half German Shepherd. Suddenly my dog jumped in front of me, tripping me. I fell on a circular flagstone and split my left knee down to the bone! I was home alone and screamed for help. My neighbor jumped over the fence when they heard me screaming. Unfortunately, on that day my ice skating, jogging, ballet, snow- and water-skiing life ended and I was on crutches with stitches. I was called a faker and forced to show my stitches to my tormentors and started to gain weight. The next sport I tried was the swim team. I walked two miles to the pool after school every day and swam for three hours five days a week. I developed muscle but never got rid of my belly. I wore a size 16 and most designers capped out at size 14. I was almost 5'8" and I had big blue eyes, long tan muscular legs, long brown hair, and I looked like I was eighteen. I got a lot of attention from grown men. It was confusing and there was a power there that I didn't know how to properly wield. I was called fat, even though I look at photos and that's patently false. The biggest cheap shot was when you call a woman fat. You invalidate her humanity and make it so that she is undesirable and subhuman. With all the attention I was getting from men, it was completely confusing. A woman's self-esteem needs to come from within, but I was ill-equipped. It's difficult when people weaponize words, especially when they themselves are overweight, unattractive, or both.

Then, when I was a junior in high school, I was an exchange student in Austria for a year and I got to date the most popular, handsome boy. He was my first true love. I walked a mile to the train which took me to school, and at the end of the day, a mile home. I ate whatever delicious food I wanted, drank wine, and smoked cigarettes (it was legal then), My body regulated itself. I was in the best shape of my life, and I believe this was because all of the food sources were local and non-GMO. It was so liberating for me as I was accepted and loved for being me and no one saw me as overweight. Sometimes, when you're from a small town, people don't give you a chance to make a new impression or evolve. It showed me that others saw me completely from a different lens. It was the dawning of deciding I was re-claiming my own self image as opposed to allowing others to choose it for me. They threw me a farewell party with over 150 people from all the different cliques, who normally didn't connect. I was so sad to come back home, broken-hearted, and missing my boyfriend and friends, Within a year, I gained almost 200 pounds. I later learned it was because I had been irradiated and contaminated by Chernobyl in 1986 when I was there. We had all of our fresh food that came from the pristine gorgeous snow-capped mountains, 100 miles from where the nuclear explosion occurred. Radiation is invisible but deadly.

It was heartbreaking to be at a Weight Watchers meeting weigh-in and aghast that I was over 400 pounds, which sounded impossible but was true. It was mind-blowing to me, yet it started me on a long-standing journey of transformational self-love.

I applied for gastric bypass surgery in 2001. People automatically assume that when you're overweight you're automatically unhealthy, but my blood pressure, my sugar, and everything was perfect. I just happened to be over 400 pounds from having been irradiated. My surgeon nicked me on the inside resulting in a bed filled with about 85% of my own blood.

An Orderly, disinterested in me, merely came in and wanted me to get up out of my bed so he could clean it. With stars going around my head, I knew that if I got up I would fall over and faint. The hospital transferred me to the ICU for five days staring at a blue mylar balloon of a dolphin. It was one of my near-death experiences. I had to have three blood transfusions.

Thankfully, as a result of the surgery I was able to release over 200 pounds of weight, and I've kept that off for over 20 years. I elected to have surgical skin revisions where I had 32 pounds of skin cut off of my stomach, my underarms, and my legs. When you expand like that, you simply grow new skin. I still have lasting scars on more than 75% of my body. I've had to come to the realization that this was my journey, to possibly help others: to inspire people to go after what they want. That is why I wanted to share my story.

Finally, in the early 1990s, they started having plus size clothing lines that were done by Spiegel Catalogs, just elegant and lovely. Clothes that weren't loud bolts of fabric. I was honored to be a plus-size model for runway shows. I immediately said, "YES!" It was really exciting to get paid with this beautiful clothing. It was also surreal to be walking in front of over a thousand people who were cheering you on! It was an experience of a lifetime.! Recently, I've been able to take up plus-size modeling again. I participated in photo shoots in the last four years, and I have been on six New York Times Square Billboards, including the iconic Coca-Cola stack cycling with Kim Kardashian's skincare line!

Being able to step into your own personal beauty, where you emanate confidence in yourself, is awesome. It's not about external validation of whether other people think that you're beautiful or not, but how you project that beautiful light—shining from within.

Recently I had someone in my life who thought that it would be funny to take me down by calling me fat when they themselves were overweight. Strangely enough, when a word is weaponized, it often loses its meaning. I felt sorry for the person who felt she needed to criticize me as it was obviously her own insecurities she was projecting onto me. If women spent more time loving their bodies and not shaming each other that energy would be added to doing good in their lives. Think about all the time we would save if we focused on our health and affirmed the wonderful things we can accomplish rather than always feeling less than or unworthy because of immutable traits. Now at 5'10", I have a large frame and that is never going to change. If I embrace that as being me, I can move confidently on and focus on more important things in my life: like how I can continue to be of service to others. Women empowering women is a powerful narrative in today's world. When women celebrate each other's successes and stand strong together against challenges, they build a network of support that transcends individual achievement. This solidarity is crucial in a world where women's rights and contributions are often undervalued.

Unlike what is often extolled, empowering women does not mean diminishing the roles or contributions of men. Rather, it involves partnering with men to foster a society that values equality and respect across genders. Men play a crucial role in this transformation by challenging the stereotypes that limit both men and women. Uplifting men in the context of a woman's essence involves encouraging them to express vulnerability, engage in caregiving roles, and step aside when necessary to let women lead. By doing so, men not only enrich their own lives but also contribute to a more fruitful society. This balance is essential for creating environments where everyone can thrive, regardless of gender. Creating a world where women are self-confident and men are uplifted requires a collective effort. It involves changing policies, challenging social norms, and educating the next generation about respect and equality. It also means advocating for equal representation in all areas of life, from corporate boards to political offices. In this pursuit of humanity, both men and women must be allies. Women need to support each other's ambitions recognizing the diverse roles they play, fostering co-collaboration and co-creation rather than the old paradigm of competition. Together, we can create a world that values and benefits from the full spectrum of human potential. In today's modern world, being a woman is about embracing the power of one's identity and transcending to influence the world positively.

It's about breaking down barriers and creating pathways for others to follow. By supporting each other and uplifting the men who share in gender equality, women can transform society into one where every individual can pursue their dreams without limitation. May words serve as a beacon for those navigating the complexities of gender roles in contemporary society, promoting a future where equality is not just an ideal, but a true reality.

Belief:

Equally important to how a woman looks is how she feels. I love to adorn my body and play with makeup, lashes, wigs, and fashion that allows me to feel whatever way that I choose.

When you're broadcasting negativity into the Universe, a person's words are casting spells. Thus we call it spelling in the English Language: it can be negative or positive.

Thoughtful words are truly a virtue. Words can be a curse or wisdom… congruence is power. So is frequency. As an energy healer: energy, vibration, and frequency are the gifts of the building blocks of the universe, according to Nikola Tesla.

Despite progress in body positivity movements, there still exists stigma and discrimination against individuals who don't conform to societal ideals of beauty. This can manifest in various forms, including body shaming, bullying, and discrimination in employment or social settings. Women, in particular, often face intense scrutiny and pressure to maintain a certain weight or appearance, which can take a toll on their mental and physical well-being. Overall, the evaluation of women's weight and beauty is deeply intertwined with cultural norms, historical contexts, and societal expectations. Beauty is your own personal concept to embrace your essence and forgive your flaws. While there's a growing recognition of the diversity of beauty and the importance of body acceptance, there's still much work to be done in challenging narrow standards, promoting inclusivity, and acceptance for all. Always LOVE your body.

Action Steps:

- Affirm yourself daily by uplifting your frequency to 528 Hz hourly: source found freely on YouTube.

- Prize the parts of your body that you like. Look in the mirror to affirm at least ONE thing you appreciate.

- When someone else harms you, use the Ho'oponopono Prayer with: "I'm Sorry.' Please Forgive Me. Thank you. I love you"—to release it from your energy field. Put yourself on a gossip diet of being above the conversation and focusing on facts.

- Keep your energy frequency as high as possible.

Barbie Layton
Scientifically Verified Quantum Healer
Manifestation Coach and Media Personality?
www.barbielayton.com
intuitivebarbie1@gmail.com
@barbielaytonofficial

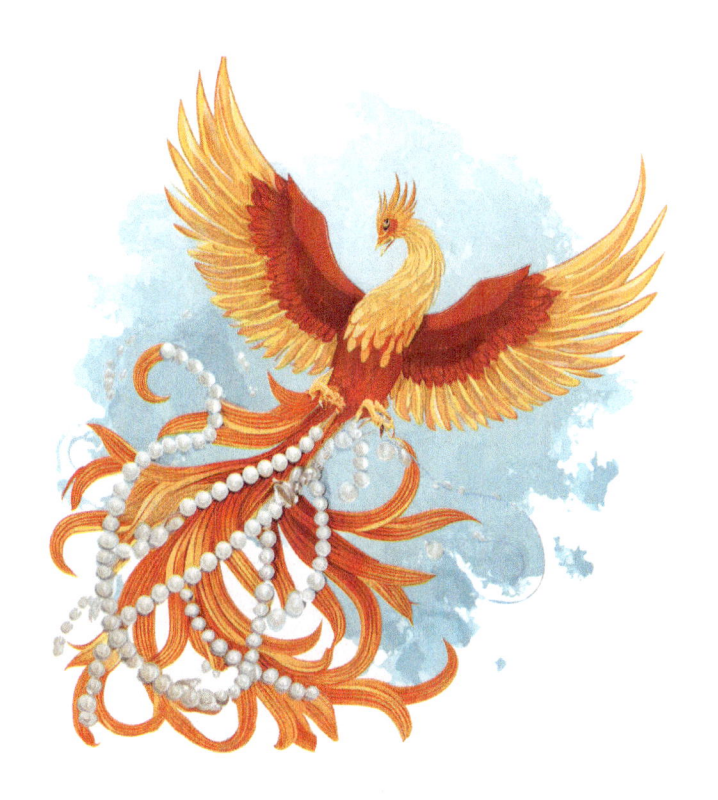

Leilani Alesh, Esq.

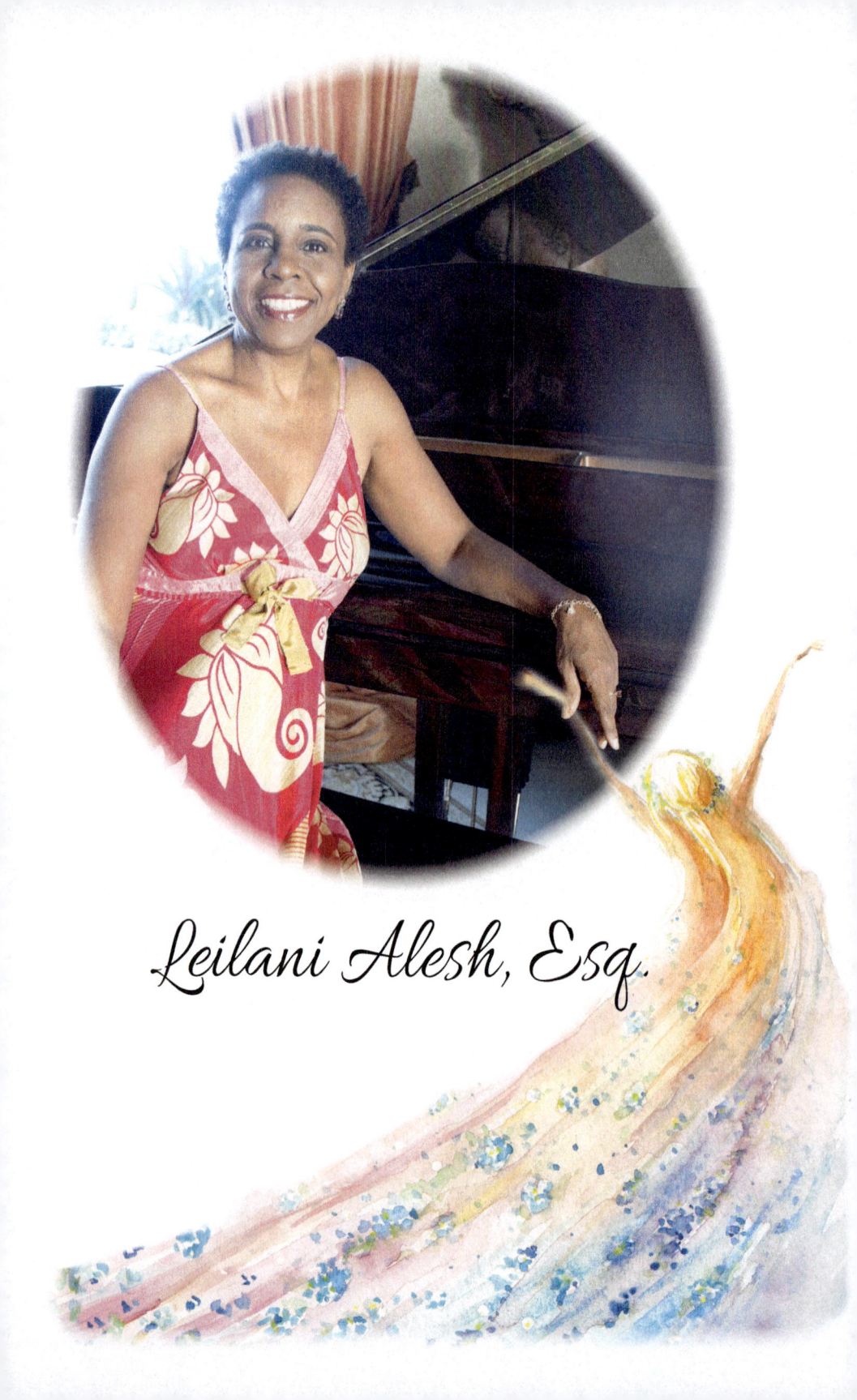

Indomitable Joy: Ours for the Taking

*"I Rejoice, in that I am spirit.
Joy is always ours, for the taking."*

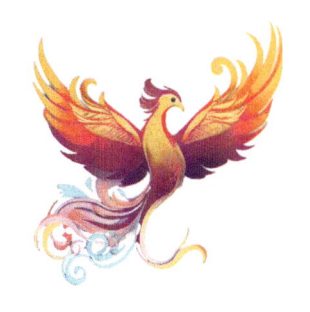

Intention:

If this story is not about you, it's about your best friend, wife, son-in-law, or maybe your boss or co-worker's daughter. You know someone who's lived in a cancer cluster, next door to a chemical plant with onerous discharge, a worker on a farm where chemical pesticides and fertilizers were used, or in a building over a landfill of toxic waste. You've traveled behind a truck that suddenly belched particles of black soot that descended and clogged your nostrils, making you tear, and maybe dizzy. The consequences appear to be temporary discomfort but can include terminal decline in health. These slow and silent killers: cigarettes, asbestos, coal, lead pipes, IUD, or hydrogenated oils. Environmental demons entering our space—Unfair. Unjust. Our inalienable right to life, recognized as sacred in the Supreme Law of this land, violated wholesale, and laid to waste with impunity, for a mere buck. Despite these takings, what of the life we still have?

Story:

I was afflicted with the malady of prolonged and severe female bleeding. Fibroids were a companion that plagued me since I was a budding adolescent. Heavy and prolonged bleeding and clotting remained a constant for nearly my entire life. The dam would burst suddenly and unexpectedly, and flow like Niagara Falls. I became a magnet for ridicule and shaming. "How could you…" as if I knew and was responsible for the poison that confiscated control of my body, my mother's, and mothers of the generation before.

At a frequency of more than twice that of women of other races, resulting in hospitalizations and hysterectomies three times more often, and myomectomies seven times more often, African American Women's symptoms can run world-class interference with opportunities, work, relationships, and social engagements. Truly a female curse, I was even dispossessed of the right to bear a child by this severe illness—all the result of chemical toxicity from an alleged beauty product.

I tried every treatment modality under the sun, desperate to reclaim my health, and holding fast to the hope of fertility. All was to no avail. Some had efficacy but required an exercise of disciplines impossible to sustain.

Others, ineffective and wasteful, such as artificially induced menopause, both exasperated my discomfort, making already awkward social interactions that much worse. Despite it all, I maintained an unrelenting determination to lead a life of indomitable joy, causing me to create my own healing exorcism.

During these travails, I nearly bled out. I should have been dead given my 4.8 RBC (red blood count). The three quarts of blood and quart of iron ordered by the Emergency Room Doctor, desperately needed, were denied to me for over 8 hours. The Creator, my ancestors, or Bessie Smith[i] was watching over me. Something and somebody declared and determined "Not again! Not this time!" I survived this attempted physical and psychological murder.

On the heels of its crime, this Kafkaesque hospital's economic assault began. For six years, I battled against the pretense of not having received payments that were negotiated. They returned checks sent to addresses where payments were previously received, then pretended to have never received them. Credits to my account disappeared. The billing was doubled. I was reported to collections, and pleas to correct erroneous credit reports based on proof submitted were fought. I thought I had relief, finally, after obtaining the US government's administrative review, finding widespread "account irregularities and abuse." Astonishing though, the hospital then changed my account numbers, and the economic assault started all over again! How much extra did I pay in insurance premiums and interest on car notes? How restricted were my opportunities for credit? I'll never know.

After several decades of battling with this illness and its tentacles, I occasionally fell into the temptation and depths of self-pity. Then I'd hear an interview of someone who'd survived genocide and learned the self-healing impact of forgiveness; a report on the plight of albinos in Africa who were stripped of limbs and sometimes life, because of archaic tribal practices based upon ridiculous superstitions. I'd learn about mass female mutilation at puberty, without anesthesia, resulting in infections, loss of urinary tract integrity, and severe pain with intercourse for life. I knew I had no right to indulge in sorrow. I was still gifted with and enjoyed so many blessings.

Around four years after the attempt on my life, I stood in my shower with, nonetheless, blood streaming down my legs and clots plopping onto the tiles. To this, I was so accustomed that it was just stasis: an anomaly not worthy of much thought. I was fixated instead, on truly indignant thoughts, hoping bitterly that a jealous adversary was suffering. I was blessed again in that moment, to have my focus pulled away by indomitable joy, beauty, and love.

Living in a beautiful, small winery in a lush, protected forest, a gently warming sun streamed through my window on this late spring day. For the first time in my life, I was deeply in love. I decided against surrendering these beautiful moments to someone whose mission had been to hurt and steal from me. "Let her Karma be hers, not mine," I said to myself. Immediately, my bleeding stopped. My understanding of a mind-body connection was jolted from theoretical to undeniably real. By redirecting my attention away from emotional wounds, I freed myself into a profound inner peace, to experience full joy, as I was allowed reprieve.

The discipline to master full focus on joy is a weighty one in a world so contaminated by brutality. I tried and even managed to become pregnant. Upon hearing from an insensitive relative, "…the thought of that white blood coursing through your veins…," I allowed myself to succumb again to indignity. My prideful warrior spirit produced a deadly chemical mix in my body, and I caused myself to miscarry.

After two myomectomies, too many miscarriages, and four decades of this illness under my belt, I sadly reported to my Gynecologist for what would be the last time, that yet again I miscarried. I finally learned that this was grace. The tumor and baby would compete for my blood supply with my baby winning. Having been so severely deprived, however, my child would have been born severely deformed, in unimaginable pain, suffering, and dying soon after birth. Finally, I resigned that my heart is forever wounded, and will perpetually weep for the children I never got to meet, as I prepared for the da Vinci removal of my womb.

Six years after my hysterectomy, I was again jolted, with confirmation of my suspicions—that this plague on Black Women was not just the luck of the draw. We were pressured, cajoled, manipulated, and oppressed by being denied participation in the economic engine lest we "tame" the texture of our hair. Our unruly naps were equated with ugliness, being unkempt, and uncivilized. We were required to pay homage to our sisters with straight hair, courtesy of chemicals the very nature of which was to destroy our reproductive capacity, that drive rampant bleeding, and clotting. A generations-long genocide, that remains largely unpunished, unspoken.

There were mass tort cases, compensating women who'd suffered as I did. But bittersweet is an economic remedy that can compensate for the consistent disruption of productive endeavors, but not for an issue that I cannot hug. What I have learned, I cannot pass on to my nonexistent children, even with all the money in the world. A damage award will not matriculate from graduate school, give me grandchildren to admire and spoil, or look after me with tenderness and caring as I age. A cash drop will never replace the end of the lineage of my unique seed. In that realization, I at times, still feel raped and brutalized out of the essence of my existence—so utterly alone.

Perhaps accidental at first, the damage being caused by chemical straighteners was eventually undeniably known. The continuation of pushing this garbage into our bodies was a willful and intentional campaign. Those responsible for these decisions should be spending the rest of their lives incarcerated. To date, I've heard not a single peep about prosecution. I feel furious and betrayed, as my right to leave heirs, part and parcel of my right to life, was crushed as inconsequential, with impunity.

But mine is not a story of defeat or bitterness. Not of fear. Not anger or some burning quest for revenge. I am grateful that my companion illness did not define my life. Nor do I long suffer myself to wallow around in sadness. I heed well the teachings that have become my own. With practice, one can and should control the mind and emotions, not the other way around. My lesson in all of this, now known without doubt, and why I rejoice, is that *I am Spirit*. Mine is a life full of adventure and traversed with gusto. The choice of how to absorb, adapt around, and respond to what happens in our environment, always remains within our dominion.

I dedicated my life to my deep passion—one for the taking—the creative process. Nothing has brought me more satisfaction than my writing and singing: whether prose, poetry, or melodies and lyrics. I find that I have something to say, that can help others more deeply feel, more clearly understand, and sometimes relate better from the heart. At other times, when I am open as a willing vessel, I find that velvet and golden words find their way through me and onto a page, or floating along a melody line. From either direction, upon completing a creative work, I feel both spent and satiated. It's the giving of myself, that has been enough. In this way, I birth my legacy and essence into the Universe.

I spent my late twenties exploring a multitude of Spiritual paths. I danced with the Aztecs, invited by their priestess into a ceremony at the Pyramid of the Sun. I lived with nature in a cabin on a bucolic Southern California ranch. I enjoyed fresh milk directly from a goat every morning in my coffee, drumming and sharing lore and song by the light of the moon, with a bonfire every night. I lived in an American Indian culture preservation center in the wilderness of the high desert behind Santa Barbara, California, sitting in sweat lodges, enduring arduous full fasts in naked solitude and prayer during traditional vision quests, and sundances. I took a year off to study with a religious historian. I can still bear witness to mysteries unfolding, making it clear beyond question that ours is not a 3D world. My varied spiritual immersions have blessed me with Fifth Dimension Living.

Through these journeys, the deep love and appreciation gained for Gaia, the beautiful, generous, and magnificent living Spirit embodied as Earth, and the care we should exercise for seven generations to come, led me to create three sustainable clothing lines. Another avenue for giving back. I expressed my creativity through the development of apparel with color symmetries, style and function selections, catalogs, styling models, set design, photography, website development, trade show booths, and boutiques—all my designing playground for most of a decade. I had the time of my life, giving birth daily to the possibility of a sustainable future for the people of this earth. I was anxious to get to my desk every morning. Whether celebrating the growth or suffering the growing pains, I felt extraordinary upon laying my head on my pillow each night, reflecting upon my baby. Running a clothing business was an effortless pleasure, never work.

These business experiences, coupled with a Doctorate in Law, and resulting work experiences in litigation and intellectual property protections, opened doors to very fun, amazing, and lucrative jobs, with the development of my writings elevated to film projects, and landing my first solo set at the jazz museum of New Orleans. In all, mine was the life I envisioned as a pre-teen. A life of adventure, feeding my fierce appetite for indomitable joy—*joie de vivre*.

Have there been misadventures? Of course. Heartbreaks and betrayals? Too plenty. Dark passages? Absolutely. But one thread kept me hopeful through all. Humility. To love and be generous without ambition for return, has a far greater benefit than strategic emotional investment. I recognize and am truly honored, to be one among the embodiments of the Divine feminine and essence of a woman. This fills me with joy, and I am convinced there is no greater victory.

What I remember mostly, looking back, are sunny days, flowers, gorgeous redwood forests, warm sand on quiet out of the way beaches, and feelings of love. Life is filled with the search for meaning, for our unique path to communing and honoring the Divine; the quest to make a difference with our choices of how to fill our days. Seeking to better ourselves requires the exercise of daily discipline to develop the habit of remaining mindful of our interactions with each person, beginning with ourselves. Of course, we falter. But how each person's acreage in the universe will surround and embrace, depends without exception, upon replicating ripples from every prior moment. Who knows who yours may touch, how it will impact them, and what they may say or do in consequence. We are weaving this world, for ourselves, and for our children.

While very happy that my body is now back within my dominion and control, but with too much of a wealth of experiences that should be passed on, I fall back to the lyrics of Burt Bacharach that I took as my mantra and dogma since a teen, from his song, "Raindrops Keep Fallin' on My Head."

That doesn't mean my eyes will soon be turning red.

Crying's not for me, 'cause

I'm never gonna stop the rain by complaining…

The blues they send to meet me won't defeat me.

It won't be long til

happiness steps up to greet me."

Belief:

So when you find yourself blue, change the channel in your head. Just sing that song to yourself. Watch a funny movie or one about victory over adversity. Take a walk and indulge in the aromatic dances and gorgeousness of Earth. Call a loving friend for coffee. Just keep looking and moving forward. Never give up on indomitable joy. It always comes back around—yours for the taking.

Action Steps:

- Remain teachable.
- Lead well when equipped to do so, in service for those who are accepting.
- Help people, as seeing them thrive: It feeds one's soul.
- Refuse to be turned cold or hard, at all costs. A tender and warm heart will always be your most valuable asset.
- Be steadfast and forgiving. Beware of revenge as a relentless seductress.
- Be honest in introspection daily, with a gentle and loving spirit towards yourself.

Leilani Alesh, Esq.
Indomitable Joy
https://sites.google.com/view/leilanialesh/home
leilanialesh@icloud.com

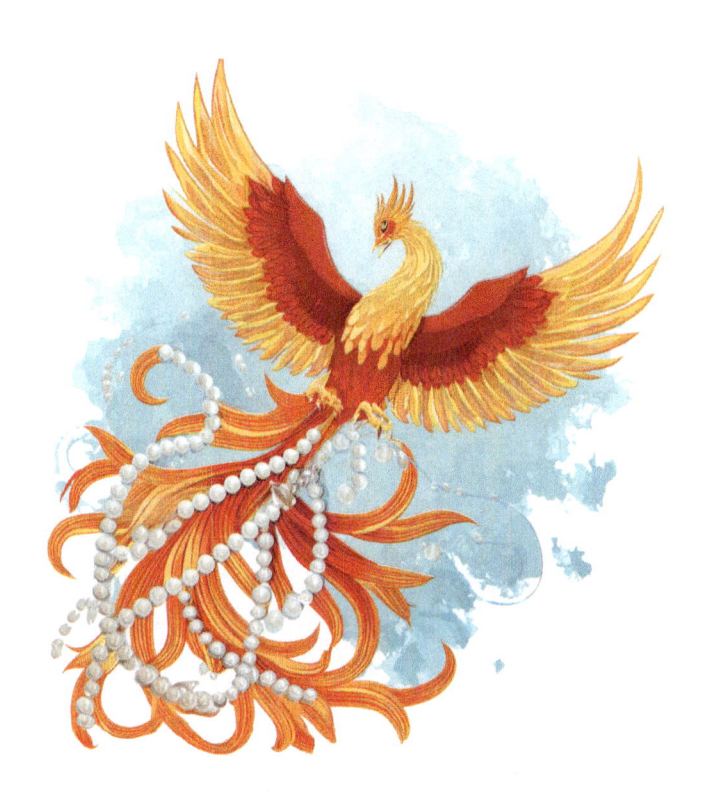

Leilani Alesh, Esq. | 213

Anna M. McKee

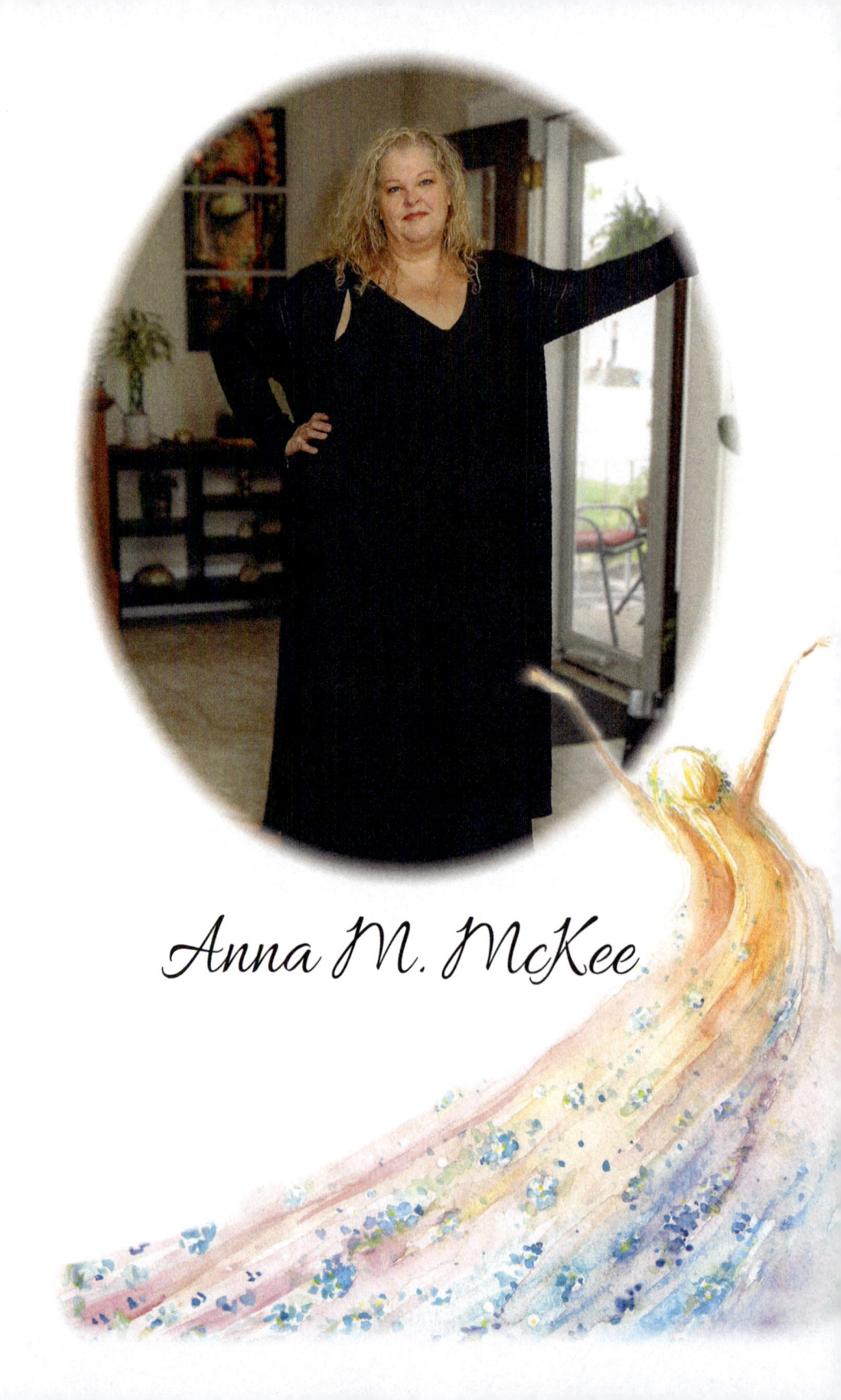

Harmonic Conversions

"Align, allow, and feel your way to inner harmony."

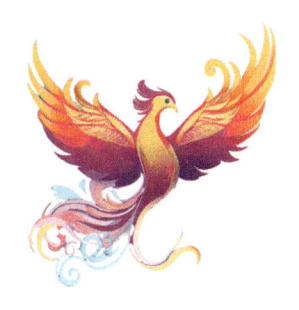

Intention:

As I stand in my light, may you remember yours and shine just a little brighter.

Story:

As a happy, open, and imaginative child, I floated through the first years enjoying the simplicity of nature, play, and childlike innocence. As I grew older, I began to feel the weight of responsibility. I felt the tension in our family home and as I witnessed those around me shift and change, I adapted to whatever role was needed to bring harmony to the environment. This learned behavior left me without a clear sense of who I was. I lacked awareness and was susceptible to whoever had the most influence in my life, which carried over into my adult relationships and choices. My parents separated when I was in my preteen years and the result was a child with a shifting foundation and a yearning for safety and stability.

Although my father and I adored one another, the love and attention focused on me contributed to the unhealed trauma my mother experienced in life. I often became the target of my mother's frustration. This taught me distorted views of women, false independence, self-sufficiency, relationships, commitment, and love; beliefs I carried along with a list of stories with similar outcomes. I watched another generation of unhealed trauma and programming passed down and taught as truth under the guise of loving and responsible parenting.

I was an only child and both my parents worked so I spent much of my time alone, unsupervised, and playing outdoors. This granted me the space to develop and learn more about myself while I connected with bugs and flowers. It also left me vulnerable to those who take advantage of unassuming young children. The innocence of my childhood was lost at an early age, and I told nobody until I was well into my adult healing journey exploring 'why bad things happen to good people.' Good and bad are simply judgments we attach to experiences, and that changes with perspective. I sought refuge in a healthier place, a natural state of neutrality, realizing that each experience we encounter is an opportunity to gain experience and growth. Sometimes we have positive examples that inspire us, and other times we have undesirable examples that show us contrast. If we learn from it, it has inherent value to us. I experienced more contrast than inspiration during the first half of my life, and while learning that what you do not want may not be a walk in the park, these encounters catalyzed my healing later.

As I sit down and share my experiences, I gently close my eyes and go inward to connect to the essence of a woman. It is a frequency that translates to a feeling that we assign words to describe. Her essence is as vast and intricate as the cosmos itself, encompassing multidimensional layers of being interwoven with threads of strength, compassion, resilience, and wisdom. Transcending the physical to include emotional, mental, and spiritual dimensions she is enriched by her experiences, and her essence is exemplified in the spirit of resilience that enables her to overcome obstacles and emerge stronger.

This feeling softens as I recognize the feeling of harmony emanating from the natural balance of the Divine Feminine and Divine Masculine within. A woman's essence is deeply connected to her wisdom and intuition, guiding her in decisions and helping her navigate life's complexities with insight and clarity. This wisdom is grounded and evident in the ability to balance multiple roles and responsibilities.

The blossoming of heart energy reflects the compassion and empathy that allows women to see the world through the eyes of others. She epitomizes great leadership, and her essence inspires others to pursue their goals and make a positive impact on the world. Women often play a crucial role in nurturing the next generation of leaders as we offer guidance, encouragement, and a boundless and transformative love that enriches the lives of those around us.

As every woman is unique, and shaped by her journey and experiences, I am no different. Raised amidst the complexities of my parents' unhealed trauma and conditioning, my childhood was a blend of joy and challenges. My experience blossomed into a story of transformation and self-discovery—a testament to alchemizing every day into growth.

I stumbled upon a window of opportunity for healing. It wasn't until I carried learned patterns of fear, lack, and unworthiness into my adulthood that I recognized the depth of my struggle. Unintentionally, I projected my unresolved issues onto partners, children, and friends, casting pain across my path. Through my twenties, the echoes of my darkest years reverberated until a profound awakening, akin to a surge of Christ-like energy, shifted my reality, leaving me bewildered. This awakening unveiled both the beauty of my energetic experience and the shadows of societal programming. The newfound frequency pulsating within me unlocked latent gifts, ushered in inexplicable synchronicities, and heightened my awareness in dream-like states. With this expanded perspective, I began to unravel the systems and structures that hindered higher consciousness, deepening my understanding of life's interconnectedness.

This glimpse of a new way of being led to an intolerance for the lifestyle I lived, and I found myself leaving everything I knew to seek a deeper meaning elsewhere. This road of discovery lasted two decades as I searched for parts of my puzzle I could see but could not figure out how to piece them together. Each time I discovered a new piece of information, I would think, "This is it, the missing piece I've been searching for!" only to realize it was just another layer leading me closer to my inner Truth.

On the path of seeking fulfillment, I encountered teachers who contributed to my growth. Each one revealed a bit more about myself and helped me piece together life for a higher understanding. Yet, none were as resonant as the one I discovered through meditation.

One year, as a birthday present my son took me to a castle overlooking a river. The water was particularly healing that day. I entered meditation with the thought, "There's got to be more to life than what I am currently accessing." During this meditation, I was led to a woman who shined her heart light so brightly that I followed her like a beacon in the dark.

A series of synchronicities led me to cross paths with Kerry K, who showed me that the woman I followed was me. I relished her "straight-talking spirituality" approach, and this began another era of my self-discovery mission. I spent years working, analyzing, documenting, and rationalizing all that I was experiencing to piece together more about myself, and hoped this time I would finally find the missing piece. I committed to a new level of change and quickly began to expand and grow with the treasure trove of added resources. I was like a sponge and could not soak up enough of the content that was weaving together my previous understanding while simultaneously creating an entirely new viewpoint. It was exciting, yet even with this upward trajectory and personal expansion, I continued to look for the easiest, fastest, and most comfortable way to the next change agent.

Most of us know what it is like to want someone to give you answers. I had access to someone that appeared to have just that—all the answers. I heard the teachings about self-sourcing and continued with my habit of seeking clarity and external validation. Eventually, it sunk in and I realized that to access the answers I sought from others, I would need to go inward. I continued to be reminded that each step was leading me back to inner harmony. It always was, and always will be. This aligned path of stepping into personal responsibility created a foundational shift. I gained a new higher perspective on my level of participation in life, and I began to see collaboration and harmony in places where I previously saw attacks, misgivings, and outright injustice. Where I once saw entitlement, I now experienced grace and compassion; challenges turned into opportunities, and I began to laugh and take pleasure in life instead of avoiding it. My inner peace started to shine outwardly.

The evolution of my inner exploration continued as I traversed the bridge between understanding and knowing. Knowing is an unquestionable truth that comes from a place of wisdom. Wisdom is the product of "walking the walk," embodying, or applying experience. There was an enormous amount of information I had collected and conceptualized, but did I KNOW it? I felt guided to apply the tools I was learning, and reflected inwardly, "Don't think about it, do it. Not to write about it, do it. Not to talk about it, just do it." As I began to feel into and embody the energetic experiences, again, the growth and expansion that followed was extraordinary!

I sought the opportunity to share what I was experiencing and began training to facilitate personal development sessions. This was a chrysalis moment for me to develop my gifts and elevate my practice. It represented my next level of personal responsibility, testing me as I shifted roles from student to teacher. I quickly realized that the real test lies in everyday life, in the choices we make each moment. It's simple: our lives are a testimony to our daily practice.

Philosophy:

I collaborate with clients who, like I once did, seek the easiest and fastest way to feel comfortable. Life is a cycle of learning, growing, and mastering. When we learn a concept, we grow and expand our understanding, field, and frequency. Once we have embodied the lesson, we achieve mastery. However, when we get comfortable, we tend to stop seeking, learning, and growing, which leads to stagnation. Have you ever encountered stagnant water? It does not support life. As infinite beings living in an infinite world, the experience of comfort is quite the opposite of what we are truly seeking in the journey of expansion into oneness.

While there may not be an easy button for mastery, I do have a few simple, and practical ways to support your development. Whether you have been working on your healing for years or are just now coming to accept change, remember: align, allow, and feel.

- **Align:** When people say, 'Follow your heart,' there is wisdom within that statement. Are you operating from your head or your heart? Close your eyes and check in with yourself. If you are thinking about it, you are not in your heart space. Relax, take a deep breath, and then just observe the breath coming in and out of your body. Feel it filling your heart space, as though each breath is expanding your chest. Feel the expansion, sit with it, and be there, in the stillness, with no thought. You can feel the energy in your body come back into alignment with the healing flow of your natural rhythm.

- **Allow:** Life is not happening to you; it is happening for you. Stop controlling and relax into the opening of the possibility of all that is. Allow the space for what is inherently available—abundance, acceptance, joy, divine love—to come into your life.

- **Feel:** When we avoid feeling and we distract ourselves—it's uncomfortable. When you feel/experience emotion (e-motion) try to remember it is just energy in motion. Let it move. The discomfort of certain energy causes us to tense or tighten up and block the flow. Notice it without judging it as good or bad and allow it to pass through. Eventually, this becomes a natural process, and you begin clearing out deeper layers of density. Remember, you must feel it to heal it. This process of identifying and transmuting energy for healing is what I accomplish with clients in 1–1 sessions.

I shared some of my path to healing and the impatience I experienced along the way. The actual shortcut is to simply go inward, develop the relationship and trust with your True Self, and self-source your answers: your heart never leads you astray. Using these basic foundational practices regularly creates beneficial habits. Eventually, we begin to self-regulate through alignment, allowing, and feeling. Until it is an automatic process for you, check in as often as you can. Set a timer on your phone, each time it goes off, check in with yourself. Where am I operating from? My head or my heart? Am I open and allowing God in at this moment? Am I feeling it? If not, you now have a new choice in front of you.

The enduring impact and essence of a woman is a multifaceted and profound concept reflecting the diverse and intricate layers of her being. We have explored various dimensions of this essence, each contributing to a holistic understanding of what it means to embody a woman's essence. My personal story of transformation and self-discovery exemplifies alchemy in everyday life. From a childhood marked by joy and complexity to adulthood characterized by awakening and growth, my journey back to me underscores the resilience, strength, and wisdom inherent in each woman.

We lead with empathy and compassion, inspiring others to pursue their goals and make a positive impact in the world. Reflecting, I can sense the essence of the Divine Feminine. The lessons I've gleaned along the way, such as embracing alignment, openness, and emotional healing, underscore the profound potential for personal growth and self-realization. My experiences have underscored the importance of transitioning from understanding to true knowing, as embodying wisdom through practice and action is essential for self-actualization. Simple practices when consistently applied, cultivate a deeper connection with oneself; a connection that embodies the essence of womanhood—marked by wisdom and intuition—guiding decisions and enabling individuals to navigate life with clarity and insight.

There exists an infinite array of characteristics to delineate the essence of a woman. At its core, it persists unchanged: it is ***love***. The radiant beacon that evokes the spark of light nestled within each of our hearts serves as a guiding light leading others home and is a gentle whisper of encouragement urging us to persevere. That love is the blossoming of creation itself, emerging like the Phoenix from within, inspiring, healing, and transforming lives while echoing the profound and enduring impact of women on our world.

I believe we each follow a path of remembering who we truly are within each step. We are our best resource and when we ***align*** to the energy of the universal flow and ***allow*** it to guide us, we can ***feel*** the harmony and balance of creation itself.

Action Steps:

- **Align:** Check-in and breathe into your heart space.
- **Allow:** Let go of control and open to your guidance.
- **Feel:** Notice the energetic communication within your body.

Anna M. McKee
Personal Development Consultant, Embodiment Coach
AM Developments
www.iamdevelopments.com
anna@iamdevelopments.com

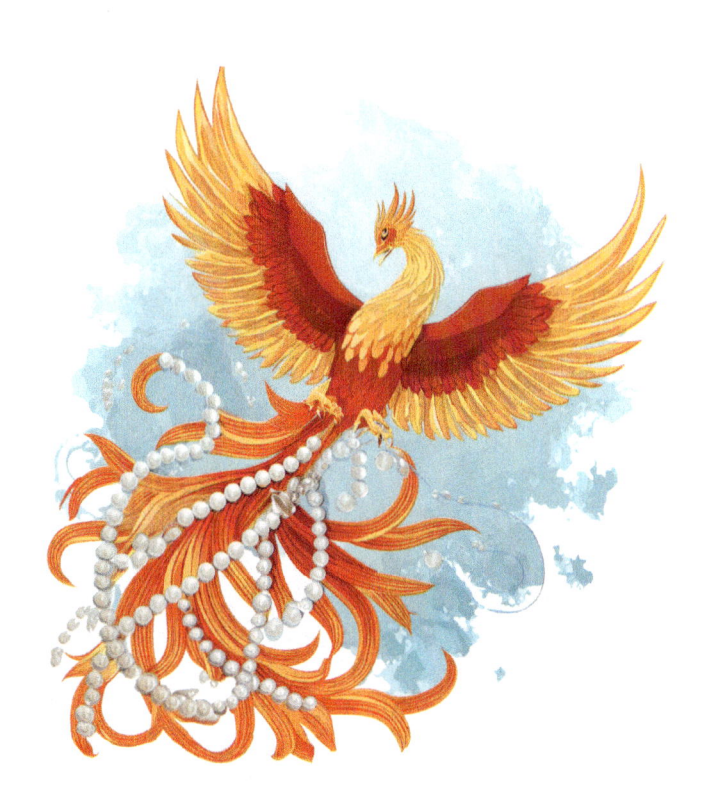

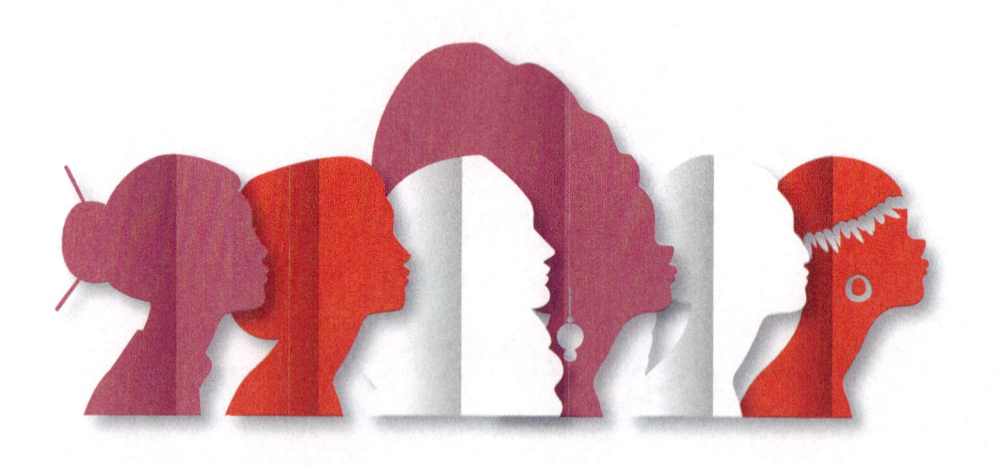

CHAPTER FOUR

Physical Pillar

"I am a dancer. I believe that we learn by practice. Whether it means to learn to dance by practicing dancing or to learn to live by practicing living... In each it is the performance of a dedicated precise set of acts, physical or intellectual, from which comes shape of achievement, a sense of one's being, a satisfaction of spirit. One becomes in some area an athlete of God."
—Martha Graham

"Beauty is about being comfortable in your own skin. It's about knowing and accepting who you are."
—Katherine Hepburn

"A woman is most beautiful when she smiles."
—Beyoncé

"Beauty is not caused. It is."
—Emily Dickinson

"Practice creates confidence. Confidence empowers you."
—Simone Biles

"Real beauty isn't about symmetry or weight or makeup; it's about looking life right in the face and seeing all its magnificence reflected in your own."
—Valerie Monroe

"To be beautiful means to be yourself. You don't need to be accepted by others. You need to accept yourself."
—Thich Nhat Hanh

"There are always new, grander challenges to confront, and a true winner will embrace each one."
—Mia Hamm

Dr. Glen Depke, ND

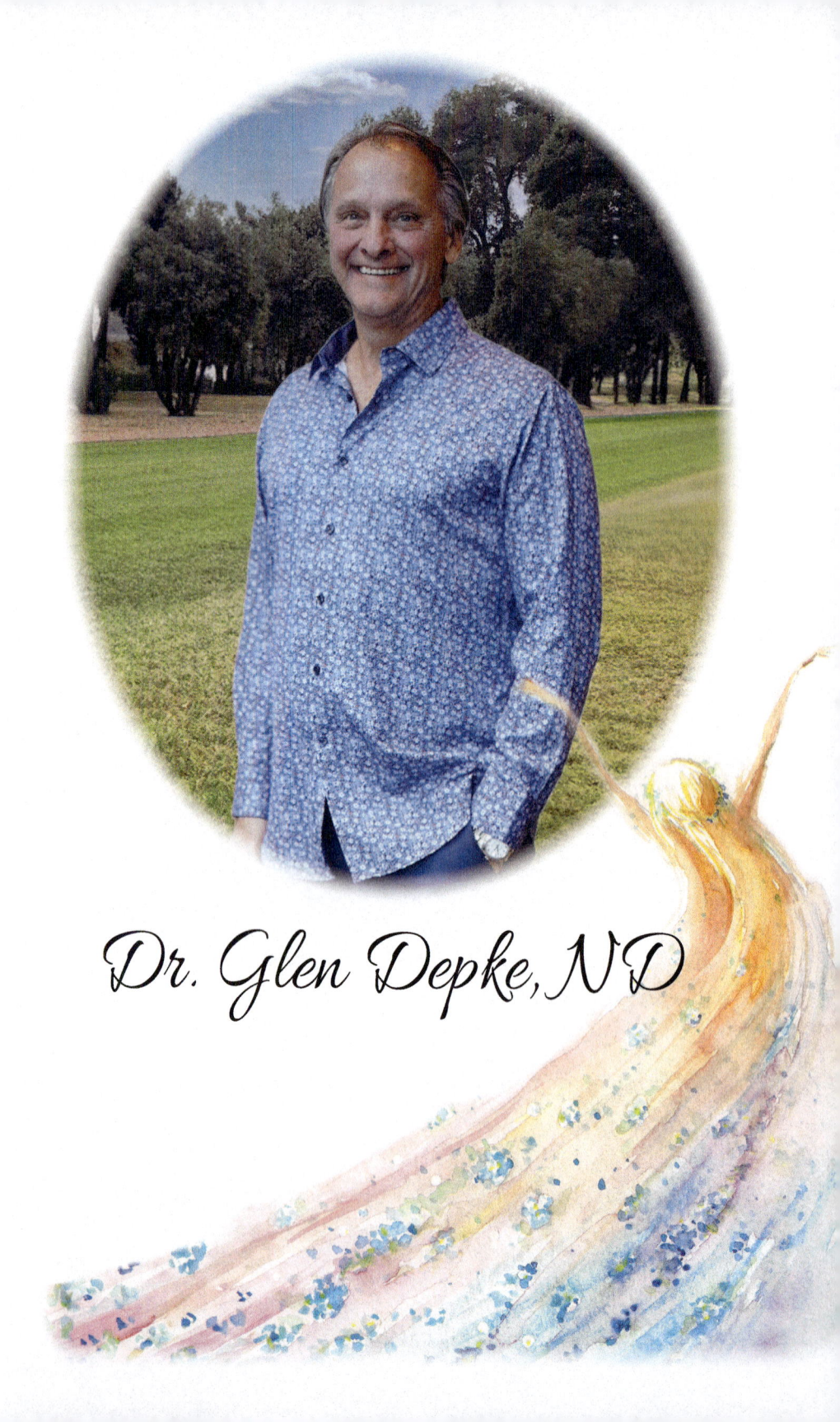

Healthy Hormones are Your Superpower

"You can turn back the clock and feel young again!"

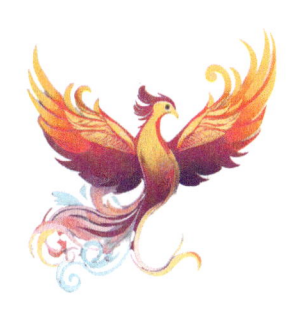

Intention:

My intention is to empower individuals to reach their health and wellness goals by addressing their individual imbalances and releasing any blocks that hinder them from achieving this goal, whether physical, mental, emotional, or spiritual.

Story:

Without understanding the impact this would have on my life, I had my first grand mal seizure at the age of 17. Little did I know that this began my journey toward health and wellness. A journey for myself and for you!

I continued to have seizures for nearly a decade. The interesting fact, though, is that every test known to conventional medicine could not produce any reason for the seizures.

So that answer was, "Here, take this pill."

That did not work so well since I still had seizures on the medication.

Almost ten years into my seizure disorder and diagnosis as an epileptic, I took matters into my own hands. I began to educate myself on many natural health practices as well as the potential dangers of prescription drugs.

With my newfound knowledge, I moved forward in changing my life with the end goal of being seizure-free and medication-free.

To make the long story short, I changed my poor lifestyle habits, removed toxins that are known as neurotoxins, shifted my thought patterns, and got off prescription drugs.

I can happily report that I have not had another seizure for more than three decades and am not concerned about having another for the rest of my life.

After working through and understanding the value of natural healing, it became my passion to teach others its benefits.

This fuels my fire to assist others in overcoming their own personal health challenges and living the lives of their dreams.

Your own personal health and happiness!

So, I continued my journey to become a Naturopathic Physician. I earned a doctorate as a traditional naturopath, a diploma level in professional holistic iridology, and a bachelor of science in natural health.

I have also been trained in many other therapies and protocols, such as the Kalish method of assessing the three main body systems, the emotional freedom technique (EFT), metabolic typing, traditional Chinese assessment tools, and German drainage therapy.

Another point to make is that I never stop learning. I believe that any practitioner who stops learning falls behind and no longer serves their clients in the healthiest possible means. This continued learning and growth continues in my own personal journey toward optimal health and happiness, as well as the journey of my clients and followers of Depke Wellness. www.depkewellenss.com.

I have also had the pleasure of working alongside some of the most prominent healers of our time, most notably Dr. Joseph Mercola and the staff at the Center for Natural Health, where I held the positions of chief nutritionist, primary EFT therapist, and wellness director. I also had the pleasure of developing the system of nutritional typing used by Dr. Mercola's clinic which is available on www.Mercola.com.

The four years at Dr. Mercola's clinic were invaluable.

With Dr. Mercola's notoriety, approximately 1,000 new patients came through the doors yearly. In four years, I assisted more people with their personal health challenges than most practitioners will see in their careers. As mentioned, this was invaluable to me and is equally as invaluable to my clients today. I was humbled and honored with Dr. Mercola's own words: *"Glen worked at my Natural Health clinic in Chicago for a number of years and consistently provided high-quality, compassionate care for our patients."* —Dr. Joseph Mercola

Philosophy:

Optimal health and wellness are your birthright, and it is of utmost importance for Depke Wellness and me to educate the public on this right. The journey for optimal wellness can begin with your first step, which was mine. Our clients frequently report that they reach their goals and do it fast—much faster than they were led to believe from other wellness centers. We keep our focus simple. The body naturally wants to heal, so by focusing on a few key fundamentals of health it allows the body to do just that!

Understand that every cell in your body has the innate intelligence to replicate perfectly.

That happens when living a balanced life; the path becomes a simple road map. This state of balance, which we call your "perfection," is simply the combined result of your focus on the fundamentals of health in your past and how you learn to apply a healthier focus to your present and future. If you're not satisfied with your current state of "perfection," you have the ability to make new choices. Your past does not determine your future perfection; your current choices do. You're always in the driver's seat—you get to choose.

Using multiple methods to teach and empower, I've created an environment to create a greater awareness of health and wellness. At our practice, we provide current health news and recommendations on products that meet our exacting standards for consistent and high-quality results. Our 30-plus years of combined experience have allowed us to develop a proven and reliable approach to wellness, leading to positive results time and time again. By addressing your personal fundamentals of health, we encourage and guide you to find your own balance. From there, the body innately knows what to do, and healing begins naturally.

And the good news? This is just the beginning! I was then led on my quest for optimal wellness in Women's Health.

You may wonder how I became the *Happy Hormone Doctor*, as Dr. Jo Dee Baer calls me.

To be candid, I did not have a moment where I consciously planned to become the leading Menopause Symptom Relief Practitioner in the United States.

This indeed grew organically, and here is how.

To begin, I have been in private practice since January 2001.

I have been specifically examining hormone results since January 2005, so at the time I am writing this, I have been working with clients one-on-one for 24.5 years and focusing on hormones for 19.5 years.

Initially, I was looking at hormones for holistic reasons rather than from a menopause perspective.

After all, the same hormone imbalances that can lead to menopause symptoms can also lead to dysfunction in any of these areas below.

- Thyroid function
- Ovarian hormone imbalance
- Pancreatic function
- Protein turnover
- Regulation of body weight and fat
- Mucosal integrity
- Detoxification pathways
- Pro and anti-inflammatory support
- Immune support
- Glucose balance
- Cellular energetics
- Bone and connective tissue turnover
- Muscular integrity
- Quality of sleep and mood
- Ability to memorize and learn.
- Neural connectivity

As I had mentioned, I was always looking at hormones due to this list above, recognizing that if you cannot get your hormones in balance, you're likely going to have issues with many of these areas of health.

And, as I was helping my clients balance their hormones and find the underlying triggers for this hormone imbalance, this would significantly assist them in overcoming their health problems and symptoms.

Now, here is the fun part!

Organically, most clients that came into my clinic were women between the ages of 45 and 55.

Their primary focus on seeking out my assistance was due to their chronic health issues. This may have been with weight gain, fatigue, poor sleep, inflammatory conditions, gut symptoms, brain fog, and so much more.

We would focus on hormone balance and the underlying hormone triggers to help overcome their symptoms.

And then, I started hearing something from a substantial percentage of the women I was working with.

They said, "You know, since working with you, I have noticed that my menopause symptoms have greatly reduced, and some even said that their menopause symptoms were simply gone."

This is when I "got it"!!!

Balancing the overall hormone system, which I refer to as the HPA (hypothalamic-pituitary-adrenal) axis, and uncovering the underlying hormone triggers was the "secret" to menopause.

Most of the women who were initially coming in with overall health symptoms never really mentioned much about menopause symptoms because they thought that was something they simply had to live with.

After all, most women are taught that most of their lives.

So, once I organically stumbled on the "secret" to menopause, that became my focus.

It made sense to me because most women were either needlessly suffering from menopause symptoms or were put on bioidentical hormones with anywhere from mild to no success, often causing other health issues.

Remember to seek a practitioner who supports you, as a woman, to achieve optimal health. All peri-menopause, menopause, and post-menopause can be in 'flow.' Keep looking and seeking until your hormones are in alignment, so, you feel happy again.

So here I am today, as Dr. Glen: The *Happy Hormone Doctor*, because I get to enjoy women finding their individual happiness by balancing their hormones and escaping their symptoms.

What I love most about this is simply the fact that I have the pleasure of helping women. It meant a great deal to me, that my colleague Dr. Johnny Bowden, agreed with me: *"Glen Depke has the rare gift of a true healer. He's a terrific communicator, a natural public speaker, and he has the one quality that can't be faked—he truly cares."* —Dr. Jonny Bowden

After all, most women have been lied to about menopause, most of, if not all, of their lives.

You are told you should suffer.

You are told you should gain weight, agonize over hot flashes, lose control of your mood, sleep poorly, deal with extreme fatigue, suffer from brain fog, lose interest in intimacy, and so much more.

Well, I'm here to tell you that your body has been created to enjoy perfect hormone balance during childbearing years, peri-menopause, menopause, and even during post-menopause.

Balance, health, and flow can begin as you unfold your personal secrets and achieve the life of optimal wellness that you deserve! It's your time, ladies. It is *your* time to shine!

Action Steps:

- Focus on improving all of your Pillars of Health, or as I refer to these, your Fundamentals of Health.
- Take the hormone assessment in the chapter to understand your potential hormone state of health.
- Test your hormone function with a comprehensive 24-hour urine collection.

- Support your hormonal system foundations per your hormone testing results.
- Assess your body signs to understand the proper testing for hormone triggers.
- Focus on eliminating your hormone triggers and supporting a healthy inflammatory response.
- Enjoy feeling young again!

Dr. Glen Depke, ND
Traditional Naturopath
www.depkewellness.com
glen@depkewellness.com

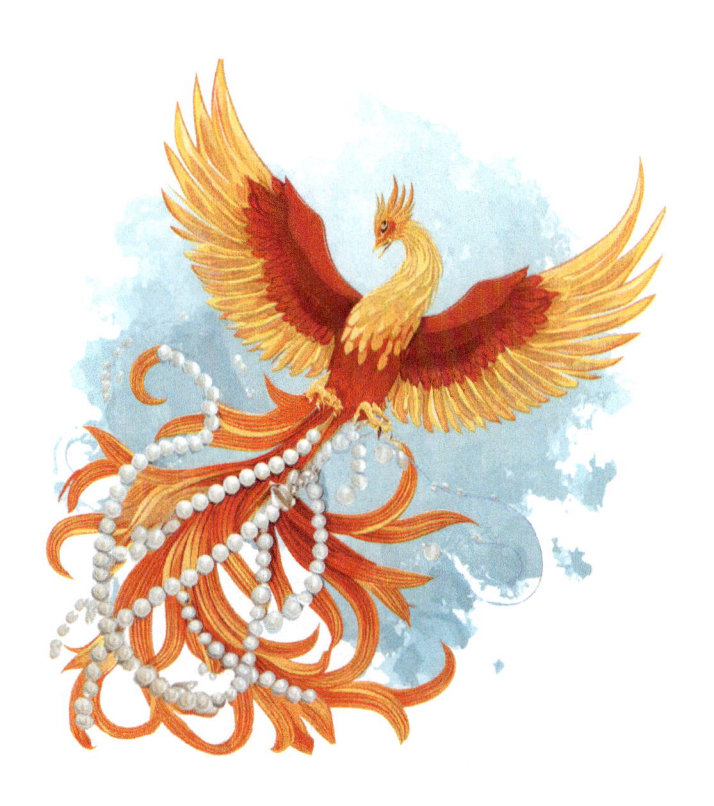

Cathy Vergara, APRN

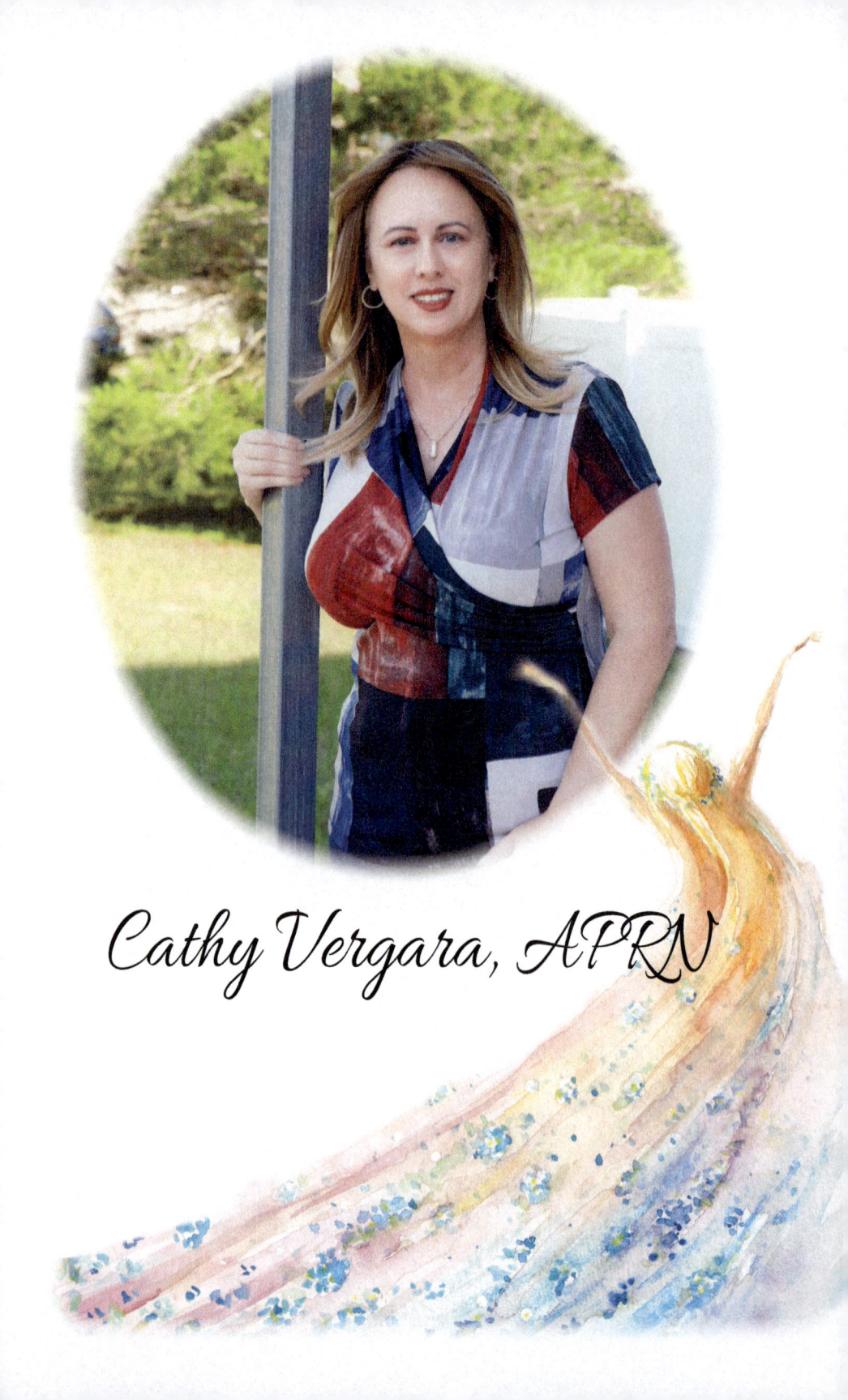

The Prescription Glass: an Unlimited Life

"Live long and strong!
Both are a prescription for a long life."

Intention:

My prayer, with my long and unique journey, is to encourage and motivate others, for you to do the same. Our world today often leaves us feeling like we are not doing enough or not giving enough—at our own expense. No matter how bad things seem, you have options. Observe and learn to see what our limiting beliefs are. So often, we feel unworthy, undeserving, and unable. *This is not true and here is a path to show you the way.*

Story:

If we were to meet today, you would see a successful nurse practitioner, full of happiness, love, independence, and strength. It would be unfathomable that at one time I was unable to stand up for myself, for the most basic subsistence in life. I struggled with basic education, suffered from poor self-esteem, had many physical limitations, with no hope for a future. A beam of light came over me, in my early 20's. I had a massive physical transformation. My body began to awaken from rubella syndrome. I went from being grossly underweight to a striving and healthy weight. Things that once eluded me now became easy. All of a sudden, as if by magic, I had so many options—but no idea where to go or how to utilize this newfound freedom.

My mother was diagnosed with Rubella, also known as German Measles, while being pregnant. In the early weeks of pregnancy, this is often considered deadly for a fetus. If one survived, it was with significant impairments. Abortion was strongly recommended for my mother. However, because of her strong personal beliefs, this was not an option for her. Most babies develop blindness, deafness, and cardiac problems. At birth, miraculously, it was believed I was a normal healthy baby, although I was blind in one eye and deaf in another. However, as I entered kindergarten, I struggled with comprehension and displayed significant cognitive challenges. Even simple concepts were difficult for me to process. I would get so irritated and it was so hard for me to be patient and wait. I just felt so out of place and so out of touch with everything and everyone. It became apparent that I also had speech and language difficulties. My teachers used to yell at me because my attention wandered. It was frustrating to my teachers but especially to me.

Providence arrived when the school decided to do vision testing. They had me put a cup over my eye. I was shocked. I couldn't see well. That was the first time my parents, teachers, and I realized I had vision problems. My mother was empowered by this new information and took me to a physician for a more formal examination. This exam determined that I was legally blind in my left eye and completely deaf in my right ear. I had attention deficit hyperactivity disorder—ADHD, learning disabilities, a metabolism disorder, and was considered developmentally delayed. It seemed my fate of limitations was sealed. This was going to be my life—physical and emotional difficulties with limited resources. The self-sufficient world of the internet had not yet been born, so eventually I dropped out of high school and earned my GED.

My time in elementary and middle school was spent as a victim, bullied because of my mental and physical disabilities. One teacher, Kathy Williams, gave me hope, with a simple rubber band and told me, "Put your hair up, so I can see your beautiful face." I didn't realize, until years later, that was my way of hiding or staying invisible.

Here I was, 20 years old, weighing 88 pounds at 5'6" with no true skills and no direction in life. The only thing I hoped for was getting married and having children. The only dream that I can really recall during those wandering and searching years, was a beautiful home—I saw while driving by—I just loved the design. I made a mental note to myself that for me success would be to have that beautiful home with those two nice cars and a husband worthy to bear my children. Inside myself, it seemed only a dream. I didn't think this would actually happen. I continued to waitress, cashier, and any other menial labor—just to pay the rent. My relationships were as unhealthy as my struggling life.

Then, a hormonal boom and explosion occurred inside my body. An unexplainable manifestation where within a 6 to 9-month period, I was able to gain weight and my weight went from 88 pounds to 120 pounds. My brain started to 'awaken.' Concepts just started to be "easy." I would spend the next several years trying to find my way to my newfound normal. I earned my real estate certification. I became a certified nursing assistant. I even became an over-the-road truck driver, and school bus driver. The next rung on my ladder of living was attending a local college to get a medical assisting degree. It was then my teacher, Mrs. Riggs, recommended I go to nursing school. I remember telling her, "That's for 'smart' people." My awakening was a massive realization that I never considered anything at a higher level. My personal epiphany and *first* massive shift had arrived. Prior to this time, I couldn't be smart enough to become a nurse. I was not good enough to become a nurse. How could I actually make this happen? It took me months to muster up the courage, but eventually, I went to the local community college and took the entrance exam. Feeling completely overwhelmed, so scared, sweating bullets, and not believing I was actually even attempting it. Somehow, I unexpectedly passed the entrance exam. I now laugh and grin to myself "this was the day" my self-esteem went from 40% to 70%!

While I enjoyed college, I still felt defeated and "not good enough." I took the "hard teachers"—as if it would mitigate my failing in class. My brain was working at full speed, but emotionally I was still impaired. I didn't feel good enough, strong enough, or even capable. I didn't recognize the shift that was going on inside of me. To my surprise, I graduated from nursing school. I remember telling my mom, "I am the greatest con artist." I didn't feel I had learned anything—until I started responding to emergencies as a nurse, and realizing I could do it! It was another boost of confidence in my prescription along my life's journey.

Timing is everything, and when I learned to walk through the doors that opened—that I attracted for me—and when they appeared in front of me—I began to discover, and overcome, challenges that I thought would always hold me back. For example, on my journey to obtaining my bachelor's degree, I went to a conference in Tampa by Louise Hay called, "I Can Do It." This was the beginning of the *second* massive shift in my life. An epiphany where I began to understand about self-limiting beliefs. I was in personal command of these beliefs that could and were influencing me mentally, physically, and spiritually.

When I look back to my humble beginnings I wonder—how did I earn a Bachelor's Degree with my physical limitation of being blind in one eye and deaf in one ear? How does one even become a truck driver with these liabilities in life? I didn't realize the self-limiting beliefs I had imposed all over me. I drove over that mountain and earned my Bachelor's Degree. I DID IT! You too can overcome whatever self-limiting beliefs or circumstances you are facing to create the life you want.

That dream of getting married and having children—I attracted into my life. I have two biological children—and have raised five other children. My husband, James, and I have been on our journey together for 25 years. I continued my nursing journey with a Master's Degree as an Adult/Geriatric Nurse Practitioner. As a nursing entrepreneur, I have the joy of working in several different specialties. Learning to own my power and find fulfilling work that provides financially for my family and nurtures my mind and spirit has truly been a gift. As a person labeled with ADHD, an office job isn't always ideal. However, I thrive in a varied and complex environment and subsequently provide care that is unique.

Of course, these life shifts had their twists and turns. I continued to hold steadfast in my commitment following the lead from my heavenly Father. I have learned how to walk through doors of possibilities. Embracing change guided me to my ultimate goals. Game-changing solutions have not always come in the form of a job. Learning about the Life Line Technique, by Dr. Darren Weissman, was a major opportunity where I began to experience seeing my world differently. We are all like a pencil, at times we need to sharpen off the parts that no longer serve us. This pencil process helps to keep us 'on point,' embracing these transitions and seeing them as unexpected gifts in wrapping paper. Changing the way we perceive what is happening so we can live with an attitude of gratitude.

Unlimited Belief—My Prescription in life encompassed by my essence of a woman. The home I wanted—I got it! The car, the animals, the children, and the lifestyle I so desired—I got it! Even now, years later, I still continue to sort through my limiting beliefs so that I may overcome and be victorious over them.

Unlimited Beliefs can have a panoramic, 360 view while even being sight impaired. Let's change the "prescription" so your view is not limited. To see the world differently is empowering and liberating.

I heard my calling and my voice in life—whispering for my ultimate life—even only hearing from one ear. Nothing needed to hold me back forever. When I learned how to see and hear beyond what I thought was possible—more possibilities unfolded. They were hiding in plain sight, waiting for me to risk stepping forward, to believe in myself, to trust my forward motion.

Mental Mindset—I overcame the prenatal physical prescription dealt to me at birth. Having been "sold a bill of goods," being bullied into believing I couldn't do it. Eventually, it became a self-fulfilling prophecy.

Graduating nursing school with honors, and even speaking at my graduation. I was only one of two speakers to do so, living on a few hundred dollars a month. Tenacity—and persistence—paid off! I was going to do it and did it! A monetary limitation was of no consequence. Why? Because I wouldn't let it be.

Philosophy:

From my semi-truck driving 16-wheeler days, 'making it happen' no matter what was just like shifting gears in a truck. Sometimes you shift easily and sometimes you grind through. It's the forward motion that counts! In my present multi-faceted nursing career, I do long-term care, physical rehab, and regeneration medicine utilizing stem cells. Each modality has its own requirements to shift in a higher gear for success in life.

In rehab, I believe the biggest lesson is taking the small steps. We can't always have great leaps and bounds. Hold steady and trust all those small steps that lead in the right direction.

In long-term care, I believe my blindness helped me to understand the importance of visualizing the long game to live long and strong. The first step in achieving a goal is to visualize the goal in detail. My dream house had floor plans, the size of my yard, and the color of my master bedroom. I envisioned myself with my future children, playing with our animals, on future family vacations, and driving in my dream car. Every year I would make a vision board with words, pictures, anything, and everything to help me actualize my goals and dreams.

Regenerative Medicine assimilates my body reset, without me really expecting it or knowing the cause. I now can utilize stem cell therapy to support my body. I have the amazing front-row seat to watch other people greatly benefit from this therapy with life-changing results. There is no better and more fulfilling opportunity than that.

From The Lifeline Technique training, I made lifelong friends. One introduced me to Kevin Lucas, owner of New Hope Regeneration, a company that offers umbilical cord stem cell therapy. Energetically I knew I must work with this company. I attracted my next greatest opportunity. I manifested all this over several years. I went through all the preliminary hoops required for a new job, with no idea what my salary would even be. We laughed when I got my first paycheck because I didn't even know when payday was! I knew in the depths of my heart I needed this—so money was not my primary focus. I got to see an advanced-age lady gain the strength to fly across the country to go kayaking with her adult children—talk about soul-satisfying work! My medical miracle came after my personal stem cell therapy. I was previously told by another Western Medical Doctor that there was strong potential for me "to wake up completely blind." My stem cell end result was an 80% improvement! Talking about a reciprocal not only helping others but helping myself.

Gratitude is everything. I've lived an attitude of gratitude. The frequency of gratitude radiates positive energy. It brings joy and light to all those around you. Just like my eight furry-fur people—they sense positive energy and energy is everything. "Infinite Loving Gratitude."

Since we only have one life, the prescription to live long and strong is available for all who choose it. Choose unlimited.

Action Steps: The Prescription from this Nurse Practitioner:

- Manage your mindset through self-awareness.
- Take small steps in the right direction. It is the forward motion that counts. Small steps in the right direction are still in the right direction.

- Believe in abundance and have anticipation for the unrecognized gifts. Check in and evaluate your beliefs. Are they self-limiting or self-empowering?

- Understanding health truly is wealth. There is power in belief and determination.

Cathy Vergara, APRN
Nurse Practitioner
www.newhoperegeneration.com
www.thelifelinecenter.com

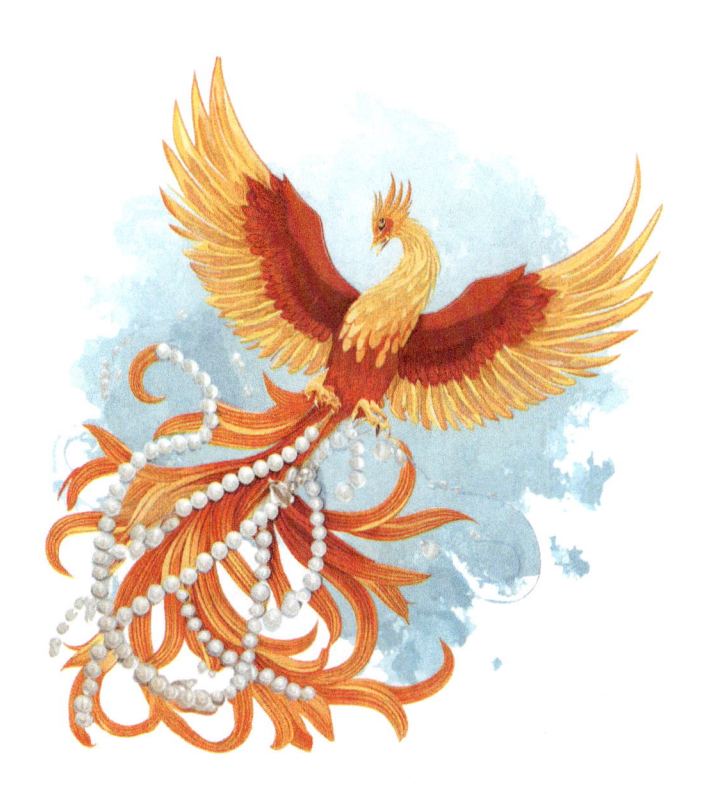

Dr. Annette Watson-Johnson

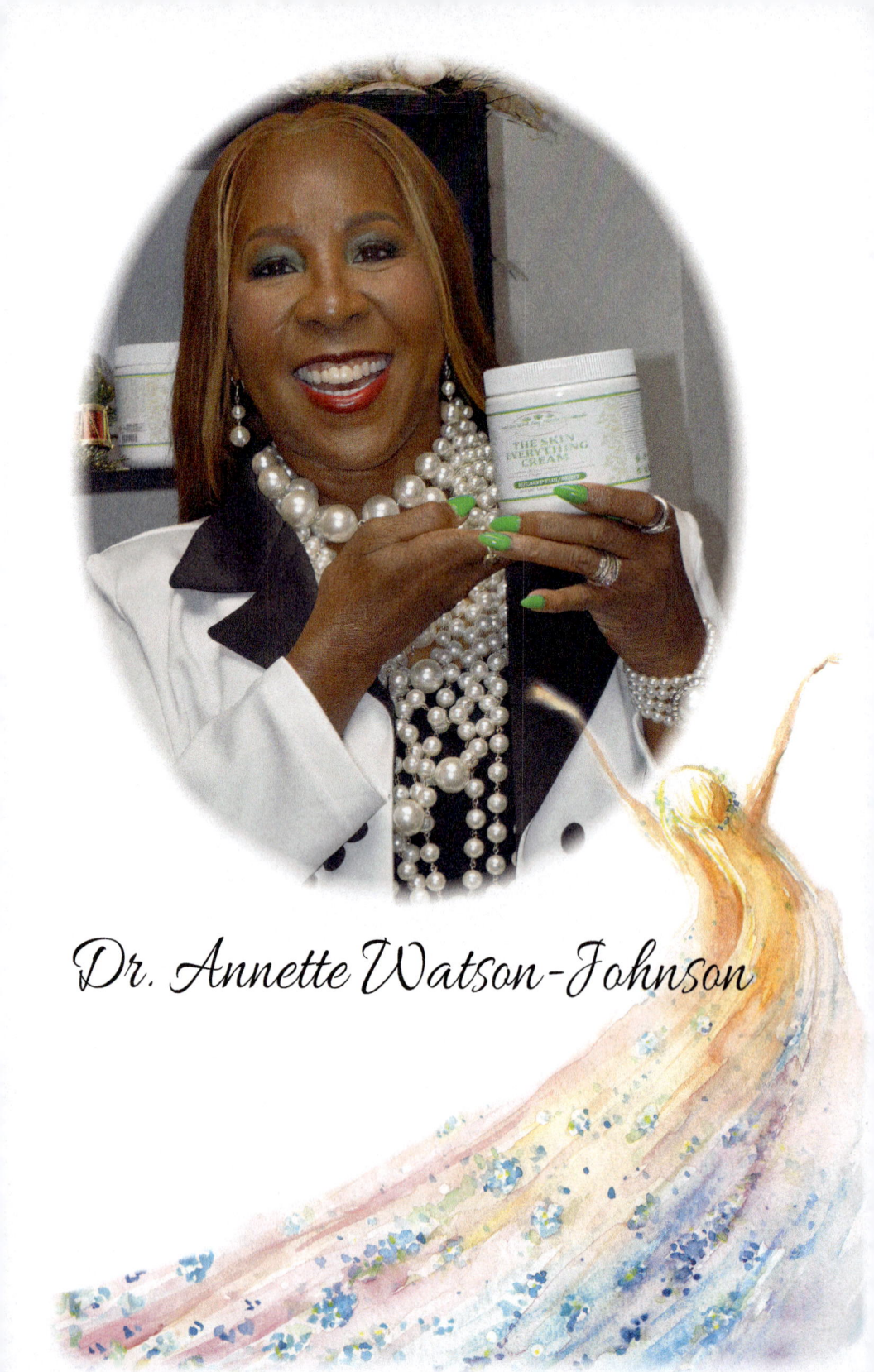

Just Get Well, The Sea Moss Way

"If you listen to your body, it will tell you what it needs."

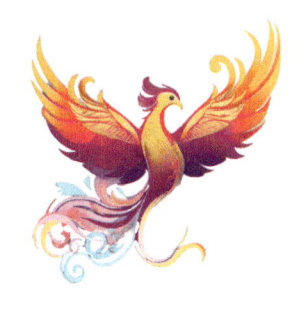

Intention:

To bring awareness of the impact that foods can have on your mental, physical, and spiritual wellness is key. Julius Erving said:

> *"If you don't do what's best for your body, you're the one who comes up on the short end."*

Story:

Women are the nurturers of the earth, so what we eat and feed our families can heal or deplete nutrients from their bodies. 1 Corinthians 10:31:

> *"So whether you eat or drink or whatever you do, do it all for the glory of God."*

We have heard the phrase *'You are what you eat'* but usually what accompanies this statement is an unpleasant picture of a person over-indulging in an unhealthy snack or the famous, oversized fried chicken leg dressed as an obese woman with an enlarged stomach. Who can forget about the new deep-fried chicken sandwich craze from a well-known franchise that caused such a demand that they sold out across the country? I have nothing against a chicken sandwich, but when you are fighting with other patrons over a space in line, ramming your car into others in the drive-thru, and threatening the employees because they sold out of these sandwiches, there is a real issue with it.

I often wondered why my African ancestors were sought after and sold into slavery. I concluded that they were not only brilliant world leaders and lived on the African continent among the most beautiful land in the world, but processed the most chiseled physiques. Africans lived, worked hard, ate from the nutrient-rich land, and traveled all over the world. They were farmers, hunters, and gatherers. They ate mainly fruit—especially figs—with some meat, fish, seafood, and eggs. They understood that the earth can supply the body with all the organic chemical elements and nutrients—proteins, fats, carbohydrates, vitamins, and minerals—to make up and create the new blood cells your body needs to survive. Once they arrived in America as slaves in 1619, they were fed different foods, which over generations changed their healthy physiques and the trajectory of their lives. Their bodies went into total disarray.

Technically my ancestors went from mainly eating organic non-genetically modified healthy fruits, nuts, vegetables, and meats, without chemical interference, to consuming garbage and not allowed access to the different markets that provided more nutritious options. They were forced to work extensively from sunup to sundown. When the body exerts energy but does not replenish the 92 minerals and vitamins needed to keep it sustained, it becomes deficient, exhausted, inflamed, and diseased. To remain healthy a diet should be fed 80% alkaline-forming foods and 20% acid-forming foods. This means consuming more top alkaline foods such as fruits, vegetables, nuts, herbs, herbal teas, seeds, green juice, melons, lemons, and seeds. In Genesis 9:3, God said:

> *"Every living creature will be food for you;*
> *as I gave the green plants, I have given you everything."*

My enslaved ancestors were deprived of these healthy foods and were only allowed to eat the leftover foods high in fat. These foods included the parts of the pigs, such as chitterlings, pig feet, pig ears, pig tails, pig skin, and discarded non-nutritious foods that the slave masters did not want their families to eat.

Since my ancestors were agriculturally savvy, they were able to plant some of the seeds that they braided into the women's hair to make it across slave ship voyages. They also reused seeds or leaves from the rotten vegetables obtained from the slave masters' foods to regrow or share among each other to grow fruit, vegetables, and herbs to create delicacies for their malnourished families—an act of survivorship. To make these foods taste better they used highly saturated oils, butter, extra salt, and sugar. They were deprived of nature's healthier alternatives. Frying the foods, adding fatty meats to the healthy vegetable meals to make them flavorful, or just skipping meals altogether—food was scarce. They were resilient and brought some of their cooking traditions with them. These foods were delicious, even though they were watered down.

Over time, this new type of food became a staple among my ancestors and was passed down to the African American slave-descendant communities. Today, it is renowned as "Soul Food." Still rooted in the enslavement of African Americans, we had to make do with whatever we had on hand. To some, *Soul Food* means food, family, and tradition. Here, nearly two Centuries after the 1865 abolishment of slavery, many African Americans continue to buy and use these same ingredients.

Although slavery affected my Ancestor's food choices, we are still purchasing, cooking, and eating these fried, fatty, high sugar, and salt types of foods—expecting a different outcome. Pondering this, I had to look at my family history. These foods have brought us together and sustained us through obstacles such as racism, political injustices, education, and job opportunities. All these factors kept us from getting a piece of the American Pie. We were denied the ability to obtain the same jobs, wages, medical treatment, communities, or essentials needed to sustain a better life as other races. This has kept us resorting back to the cheaper foods and recipes that our ancestors passed down to us because these brick walls suppressed us into poverty. However, we have prevailed through depressions and pandemics, and that has given us the resilience to build legacies.

So, I cannot blame my ancestors for passing down these disease-causing recipes because our descendants would not exist if they had not! Genes and DNA play a role as well. So does the environment in which people live, socioeconomic status—and, yes, again racism. As a result, many in my family have succumbed to the diseases that these foods may have caused. My late father insightfully stated, "We don't have to eat like slaves anymore." His intent was to break a generational curse so that we can eat more of the foods God created for us to eat. Some of these garbage foods have caused diseases disproportionately within the African American community to include health disparities: diabetes, high blood pressure, heart disease, asthma, stress, mental illness, high cholesterol, some cancers, and higher mortality rates. In my family, I see that every generation has suffered astoundingly from these ailments.

As a slave descendant, I had to learn how to prioritize and make better food choices for two important reasons: To educate my children so that they can stay well, and to keep me within my wellness journey so that I will not live a lifetime of prescription medications. Traditionally, women have been the stewards of their kitchen and usually make the decision on what foods to buy and what meals to cook. As a woman of power, I chose to break the tradition of not serving my family disease-causing foods.

Already personally predisposed to some of the ailments that are prevalent in my family. I advise everyone in my path to listen to your body and what it is telling you. Your body will give you warnings when something is not working right, yet we often ignore it. If you become ill after you eat sweets, pork, dairy, etc.—don't eat it or eat smaller portions. After the Easter, Thanksgiving, and Christmas Holidays—those needing prayer from the request list at church always gets a little longer. It is safe to assume that several saints are eating and not practicing portion control, which can trigger episodes or conditions of many diseases. Due to healthcare disparities, we in the black community must be an advocate and demand the same amount of attention for our healthcare needs. We need to pay more attention to our wellness needs and break the negative tradition of eating foods that are not beneficial to us and our families.

I have been consistent with going to my annual doctor's exam. About seven years ago, I asked my doctor to review my blood work to ensure I do not have any vitamin deficiencies. I was surprised when she told me that I was vitamin D deficient. I was at a loss for words. I immediately added this vitamin to my daily intake along with my multivitamin without hesitation. Lack of vitamin D effects bone metabolism leading to osteoporosis, muscle weakness, and increased risk of fracture. Conversely, proper amounts of vitamin D may decrease the risk of cancer, colds and flu, cardiovascular disease, and infection. Recently it was determined that many are deficient in this vitamin, but are unaware. I would advise everyone to get tested.

I love buttered rolls, sweet potato pie, caramel cake, and pecan pie, but I know these types of foods can cause blood glucose to spike and, if unchecked, eventually lead to diabetes. So, I eat them sparingly using portion control methods.

Belief:

There was a reason First Lady of the United States Michelle Obama fought to allow black kids to have options other than milk with their school lunch and planted a garden at the White House. She knew the importance of our health struggles and was a great advocate for wellness. She started the "Let's Move" initiative to decrease childhood obesity. There are so many healthy food alternatives for every food we eat.

It is said that what you put into your body is what you get out of it. I realized I had to remove certain foods from my diet. I craved certain foods during my menstrual cycle but correspondingly altered my emotions. Each month I started to choose healthier foods and became a mentally balanced woman. Unknowingly hurting myself and putting my family into a state of chaos, I lived out this true statement: *"If momma ain't happy, no one is."* Olivia Newton-John said it best, "Listen to your body." Be aware that you can eat the healthiest foods, but without physical exercise, it's impossible to maintain stable stress levels—especially with a woman's work-life balancing act. I have always been the wellness ambassador for my family. I make sure that everyone is taking their vitamins and is doing their best to stay healthy.

Now that we witnessed the detriment of a deadly pandemic such as the COVID-19 virus that compromised the immune system, it is obvious that the health disparities caused by over 400 years of systemic bias and racism have tormented many in my community. We've inherited diseases that we were predisposed to, so this virus affected many of us with these pre-existing health conditions, which in turn compromised our inherently low immune systems.

Intuitively, I began making products with sea moss in 2019 which was before the Pandemic. Sea moss helps to keep your body alkaline. Wild-crafted sea moss contains 92 of the 102 vitamins that a body needs for sustainability. Sea moss contains high amounts of certain nutrients, including folate, vitamin K, iron, iodine, magnesium, calcium, B2, B12, zinc, chromium, and much more. It provides the body with key nutrients the way God created it, in its original essence. Sea moss helps in maintaining mental and physical health. It is also a rich source of minerals, including iodine, which helps in hormone production.

This all started after God came to me in a dream in 2019 and said, *"Just Get Well."* Out of obedience, I humbled myself to Him, and I allowed myself to be led into my kitchen. I heard the words; sea moss, and immediately began formulating and creating sea moss infused products using my gift of herbalism. This ability was unveiled to me, for I was unaware: 1 Corinthians 15:44 says:

> *"It is sown a natural body; it is raised a spiritual body.*
> *If there is a natural body, there is also a spiritual body."*

Educating everyone on the benefits of sea moss and the fact that God created the body to heal itself, is now my life's calling. However, it can only heal when provided with the proper nutrients.

My company, Dynamic AWJ Products LLC, has created and formulated over 65 organic, plant-based, vegan, and cruelty-free products. All these products can be used by all races, but I initially began targeting those in my family, church, and community because we suffer the most from generational ailments. My company's product line includes gels, capsules, creams, oils, baths, and other body care essentials infused with sea moss, teas, and herbs for the internal and external body. When you are not mentally, physically, and spiritually sufficient you can easily be distracted because your imbalance is causing you to miss what God is trying to tell you. The song from *"The Color Purple"* movie called "Maybe God is Tryin' to Tell You Somethin'" is one of my reminders to stay holistically balanced. That is probably why many of us cannot sleep at night—because we are not well enough to hear him.

Being a healthy mature woman is paramount for me to stay on my wellness journey. My advice for every reader is to feed your body the right foods so your body can thrive. I own my physical journey and continue to take one day at a time with reminders to self-care because God has blessed me with a gift to create products that heal and yield testimonials to help others. Therefore, as women, we must continue to eat foods that will nourish our bodies. Our essence as women is to keep our mental, physical, and spiritual presence strong.

Our body's immune system can become deficient due to the foods we consume, heredity, or environmental factors. My company's Skin Everything Body Creams, Hair Cream, Body Wash, Sea Moss Gels & Capsules, Herbal Bath Teas, Healing Oils, and Detox Scrub products contain all-natural ingredients made by God but formulated by us. They will provide the body with both internal and external max nutrition to keep the body well nourished. We are now in the post-pandemic phase yet using our products can help to build a healthy internal and external immune system. Here is a list of ways recommended for you to begin your wellness journey.

Action Steps to Just Get Well:
- Listen to your body.
- Take "Just Get Well Sea Moss" to provide the body with the key nutrients.
- Make healthier food choices that can energize and heal the body.
- Include skin care for the skin, using the "Just Get Well Sea Moss" skin care products or equivalent to heal, protect, and fight against skin ailments.

Dr. Annette Watson-Johnson
Health Coach
www.dynamicawlproducts.com

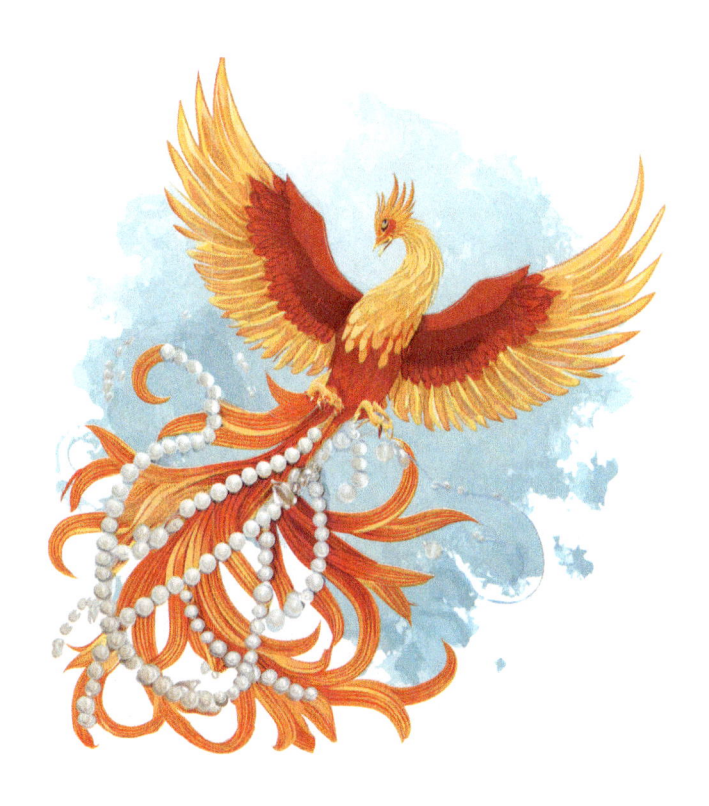

Dr. Hepsharat Amadi, MD, LAc

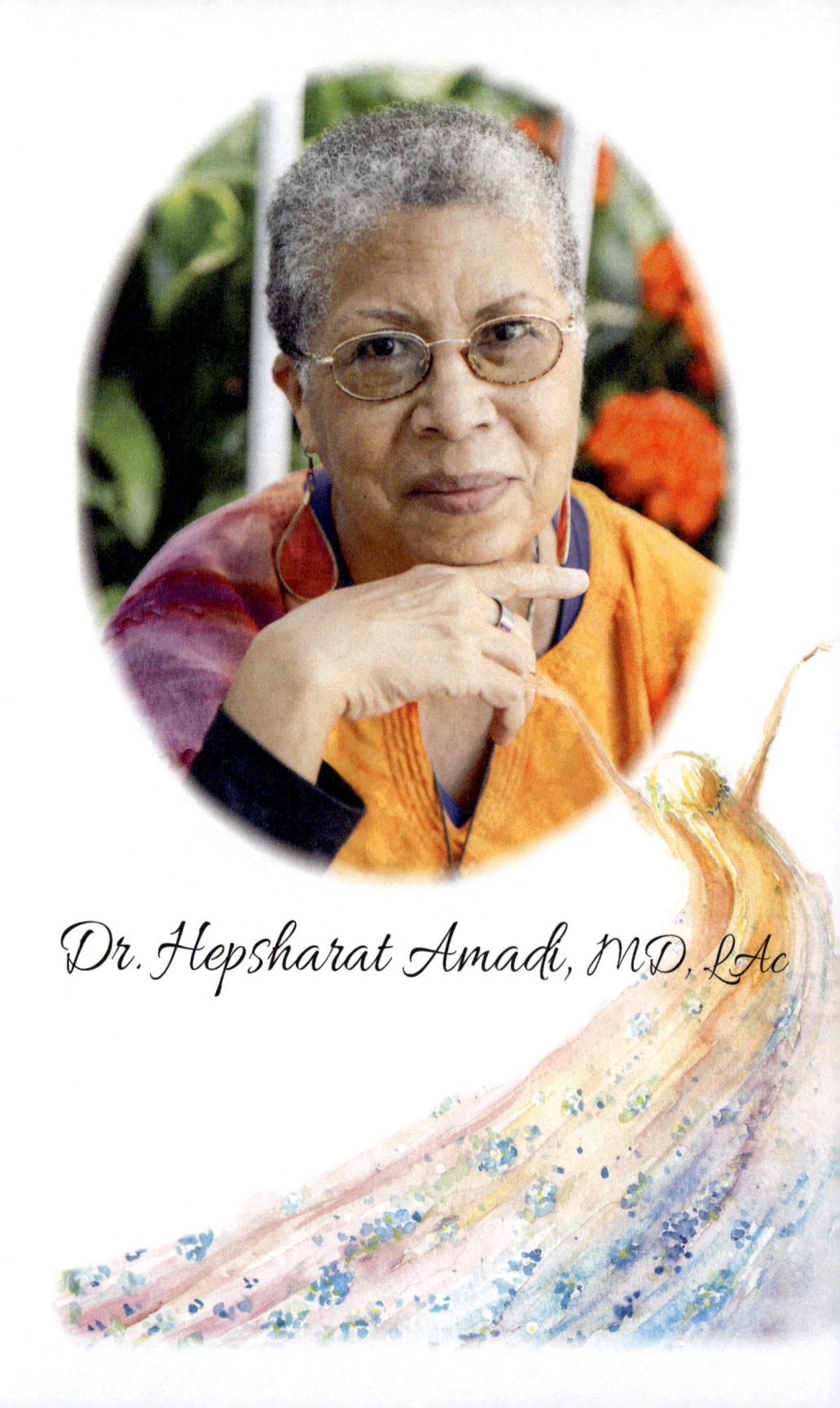

Natural Hormone Balance at Any Age

*"Hormone awareness:
Live life—in harmony and balance."*

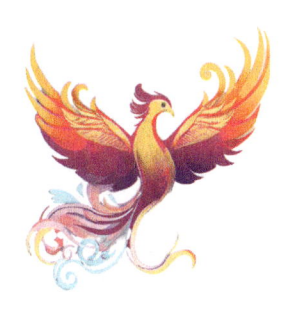

Intention:

Hormone balance affects everything in a woman, including a woman's overall well-being. May you unlock the simple secrets to your abundant health at any age with a simple and applied purpose.

Story:

Hormone balance affects the immune system, libido, digestion, sleep, fertility, energy levels, mood, metabolism, connective tissue, hair, recovery from injuries, cognitive functioning—your entire body. That exhaustive list covers almost everything!

Finding your best hormonal balance at any age requires awareness and the ability to be assertive in requiring your Healthcare Practitioners to do the right tests to determine your hormonal status. They can then help you balance it with the appropriate nutrition, bioidentical hormones, supplements, herbs, and/or homeopathic remedies.

The most common hormonal imbalances I see in my functional integrative practice are estrogen dominance (having too much estrogen for how much progesterone is present), hypo adrenal (low in cortisol), and/or hypothyroid (low in T-4 or T-3 or both), oftentimes some combination of the above. Tests that would reveal a lot about a woman's hormonal status are the following: Free Progesterone, Free Estradiol, Free Testosterone, TSH, Free T-4, Free T-3, and serial cortisol levels in saliva.

If hormone testing reveals a woman's hormone levels are unbalanced, the most direct approach to resolving that problem is giving her bioidentical hormone replacement. This can consist of progesterone, estrogen, testosterone, cortisol, T-3 (liothyronine) or T-4 (L-thyroxine), or some combination of the above. A relatively small number of women have hormones that are inconsistent or who personally reject the idea of taking hormones. For these women, an approach that involves herbs, glandular supplements, or homeopathic remedies may be a better option.

Nutrition influences hormonal balance as well. Certain nutrients nourish different glands. For example, vitamin C, vitamin B5 (pantothenic acid), and calcium help nourish the adrenal glands. Iodine is necessary for thyroid hormone production. My favorite 'female' herbs are Vitex (also known as Chasteberry, which supports the progesterone system) and Dong Quai, which is often useful for symptoms of menopause such as hot flashes, including night sweats.

Homeopathy is a medical philosophy and practice that is the opposite of allopathic Western Medicine. With this philosophy, the higher the dose of something, the greater the effect it is expected to have. In Homeopathy, it is the opposite: The more dilute the remedy, the more powerful it is expected to be! Homeopathy is energy medicine in that it imparts the frequency of a substance into the remedy to strengthen and support the functioning of an organ functionally. I am not a classical homeopath, so I use remedies that support the working of an organ functionally in order to help support their ability to produce certain hormones. For example, I promote Kidney, Ovarian, and Adrenal homeopathy as a remedy to support the functioning of all three of these organs in synchronicity.

Hormones, especially those of women, are the chemical messengers that help to keep our bodies in homeostasis even though our external environment is constantly changing. *Homeostasis* means maintaining a stable internal environment. For example, the internal body temperature tends to remain constant even though the temperature outside the body goes up or down.

Hormones have been my adult life and passion; however, when I think back to how I got started in all of this, I was just 15, and I was already torn as to what I wanted to do as a career. It was a diametrical choice of *'heads or tails'*—between being a dancer or a doctor. The doctor's side of the coin obviously won. My reasoning at the time was that everyone knew and understood what a doctor did and was willing to pay for some kind of healthcare, but not everyone understood the artistry of a dancer or was willing to spend money to support the art. I learned that medicine was also an economically driven art and I could be performing its gift for humanity.

Humanity was integral in my focus, for I have always been interested in animals, plants, biology, and psychology. I wanted to be an orthomolecular psychiatrist—one who balances the psyche naturally using diet modification and supplements instead of pharmaceutical medications. However, when I shared my desire with people, they informed me that first, a psychiatrist has to go to medical school. Along the path of preparing myself for medical school, I found that I was just as intrigued with physical ailments as I was with mental illness. When I got even further down the road in my training, the body was a whole entity. You can't have one without the other.

The integrative approach with mental issues being intertwined with physical and vice versa was key to my philosophy as much then as it is now. This is ultimately why I was destined to become an integrative family physician. This specialty encompasses dealing with both physical and psychological health issues in individual patients and within the context of their social family dynamics.

Even in Medical School, I instinctively integrated Functional Medicine into my studies and training. In my last year of residency, I designed an elective for myself to observe functional medical practices that incorporated Acupuncture, Homeopathy, Chinese Herbs, and various Physiotherapy Modalities to address the broad spectrum of conditions that primary care treats. After I saw the astounding results, I was inspired to be able to offer this therapeutic menu to my future patients, providing both natural and conventional methods that give them optimal results. One of my mentors whose office I hung out in during that month-long elective told me something so profound that it resonates with me today. He said, "If you go into private practice, you can make a difference.' With these encouraging words, *I did just that!*

I have been an Integrative Medical Healer for three and a half decades. During the last year of residency, we were required to take one month of 'Practice Management,' during which we observed a doctor's office that worked with insurance to learn about the practical aspects of the business of medicine.

During this time, under the leadership of Kaiser-Permanente, HMOs were just starting to become the dominant model in this so-called 'health care delivery' system. Although Kaiser's original concept helped to shave some unnecessary medical expenses that insurers had to pay, the end result unfortunately occurred that the HMOs were no longer run by the doctors who actually gave the care. Medicine became controlled by corporations with much more interest in their *bottom-line profits than the personalized care their patients needed.*

Accelerating to the present day, the corporatization of medicine, hospitals and group practices are being bought up by corporate entities. Much like a business merger and acquisition—concentrating power in fewer and fewer hands. Instead of trained doctors making the decisions that determined what medications, testing, and specialists a patient had access to, a person who worked for a health insurance company, with no medical training, was in charge of making these decisions! The number of solo medical practices began decreasing, which is a tragic trend that continues.

People used to stay in one job for a long time and get to know their family physicians. Over the years, the trend has been that people change jobs more frequently, and companies change healthcare plans more often, so people often end up bouncing around and consequently changing doctors. The unfortunate result is that the new doctor doesn't know the patient or their family history. It became like the game "musical chairs." In some places, healthcare has been reduced to how many patients you can see—often asking doctors to spend 10 minutes or less on a daily conveyor belt moving on to the next patient. This means that patients are, in general, not getting the basic and proper care from strangers who don't know them, let alone their medical history, not to mention the 10-minute consultation rush.

Another aspect of this medical corporation phenomenon is that patients are usually unaware—doctors who are 'in-network' with HMOs are constrained from ordering tests and referring to specialists—even if they think it is medically appropriate. Afraid of being dropped as a Provider under these plans because they are labeled as an 'over-utilizer,' whether the tests or referrals are medically justifiable or not. The HMOs just don't want to pay for certain things, period. Doctors who are a part of HMOs know that part of the 'price' of providing service through HMOs is that they have surrendered a certain amount of personal medical autonomy.

For all of the above reasons, I have remained clear and focused on 'the whole patient' not as a number or a disease entity but as a unique human being that has psychological, emotional, social, and spiritual aspects to them. The quantum biofeedback device that I use allows me to interact with all of these aspects (even those within their emotions and psychology that they may not be consciously aware of). I receive their frequencies, which identify the current trends that are going on with the patient in all these areas, and I can send frequencies to them that help to balance them subtly and non-invasively.

This device also allows me to test for what I should prescribe energetically. It tells me whether these substances would be harmonious with the patient's acupuncture meridians (the pathways of electromagnetic energy that flow in the body) or not. This is how I am guided as to which hormones to prescribe for my patients who are on bioidentical hormone replacement.

Unlike other doctors who do bioidentical hormone replacement, which most doctors don't do, I do not base my prescriptions solely on lab results. Lab results can tell me the levels of hormones that a person is making, which is one of the two very important aspects of hormone function, but lab tests cannot show me how their hormones interact with their receptors. That is the other crucial aspect of hormonal balance that they did not teach us about in medical school or residency.

Quantum biofeedback is another tool I use with my patients. The lab results tell me if a patient is deficient in certain hormones or produces too much. My biofeedback tool tells me the status of one's hormonal function (normal, hypo, or hyperfunctioning). To determine the patient's best hormonal prescription it is also important to understand how the patient's receptors are interacting with the hormones. This is not taught in medical school.

Philosophy:

Many times, I have met women who suspected their health issues had something to do with their hormones and yet were not helped when they consulted conventional medical doctors. For one thing, most doctors are not oriented toward considering a person's hormonal status, so most of the time, they do not even order hormone tests, and when they do, those tests are often incomplete. I once had a patient tell me that she actually requested that a doctor test her hormones. Still, the doctor blew her off, saying that he "could tell just by looking at her" that she had no hormonal issues and, therefore, was not even going to order any hormone tests for her!

Women in corporate medicine often have their symptoms overlooked or just attributed to "stress' or "depression," or malingering/just wanting attention. Men would not be looked at in the same way by doctors if they presented themselves as having some of the same issues that women can have when their hormones are unbalanced. Men are often given much more credibility and taken seriously, whereas women are often gaslighted and made to feel as though "it is all in their head." Sometimes, patients have even been offered medication for anxiety or depression or have been referred to psychiatrists for symptoms that are the result of hormonal imbalance. Their hormonal imbalance may have begun because of stress, but having begun, it needs to be addressed hormonally in order to put a stop to the vicious cycle of stress causing hormonal imbalances, which then cause more stress. Here are *Eight Indicators* of women's hormonal balance:

- Bone density test—Will reveal conditions of osteopenia or osteoporosis.
- Digestion—Digestive symptoms, fatigue after eating, or trouble with regular bowel movements.
- Sleep—Adequate sleep at regular hours is crucial to overall health.
- Energy levels—Do you wake up feeling tired or rested? Is there inconsistent energy throughout the day?
- Immune system—Are there frequent colds, infections, or other immune challenges such as autoimmune conditions or cancer?
- Mood—Irritability, anxiety, or depression could be related to hormonal imbalance.

- Libido—Sex, at any age, can be great with hormonal balance both systemically and locally. When needed, hormonal preparation can strengthen and lubricate the vagina.

Medical marijuana can be used to help with issues related to insomnia, anxiety, and depression. As such, it can be used to help prevent those emotional triggers that could lead to hormonal imbalance if they are not addressed in time.

Medical marijuana can also be used to help women with menstrual cramps as it counteracts muscle spasms, such as the smooth muscle of the uterus. The following are two case studies, a typical cross-section of my practice:

One patient was always tired, even after waking up in the morning. She was hypoadrenal and perimenopausal. I gave her a small amount of progesterone 20 mg. along with cortisol 5 mg. After taking this combination for a week or two, she noticed that she had more energy and slept better.

Another woman, who was never able to conceive, was able to get pregnant after starting on a small dose of progesterone and 1–3 mcg. of T-3. Her daughter is now six years old and very healthy! Her parents were delighted because they had thought that pregnancy was not an option.

Lastly, I've been heralded as a pioneer in Quantum Energy Work. It has been a staple of mine for half of my practice. When I see a new patient, I evaluate them on three levels. The quantum biofeedback device helps measure what is happening at the electromagnetic level. Lab results measure the biochemical level. Doing their physical exam and reviewing the results of their X-rays or scans helps me evaluate them on the structural level.

- After their initial visit, patients receive a written assessment and plan to help them remember what is causing their issues and suggestions about what they can do about it. This would include bioidentical hormone prescriptions when those would be helpful.
- I do follow up monthly to make sure that the hormone prescriptions I originally gave them are still optimal for them. I have noticed that most people's best prescriptions tend to change over time.

The joy, satisfaction, and fulfillment of supporting, educating, and empowering these women have been a key to my professional essence as a woman. Seeing women in balance in all six pillars of health and discovering their 'wholeness' in health has been beyond rewarding. Within physical homeostasis, with the ebb and flow in harmony of the abundant dance of life, we each truly become the essence of who we are, an artistic living masterpiece.

Action Steps for Hormonal Health:
- Eat organic foods and stay well hydrated.
- Be aware of and manage stress levels.
- Seek a functional practitioner for optimal health.
- Maintain your digestive and overall health by having routine colonics.
- Focus on proper exercise and quality sleep.

Dr. Hepsharat Amadi, MD, LAc
Medical Doctor, Licensed Acupuncturist
www.greatnaturaldoctor.com
www.dramadi.com
dramadi@dramadi.com

Dr. Tyra Good

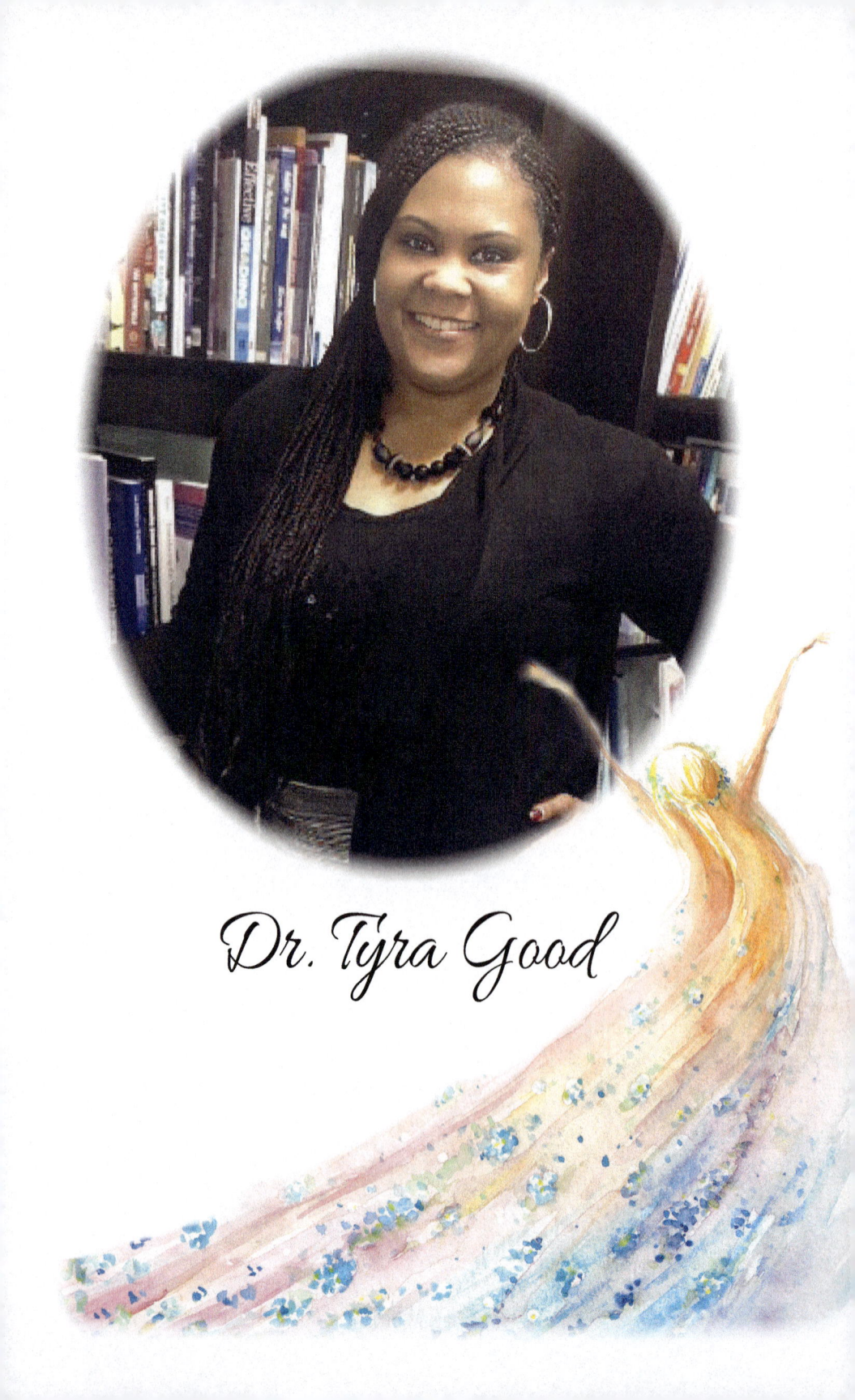

My #GOOD and Lasting Healing

"When you stop getting better, you stop being your best version of #GOOD."

Intention:

Your #GOOD and healthy life begins when you turn your personal door key, unlocking the door to your wholeness in health. May you become your own personal version of lasting healing so that you can become your best self. You will be, Oh! So #GOOD!

Story:

It was a brisk winter day in New England as the blue jays harmoniously awakened the universe to the splendid golden rays of God's morning dew of new hope and possibilities. Thump! Suddenly, from the couch I collapsed to the floor, feeling a slight shock of electricity going through my veins and pulsating in pain as my body overheated like a raging inferno. As I hit the ground, I heard the sounds of my family running downstairs to my rescue. They exclaimed," Oh, no!" My heart was pounding, faintly, as I gasped for air. I lay helplessly. The room seemed like a spinning top, as though I was riding an endless Merry-Go-Round at the county fair. Like a daring flying trapeze swaying through the air, my blurred vision mirrored a vibrating tuning fork and pendulum swaying to and fro. What was happening?

"Waaaaaahhhhhhh!" "Waaaaaahhhhhhh!" "Waaaaaahhhhhhh!" The resounding siren sound and flashing lights provided a glimmer of hope, yet scary realizing that the ambulance was pulling up in front of *my* house. Moments later, I was strapped onto a transitional chair, and then onto the stretcher. Neighbors were coming out from everywhere witnessing this alarming sight just to see what was happening—watching in dismay that I was being rolled into the back of the ambulance. The illuminated flashing lights of the emergency response vehicle intensified and exacerbated my excruciating pain. The team of paramedics was incapable of administering an IV into my veins because I was so severely dehydrated from excessive sweating. In a perpetual conundrum of inflammation throughout my body, this was my third trip to the hospital in just two weeks. The internal swelling was penetrating my veins and what once seemed like a flowing melodic river inside my body was turning into a lake of stagnation yearning for its freedom to even live!

Something was definitely wrong. I was in a struggle for my own survival to unlock this mystical version of the broken pieces of my health that would restore wholeness and peace to my body. It was a battle for my life at every turn. You see, my name "Tyra" means God of Battle, so I was born ready to fight the #GOODFight of faith for victory. Who knew that the battle I now was fighting was for my own life? God Knew! My prayer warriors, led by my mother, were locked in position and ready for battle. This was a war cry and my prayer warriors were ready to take charge!

My family's prayers were unlocking my physical healing into motion. Finally, after many extended stays at the hospital, the cardiologists found the source of my enduring pain and labored breathing through a CT scan. I was afflicted with massive blood clots throughout my lungs, heading to my heart. Once I became lucid again, questions swirled through my mind: How did this happen? When will I get better? Will I even get better? What in the world am I going to do now? Where are YOU, Tyra, in the midst of all of this? Alas, I had no answers, just clinging to faith and hope.

After a 2-week stay in the Intensive Care Unit with around-the-clock care, I was wheeled out of the hospital—yet the wheels in my body were not beginning to turn yet. Accompanying me at home were a walker, an Occupational Therapist, a Physical Therapist, and a Home Health Care Nurse. *No Way* this could be my path and quality of life now! I thought this couldn't possibly be what God meant in His word when He said:

> *"I know the plans that I have for you, declares the Lord, plans to prosper you and not to harm you, plans to give you hope and a future."*
>
> —Jeremiah 29:11 NIV

Or was it in His plan?

His present plan now came in the loving form of my Mom who moved in with me and once again took on the role of my caretaker and advocate for the next three months. It was then that I attended Dr. Jo Dee Baer's Virtual Class: "Five Weeks to Foundational Health" whose mentorship, coaching, and depth of knowledge changed the path and trajectory of my health. I experienced her health wisdom and easy plan for daily implementation—a plan that even in my unhealthy state was one I could execute. When she said in such a cavalier way that "inflammation was the cause of all disease," she unlocked the keys to my recovery, and I was able to open the door. She concluded with an encouraging promise: "The body is a miracle-making machine. It can and will heal itself." No wonder why they call her America's Top Foundational Health Coach. My spiritual beliefs and personal walk with Christ kicked in as well for my foundation. I have always had a positive mindset. I was living right, but not well. Now, at last, I held in my hands a healing path for mind, body, and spirit. I knew in my heart that I would become #GOOD again.

It took nine months to birth this #GOOD body back to health again through prayer, fasting, and rehabilitation services. As a Mother, it took nine months to birth my son, so why not me? With an assisted walking device, I was finally able to return to the university campus, which has been at the intersection of my life's work for nearly two decades. Teaching is my form of ministry and mentoring the next generation to become transformative educational leaders embodying faith, community, justice, and excellence. As I engaged in this work again, some of my less-than-optimal habits for self-care reemerged. I brushed some of my rejuvenating health practices aside and allowed my work demands to take precedence over me. Adding my predisposition and tendency for perfectionism, and my over achievement to rule the day, I reverted again to a less-than-optimal version #2 of myself—my full plate of responsibilities was overflowing again.

Ironically, as a university professor, one of the courses that I teach focuses on trauma-informed advocacy and creating equitable learning spaces where individuals—teachers and students alike—are able to thrive. I guide my students to look at themselves first, so they can be better equipped to help their students. Without our own inner work, we may miss key pieces of helping to eradicate social injustices and eliminate cultural oppression. We need to show up as the best version of ourselves. We are always in the process of learning, unlearning, and relearning, and my personal and professional life experiences collided to become the curriculum. I was living out loud the pages in my own book. Was I going to pass this open book test of unlocking my past traumas to my wholeness in health? What an oxymoron in and of itself!

Now, in addition to becoming a self-educated Professor on this roller coaster ride of personal health, I discovered another twist and turn pertaining to the unseen labor and pain of Black Women. I discuss and teach about issues related to racial, economic, and societal biases in my classes and it wasn't until I experienced these alarming health issues myself that I began to ponder about the biases in healthcare, especially women's health, in a deeper way. Some of my life's work in the field of education including teacher preparation, youth development, out-of-school time learning, and school-family-community partnerships, over the last two decades, has centered around DEI: Diversity, Equity, and Inclusion. It was now time to teach myself my personal Health DEI of Diversity of *Daily Habits*; Equity of *Everyday Self-Care*; and *Inclusion of Me* first in my life!

On a broader scale, to better address inequities in women's health, it is vital for healthcare providers and patients alike to understand the myriad of ways bias affects the quality of care and contributes to health disparity: Health DEI. Another layer of health advocacy began to unfold.

There was more than a tap on my shoulder. It was time for a #GOOD and lasting change. How could this be happening to me, Dr. Tyra, in less than a year after my third stint of weeks of overnight hospital care, when I heard the Doctors say in the emergency room that, "She made it just in time, and wouldn't have made it through the night." Here I was, in the middle of this abyss and back, living my name of origin again, re-discovering my health, for I was reverting backward quickly. I found myself once again, no longer being the best version of #GOOD.

Research has shown that women, due to our physical constitution, experience a higher prevalence of chronic pain. Due to medical bias, women's chronic pain conditions sometimes go untreated, which only worsens health disparities. Adding the component of Black Women who may experience even worse outcomes because of the combination of gender and racial bias that leads to further health disparities. A *'Healthy Women'* report noted that several conditions linked to chronic pain are experienced at a higher rate by women. These women are more likely to be dismissed and have their symptoms attributed to mental, psychosomatic, or emotional issues. There is such an undeniable systemic impact, mentally and economically, when the pain that women experience goes unaddressed.

When I think back to that fateful night in the hospital, I revert to that mental and deep physical pain that I was trying to ignore, until it almost took my life. I knew I immediately had to kick into my spiritual foundation and faith to overpower the words that were constantly echoing in my ears of the doctors saying, "She wouldn't have made it through the night." While I was in the hospital, I created an atmosphere of spiritual healing by playing bible verses and prayers accompanied by the healing frequency of music in my head, and in my heart, shutting everything else out. As I look back, I know that my belief in Jesus Christ and following the inner knowing that this situation, on human terms looked pretty dire—but on God's terms, anything is possible! I chose to believe in my master healer, God, as I faced this unthinkable time. The two years following this traumatic and life-changing experience were met with perplexity and amazement from various medical professionals as they assessed my original diagnosis and subsequent progression of healing. I meditated on this verse in my mind and heart:

> *"Beloved, I pray that in every way you prosper and enjoy good health, as your soul also prospers."*
>
> —3 John 1:2 BS

One of the ways that I have recently been able to prosper is by sharing my voice and wisdom in being the Co-Editor of *'Black Women Navigating Historically White Higher Education Institutions and the Journey Toward Liberations.'* This publication provides a collection of ethnographies, case studies, narratives, counter-stories, and quantitative descriptions of Black women's intersectional experience learning, teaching, serving, and leading in higher education. It also provides an opportunity for Black women to identify the systems that impede their professional growth and development in higher education institutions and articulate how they navigate racist and sexist forces to find their versions of success.

My health challenges woke me up. It kept tapping on my shoulder, eventually pounding, until I could no longer ignore the importance of taking care of my own health—self-care. Me first, became my echoing daily mantra; crescendoing to a physical and spiritual war cry. On this battlefield, there was a bomb lying within my own body. The pain that was sounding the alarm to alert me that I was in a dangerous territory, needed to be dismantled.

Where has that taken me? The second time around cementing my personal health-first daily routine has unlocked and flung the door wide open for me to transcend the university classroom, widening my social net with DEI, and elevating me to live my mission of helping women worldwide understand their pain against the backdrop of societal injustices and ways to unlock their #GOOD within. Allowing me to flow as a vessel, and to help and support them to reduce their stress and to advocate for themselves—personally and professionally—has given me the platform to advance the framework of the United Nations 17 Sustainable Development Goals. These global goals, designed to transform our world, are a universal call to action to ensure that people enjoy peace and prosperity while addressing a range of social needs including education, health, economic, and environmental sustainability; as well as to end discrimination against women and girls. This work has allowed me to connect with the United Nations Commission on the Status of Women through Trimm Global Charities to advocate for education, health, and gender equality around the world.

You can choose to be the Phoenix rising instead of the woman who ignores the sirens. Do not ignore the signs of your body, especially if it is screaming at you. Use your voice to help transform your life and the world!

Belief:

Listen to your body. It perpetually tells you a story. The story version will be clear when you listen with your heart and mind. Communicate with it for your best life of everything and everything will be Oh! So #GOOD!

It's possible to unlock the door to your own personal health, and when you do this with as much passion and purpose as the air you breathe, you become the best version of yourself and can live out your mission most effectively.

> *"Ask, and it will be given to you; seek, and you will find; knock, and the door will be opened to you."*
>
> —Matthew 7:7 NIV

My life mission statement is one I wish for all women to feel and experience their true essence. Just as I was lying alone in my hospital bed, I unleashed the soul of my life that begins and ends with faith and hope.

> *"I create radical spaces of hope that bring GOODness, prosperity, and progress to the world."*
>
> —Dr. Tyra Good

May your lasting version of your best self in mind, body, and spirit be lasting and eternally—Oh! So #GOOD!

Actions Steps for #GOODHealth Advocacy:

- **Diversify Daily Habits:** Leaning into Lifelong Learning: Learning, Unlearning, Relearning.
- **Equity of Everyday Self-Care:** Emotional Regulation of Self: What are you saying Yes to and what are you saying No to? Knowing your boundaries: How much energy are you exerting in the different spaces that you are in? Walking away if a situation no longer serves you.
- **Inclusion of Me First in my life:** Self-Awareness and Self Advocacy: Reaffirming your identity and not losing yourself. Check-in with Me moments: Pausing, breathing, and reflecting. Using your voice to speak up.

Dr. Tyra Good
Associate Professor of Education
GOOD Knowledge Connections, LLC./ Elms College
tyragood@gmail.com

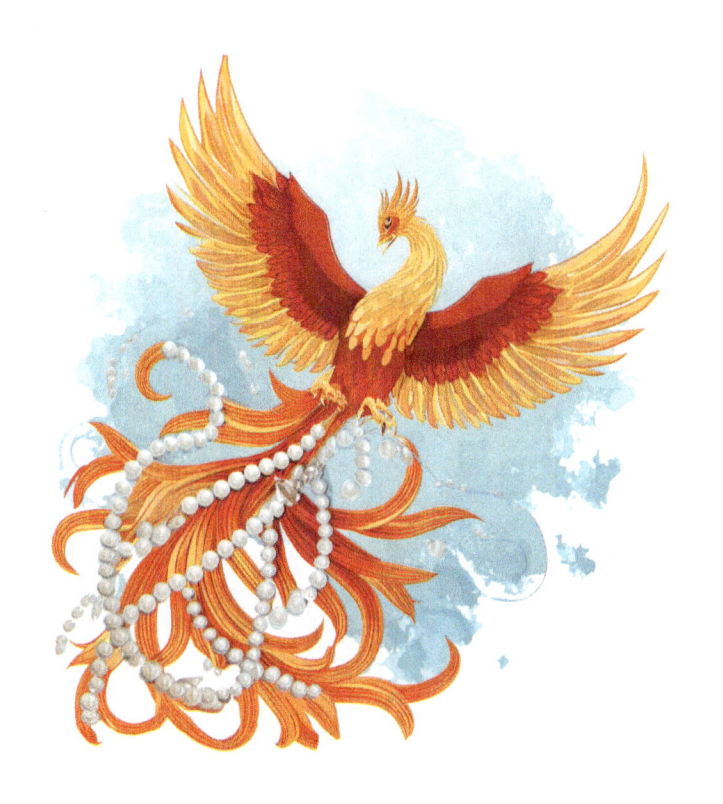

Dr. Tyra Good | 275

Dr. Golda Joseph, PhD

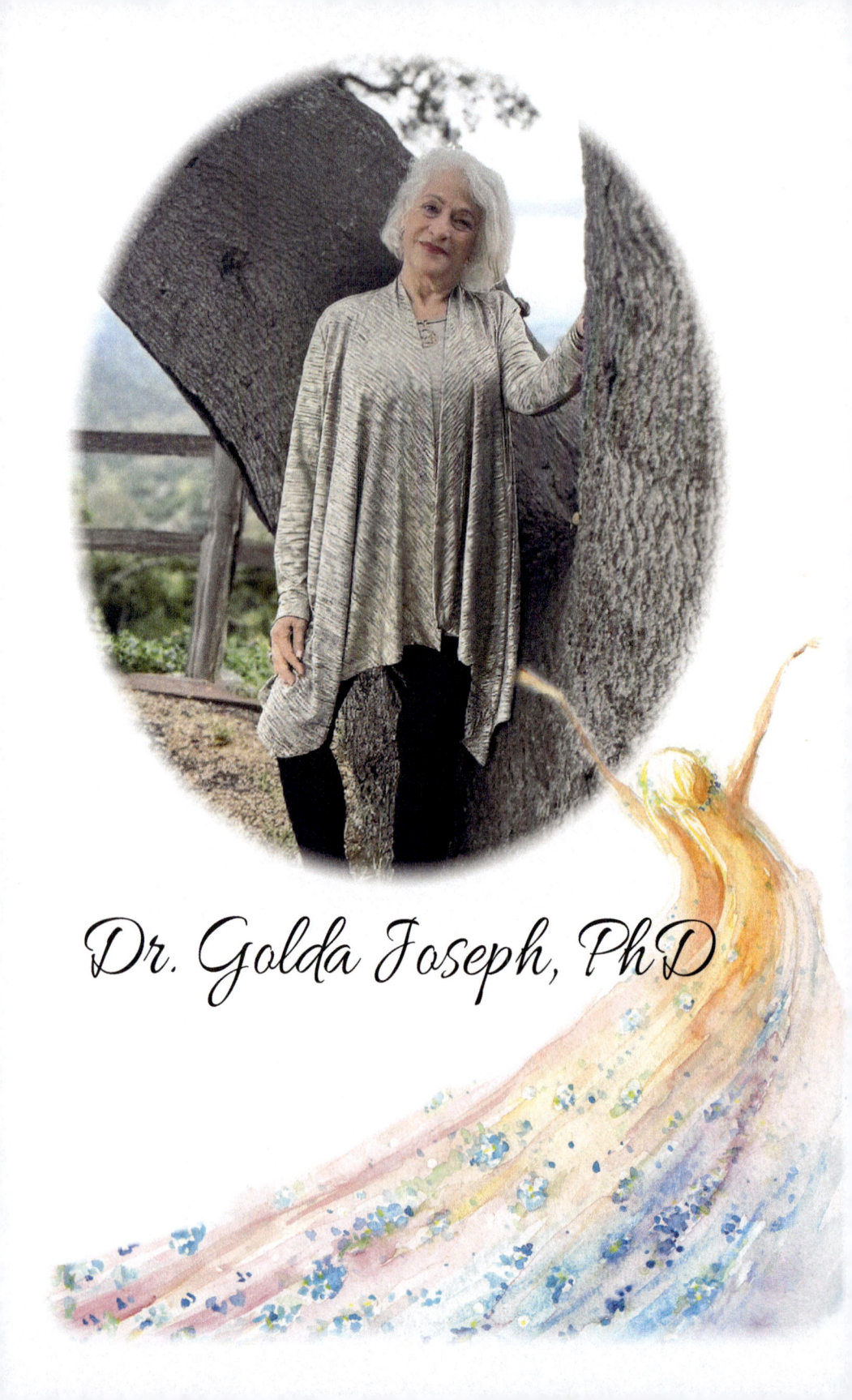

She-oric Journey Through the Circle of Time©

"Awaken your body and soul.
It's never too late to regenerate!"

Intention:

My work and "The Circle of Time"© (COT) book uses the Age Interpretation Method© (AIM) to guide your 'She-oric' Psycho-Somatic-Spiritual Journey. Now you can strengthen your body, empower your soul, and align with your true "I Am" essence. View life crises, transitions, trauma, and suffering, more objectively. May you triumph *"from womb to tomb"*!

My Story:

I was born into a Jewish family that survived the holocaust. My parents were first cousins who lost over 140 family members in World War 2. I grew up knowing this travesty. In my Jewish family, being born female was relegated to second rate. At birth, my father was angry that I was not a boy. I was a failure from the beginning. Marked psychologically as inferior solely because I was not born male.

My mother was encouraged, because of her cesarean, not to nurse or bond with me. My postnatal trauma was a very lonely beginning for me.

Today, both leading world powers and third-world countries concur that gender abuse and oppression of women and girls is a core moral issue.

In my theta state, during the first 7 years of my life, I learned to identify with my father. He led the family, often overpowering my mother's voice. I was emphatically attached to my mother's grief, loss, and trauma from WW2. My highly intuitive clairvoyant perception, even as a child, led to me being called 'the stupid one' by my family. By the 2nd grade, I was branded with moron intelligence based on a now arcane, anti-Semitic 1950's IQ test. I learned that IQ tests were written to exclude Jewish children from Ivy League Universities. However, I broke through both IQ and racial barriers in the 5th grade. I became a straight-A student. What persisted and remained, was the inferior stigma in my school records and family.

My 'She-oric Journey' began with an initial separation from feminine values. I sought recognition and success from the patriarchal culture and Jewish family values. I lost my true power, the essence of my womanhood, and the spirit of my sacred feminine. These early life experiences set the stage for my life's trajectory and professional path. I unconsciously chose to separate from my innate feminine values, and then identified as weak. Such a shame that my mother always talked about being a slave. My unconscious wish was to separate from the societally prescribed, marginalized, disempowered, female roles of womanhood in the 1950's and 1960's. I wanted to be "free" like my father, to become a truly liberated woman in "Freehood."

Entering my early adolescent phase, I desired to go to work with my father. He loved the stock market. He could educate me about his world. I wanted to identify with his successful and masculine ways. I was driven to embrace a new way of life and compelled to fight the projections against becoming an empowered woman or enter the masculine, dominant identity that also defined success for women. This internal conflict raged on for years. I remember the Rabbis wouldn't translate my Hebrew studies because I was a girl. I was rebellious against the negative and powerless qualities associated with being a Jewish young and gifted woman, yet I felt second class.

Deep within my soul, I yearned to associate with the feminine positive qualities of nurturing, intuition, empathy, creativity, and spirituality. These languages of Empathic Wisdom© and deep somatic feelings naturally perceived by women, were seen as less valuable than masculine analysis. As I entered adolescence, life gifted me my first solution. I began meditating, doing yoga, and reading spiritual Eastern and Western philosophies while practicing humanistic and transpersonal psychologies.

Emerging as an empowered teenage young woman, my family resisted my wish to go to college, and new found self-actualization. Overcoming their resistance, I made it through undergraduate college. I was the first woman in my U.S. family to get a bachelor's degree. I entered graduate school at 21 to receive a double master's degree in Marriage, Family and Child Integral Counseling, East/West Psychology, and a PhD in Philosophy of Nutrition. Breaking through these brick walls of education and achievement was exhilarating. I was driven to achieve success as a conscious creative woman.

At long last, I was in tune within myself. I chose a career in humanistic and transpersonal counseling, East/West philosophy, and holistic nutrition. I could use my intuition, expressive art therapy tools, and somatic healing to teach lifecycle wisdom throughout "The Circle of Time"© and to earn a living. I followed my spirit and true soul's purpose. However, still geared toward leadership and achieving prestige, I became an Organizational Transformation (OT) consultant to top executives and strove for financial equity as an empowered young woman.

Definitely caught up in the myth of romantic love, I thought I needed an outer masculine partner to complete my life and fulfill my parents' wishes. I maintained an inner attitude that a male partner would help me actualize my destiny. I was motivated by my mind and lived by my heart. Working on the developmental tasks necessary to be an independent adult, I separated from my parents and established a new identity as a woman in the world. I was deeply programmed and re-programmed to be dependent on a man, to disregard my need for independence, to have children, and to empower my male partner to always be successful like my mother did. Wish accomplished, I married.

During my early psychological maturity phase, I had the honor to serve Dr. Rina Sircar for four years to establish the Buddhist studies department at the California Institute of Integral Studies (CIIS). Dr. Sircar and I created her department while I completed my double master's degree in East/West Psychology and Integral Counseling at CIIS.

My multi-faceted success as a psycho-spiritual, somatic-based art therapist, regenerative nutritionist, and motherhood filled my heart and soul. My first daughter arrived while opening our first holistic health centers in San Rafael and San Francisco, California. I was now the chiropractor's wife, marketing and managing two clinics and Independent Medical Evaluation (IME) consultancies full-time. I could do it all!

On the inside of my soul, the internal conflict remained, because my husband wanted more children, yet I desired to focus on building my career as an Organizational Transformation (OT) consultant, psychosomatic art therapist, and regenerative nutritionist. My life included private clients, consulting with top management, managing two clinics, being a serial entrepreneur, and our IME consultancy in two states, while nursing our first daughter for three years. We were very successful!

Reluctant yet eventually willing, I let go of my OT top management consultancy to fulfill my husband's wish and had two more children. I became dependent on my husband when we moved to Hawaii.

For the next 35 years, I followed my husband to Hawaii and eventually to Panama. The geographical shift was his wish. I lost my independence yet gratefully devoted myself to conscious parenting and grandparenting.

On a spiritual level, I learned a great deal about surrender and service, yet in the process, I lost my childhood wish to be like my father, I regressed to being like my mother. I became her and prioritized my husband and children over my desire to build my independent career.

Leaving the executive coaching world, I found a way to empower groups of young mothers and taught "MaMa Please Understand Me"© courses while the children were in school. In addition, I established several community initiatives and spent 15 years in Waldorf teacher training, while I raised my three children at the Honolulu Waldorf school. I was fortunate to have my daily meditation and deep Spiritual Scientific study of Anthroposophy and Applied Psychosophy based on Dr. Rudolf Steiners' wisdom.

My 'Noble Quest' to actualize my masculine strength in the world was somewhat swallowed by my devotion to my husband and children. My journey for outer success and "freehood" turned inward as I healed myself. I continued to study Applied Psychosophy and relished teaching Empathic Wisdom© to small private groups and organizations.

In the name of family first, I held my family close with unconditional love and surrendered some of my personal ambitions to put their daily needs and desires first. Perhaps this was an essential life lesson and challenge to completely surrender and selflessly serve others with gratitude and reverence.

All the while, I consciously raised three children, co-founded a Waldorf High School, established a holistic health center at Unity Church, taught "Circle of Time©" biography seminars for elders, and facilitated groups of new mothers. My plate was full, sometimes overflowing.

I was constantly searching for new ways to integrate my passion to serve women and be a leader in holistic healthcare. I attracted great fortune as the CEO of our Managed Care Organization (MCO), facilitating thousands of clients alongside my husband. We doubled his capacity by bringing me into each consultation to perform client intake, lifestyle coaching, and offer private psychosomatic counseling sessions. I found a way to serve both my inner hero and outer 'Sheroic Journey.' I was very content being immersed in the present moment, balancing the needs of my family and community.

My inner masculine hero's journey actualized! I did all the marketing, management, bookkeeping, business strategy, executive consulting, and served on the Long Term Care Committee in the Hawaii Senate. We were highly respected and successful as Independent Medical Evaluators (IME) in California and Hawaii. I realized I could navigate a man's world and nurture as a woman in my home and community. The inner spiritual marriage between my masculine and feminine qualities bonded during this profound spiritual maturity phase.

Almost victorious as empty nesters, our managed healthcare company, unfortunately, kicked us out of our comfortable lifestyle and destroyed our IME practice. My husband went into despair. He wanted to drop out of life and leave the U.S.. My wish was to stay was devalued and completely discarded. My two choices became clear: remain in the marriage and leave the country with him or separate the family. Reluctantly, I chose to move with him. What followed were extreme economic, cultural, and social challenges.

Lost and alone—eventually tossed and discarded by my husband, I did not have the courage or wish to break up my marriage or family. My courageous sacrifice was to just let go and follow his lead.

We ended up building the first organic, holistic health and beauty spa in Panama City, Panama with our eldest daughter called Alta Vita Spa eighteen years ago.

Our geographical and hopeful transformation was our move from Hawaii to Panama. Hardly a transformation, I fell into an intense hormonal stress-related breakdown. My estrogen and DHEA (Dehydroepiandrosterone) levels were dangerously depleted. It was a very physical and emotionally challenging time.

My greatest challenge became finding a way to overcome my perimenopausal symptoms, debilitating anxiety, hot flashes, and brain fog. I was desperate to find a natural hormone replacement therapy that worked to regain my health and find a new balance.

Good fortune and regeneration came in the form of meeting a U.S. naturopathic medical doctor, who had a functional medicine testing laboratory and manufactured quality nutriceuticals to specifically target hormonal, stress, metabolic, and genetic imbalances. This specialty lab formulates precise, personalized nutritional protocols for menopause and numerous imbalances. This team of trusted researchers and doctors offered me their unique approach. Based on my precise biochemistry and genetic lab results they could customize transdermal creams and personalized powders to reduce my stress, balance my hormones, and reset my metabolism. This scientific 'Metabonomic Model' and protocols restored my health. I was my own first client. My results over the last 33 years have been phenomenal.

Each specific prescription our team now formulates meets the needs of each individual client I facilitate. Based on personalized biochemical and genetic lab results we can formulate hormone replacement and regenerative nutrition protocols from comprehensive home-testing kits. As a regenerative nutritionist, I can provide specific nutraceutical support programs that enable my clients to regenerate and improve the quality of all aspects of our lives. Now as a part of this holistic health movement, I can offer hormonal balancing and regeneration through "The Circle of Time"© to the whole family.

I am grateful to enter these 'Years of Grace' realigned with my true sacred feminine nature, regenerated and hormonally balanced. The Empathic Wisdom© I teach lives deep within my body, soul, and spirit.

The creative impulse of this transpersonal maturity cycle gives me the incentive to be productive far into elderhood. Over the last 20 years, I was able to regenerate my health hormonally and reverse degeneration. I envision a positive future, devoting myself to living enthusiastically, as I continue to express my creativity and help others to do the same.

Each hero and heroine returns home transformed and changed by life experiences, armed with the wisdom and insight to benefit humanity holistically.

I feel blessed to call upon a whole lifetime of being an intuitive, empowered, entrepreneur, counselor, art therapist, nutritionist, friend, mother, grandmother, teacher, and wife. I am honored to represent my multidimensional 'freehood' as a global citizen of the cosmos.

I've returned to the U.S. deeply committed to offering my specialized functional health labs and precision, personalized, nutraceutical and cosmeceutical protocols to regenerate your body-soul-spiritual health and optimal well-being. I am a living testimony that "It's never too late to regenerate!"© I still practice and teach psychosomatic expressive art therapy and regenerative nutrition to support families *'from womb to tomb.'* My sacred feminine Empathic Wisdom© coaching and courses offer *'Ancient Wisdom for Modern Times©'* throughout "The Circle of Time."©

Philosophy:

As a spiritual initiate, new possibilities for intuitive development previously unattainable awaken. I am grateful for each new day. This is my time to penetrate the secrets of life. Now I can cast off undesirable qualities, give up attachments, allow transformative influences to free old patterns, and prepare for rebirth. I know the right use of my thoughts, feelings, and will are essential to make this transition joyously.

Now I know that all heroes and 'Sheroes" can live in 'Freehood' when consciously prepared and spiritually initiated. I can live happily ever after in an evolved state of hormonal balance and inner peace while embodying Empathic Wisdom.© My "Psychology for Freehood"™ programs offer a psycho-somatic-spiritual-scientific-artistic approach for body, soul, and spirit integration *"from womb to tomb."* My powerful and impactful Regeneration Way© can guide every feminine soul's story, across cultures, through "The Circle of Time."©

I invite you to embrace both your feminine and masculine body, soul, and true 'I Am' spirit. It is important to remember you can always regenerate and transform your unique body and soul to attain higher spiritual development and 'freehood' based on *'Ancient Wisdom for Our Modern Times.'*© Now is the time to regenerate your body, soul, spirit, and our planet! Remember: *It's never too late to regenerate!*©

Your Circle of Time©—Action Steps:

- Write your own biography for each 7-year cycle.
- Share your biographical review with another woman you trust.
- Acknowledge breakthroughs from each 7-year life stage.
- Let go of past trauma and regrets.
- Celebrate the awakening of the new you.
- Step into your future Higher Self.
- Describe how you will create your new reality.

Dr. Golda Joseph, PhD
Holistic Nutritionist
Regeneration Health, Inc.
www.regeneration.com
drgolda@gmail.com

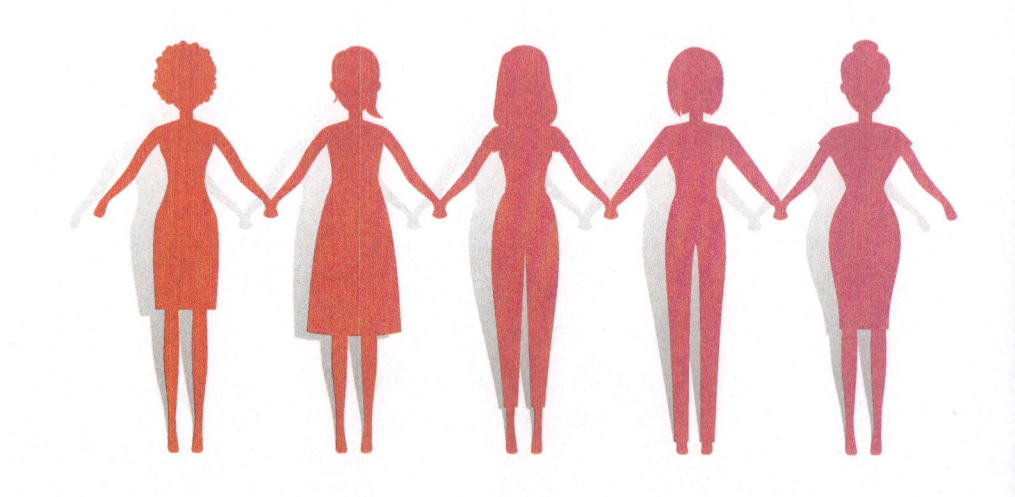

CHAPTER FIVE

Financial Pillar

"A beautiful woman is a beautiful woman, but a beautiful woman with a brain is an absolutely lethal combination."

—Prabal Gurung

"Women are the largest untapped reservoir of talent in the world."

—Hillary Clinton

"The most beautiful thing a woman can wear is confidence."

—Blake Lively

"A girl should be two things: classy and fabulous."

—Coco Chanel

"The most beautiful thing a woman can wear is her dignity."

—Unknown

"In every woman there is a Queen. Speak to the Queen and the Queen will answer."

—Norwegian Proverb

"When virtue and modesty enlighten her charms, the luster of a beautiful woman is brighter than the stars of heaven, and the influence of her power is in vain to resist."

—Akhenaton

Dr. Shirley Luu

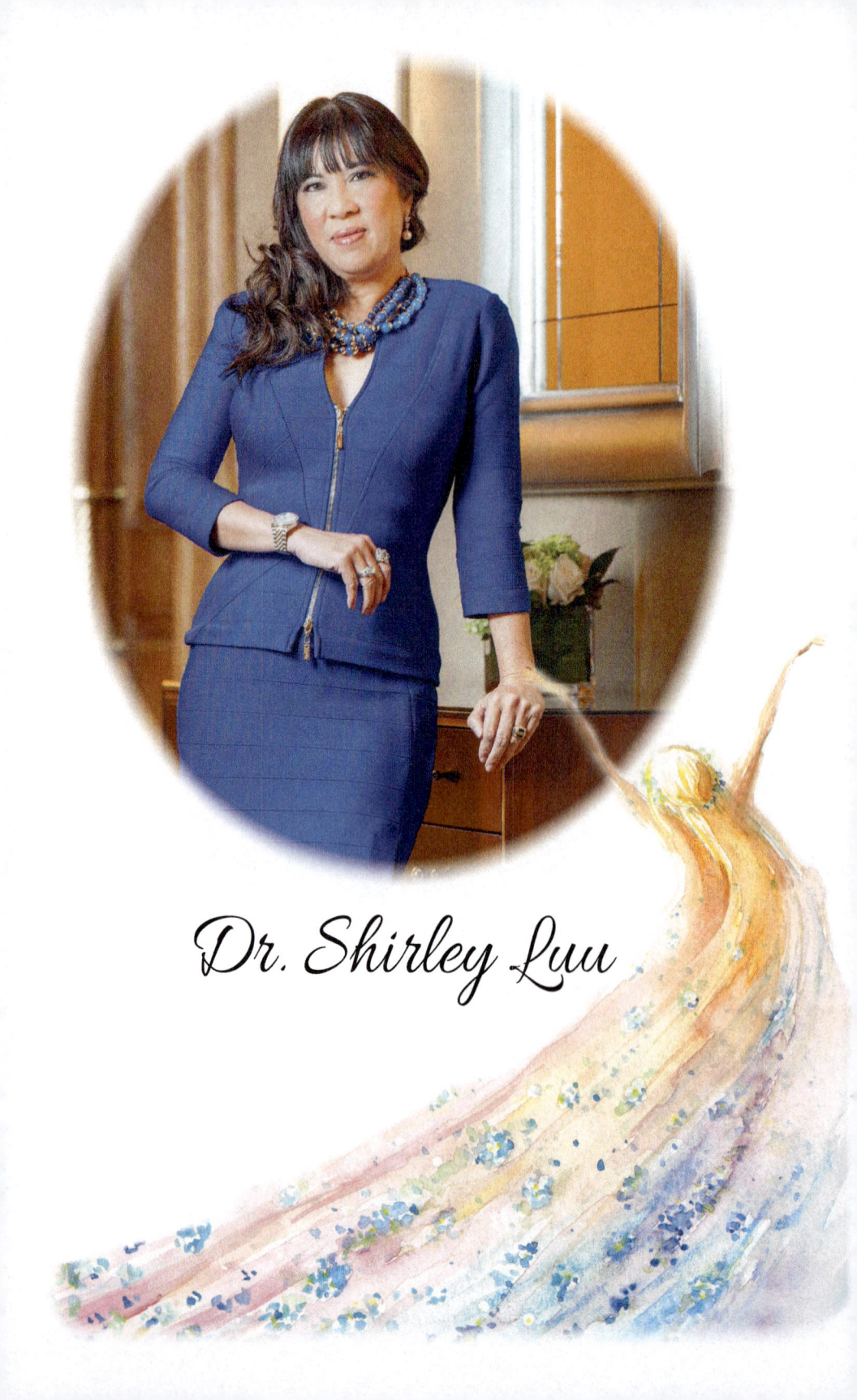

How to Win the Financial Health Game of Life

"In life and finance, live the A.S.A.P. way."

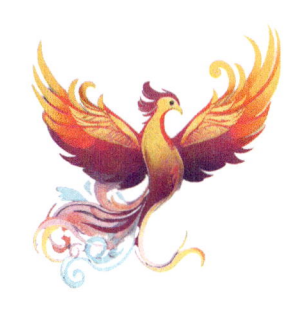

Intention:

I am noted and quoted for the following quote: "When you feel life is pushing you toward the cliffs, you either learn how to fly or die. You always win when you choose to fly." May you fly in life with all things in health and finance.

Story:

Tragedy struck in my life in the unexpected loss of my husband almost 20 years ago in my home without having life insurance to protect our family. I turned to my spirit of courage and faith. As a single mom facing homelessness, I realized my options were limited. I was working in the mortgage industry, as the economy was facing its historic decline, causing the housing industry collapse to all but lose its footing, I knew that if I had to provide for myself and my three young children, I had to embrace a new direction.

I knew one thing for certain. Life is a gamble like a roll of the dice, and challenging times do not discriminate. At any time, any one of us may face adversity due to an unexpected and devastating event. If you do not proactively plan your finances to include a healthy foundation for your retirement, and, most importantly, life insurance, the prospect for success of turning it all around is bleak, at best.

Completely feeling helpless when my daughter called me one day and asked. "Where will we go, Mom, when we can't go back into the house?" You see, my husband had just committed suicide in our own home, and at that moment, my world was shattered. I felt despair, unlike anything I had ever known, wondering how in one moment, I could have everything and, in the next, lose it all.

Instantly, in the midst of all this overwhelming grief and confusion, my *Maternal Women's Essence* kicked into overdrive, and I knew I had to find a way to keep my children safe. I told her, "Go and sit at McDonald's until we figure out where to go." And that is what she did.

It was the only place I could think of that was open and familiar, a small refuge within the tsunami we were tragically thrust into. Even though

I felt devastated and broken into a million pieces, I had to focus on what needed to be done next. My instinct was to protect my children through those traumatic moments, who were ages one, fifteen, and sixteen at the time. Desperate to find some semblance of stability, even if it was just sitting at a McDonald's.

Having been thrust into the role as the sole provider for a family of four, I faced significant financial challenges that underscored the critical need for thorough planning and protection. But I had none and was looking anywhere for a place to turn. This personal tragedy ignited a deep-seated passion to explore the possibility of life insurance and financial planning for myself. This transcended into a strong calling whereby I could safeguard others from similar uncertainties.

My decision to pursue this path was not only influenced by my own experiences but also driven by a desire to empower individuals and families with the knowledge and tools to secure their futures. I am grateful and thankful that through my personal story, I can authentically share my personal insights and practical guidance, ensuring that others can avoid the financial hardships I encountered and navigate life's uncertainties with confidence. Being able to traverse the bridge to a healthier financial model for each client I encounter has been as exhilaratingly high as the depths of where I came from with my three children. Remember that poverty does not discriminate.

While I am proud of what I have accomplished professionally, my heart truly lies in service and giving back to others. It is my purpose and passion in life to share my gifts and insights with others. I believe that by especially empowering women and our community, in general, we can help save and build the foundation for our families now and in the future—by navigating a healthy financial plan.

Today, I am an award-winning financial advisor, bestselling author, hands-on trainer, national speaker on financial literacy, and a renowned wealth guru. Accumulating over 20 years of expertise in the financial services field, and as a philanthropic influencer, I am now one of the industry's most notable authorities. I was recently selected by *Forbes 50 over*

50 as one of the most influential women in finance and a 3-time winner of the *Washington Business Journal's* Fastest Growing Companies in America today.

Having experienced the unique and seemingly impossible challenges of tragedy and unexpected loss raising three young children, I discovered my life's passion in not just finance, but financial health and security which transcends true financial freedom. My deepest desire is to prevent any other single mother—or parent—from struggling through the mire of what I went through.

Belief:

One of my favorite quotes from Althea Gibson is as follows:

"I've always wanted to be somebody. If I've made it, it's half because I was game to take a wicked amount of punishment along the way, and half because there were a lot of people who cared enough to help me."

Like Althea Gibson's famous quote, I endeavor to educate women worldwide to "know the health and sustainability of their money." Today, I conduct and train people in various educational institutions, organizations, events, and community enrichment programs.

Founder, Phil Gerlicher, from First Financial Security gave me my first opportunity and changed my professional trajectory in life. He shared that his company had a vision and wanted me to help carry it out. He was there to support me, as a mentor, but it was my personal responsibility to make it happen! The company provided the materials and believed in my ability. True mentoring and mentorship sometimes evolves collaboration, for I have, in turn, made their vision a reality.

This is where my passion was born. I love working with and helping people. I especially enjoy educating and empowering women to know their money: who has it, who keeps it, and where it comes from. I hold one of the highest executive levels with my broker, First Financial Security. Now, they run one of the top teams in the U.S. for any financial company. I am honored that I helped launch them all those many years ago. My organization includes over 6,700 agents across the country, and within it, over 80% minority and women.

With the depth of my organization and the power of First Financial Security behind me, we simply create wealth for families, with the desire to make their dreams come true: whether that means saving for retirement, protecting the family, accumulating tremendous wealth, or taking full control of your finances. My company, Shirley Luu & Associates, brings the latest technology and expertise in financial services, concepts, and products to improve the saving habits of our clients. My dream has become a reality by creating a one-stop shop with clear personal goals in mind to help our clients achieve their wildest dreams.

Retirement planning is crucial, and starting early in life is key, even if you think you don't have much money to invest. Following are three essential steps that you need to consider. **Health Coverage:** Insure yourself with adequate health insurance and savings for medical emergencies. **Retirement Needs:** Plan for your retirement by setting financial goals and estimating future expenses. Consider consulting a financial advisor. **Life insurance:** Make sure you protect your family with a life insurance policy to provide financial security and leave a legacy. The trifecta of the previous steps will help secure your future and safeguard your family's well-being. Be aware of the following common retirement planning mistakes—and how to avoid them: expecting the government to look after you, counting on an inheritance, not having an estate plan, not accounting for healthcare costs, forgetting about inflation, paying more tax than you need to, not being realistic. Embrace your future.

If you are going to be successful in life and business, you need a partner, mentors, and people who believe in you. You need someone on your team who you trust and who supports you. AND you don't need a lot of money to start—but you have to start. The sooner you do, the better you will be. Effective financial planning includes three essential components.

1. **Guaranteed Income**—Ensure you have reliable income through retirement through:

- **Social Security:** Maximize your benefits by carefully choosing when to start claiming.
- **Pensions:** If available, use traditional pension plans.
- **Annuities:** Purchase annuities for consistent retirement income.

2. **Living Benefits**—Protect yourself against health issues with:
   - **Long-Term Care Insurance:** Covers costs when you can't perform daily activities independently.
   - **Chronic and Critical Illness Coverage:** Financial support for severe or chronic illnesses.
   - **Critical Injury and Terminal Illness Benefits:** Provides funds if you suffer a debilitating injury or terminal diagnosis.

3. **Leaving a Legacy**—Build generational wealth. Ensure your family's well-being by:
   - **Life Insurance:** Offers a tax-free death benefit to your heirs.
   - **Estate Planning:** Wills, trusts, and proper beneficiary designations.
   - **Tax-Advantaged Accounts:** Use Roth IRAs.

My success led to incredible opportunities to educate a broad range of audiences, from my TV Show: *'The Real Secrets of Money',* to my feature on Sirius XM Satellite Radio, I've been blessed to have contributed articles in finance to newspapers and magazines, including *Forbes, Oprah, New York Weekly, World Reporter,* and *Entrepreneur.* I am the proud author of *I.U.L. ASAP,* an Amazon Bestseller in seven financial categories, and the new Financial Anchor host for Fox5 PLUS. Another Financial Strategy Book will be launched in the summer of 2024: *'FIA: ASAP'* to guide you to financial health.

Service in philanthropy has always held a special place in my heart. I am passionate about my community outreach work. My chief focus within that mission is the LiSA Initiative: a grassroots movement founded by Debbie Gerlicher of First Financial Security. The LiSA Initiative informs, educates, and empowers women and their families about financial security.

This project is near and dear to my heart as I know firsthand, as a woman, it is not a matter of IF one will be solely responsible for their finances, but ***when***. Through the LiSA Initiative, women gain confidence to take stock of what they currently have or do not have financially and take control of leading their path to financial health.

I am also grateful for the opportunity to partner with Shelter House, Inc. and Women of GoodWorks. I provide financial support and housing supplies for women and children as they transition into the gift of a home to start new lives. I thrive when helping others. I am excited about the work that Shirley Luu & Associates does in partnership with many nonprofits to make a difference when it comes to philanthropic responsibility.

Empowered women living in their truest essence must continually play an active role in their finances—now and in the future. My advocacy is rooted in the belief that women can support and uplift other women to champion in the workplace and in life. Financial literacy then, is truly the 'unleashing' of their financial feminine soul.

Inspiring changes to advance women in business is part of my daily routine operations. Whether I attend a women's event or job fair to hire women on my team, advancing women in business is what I live for in my professional mission. Even everyday women, like I was, deserve to have opportunities to shine their gifts bright in this world.

Take my tactical and practical advice to heart—for it was exponentially shaped by my own experiences. Don't let another day slip by without planning for your financial future. Tomorrow is unpredictable, but through proactive planning, we can be prepared for whatever lies ahead. And if we do choose, the future is very bright and *we all fly*.

Action Steps for Financial Health:
- Know your money:
  - **Budget** for savings.
  - **Gather your important documents** and keep them in a safe place.

- **Leverage** IUL's ASAP and FIA's ASAP.
- Utilize these retirement planning steps:
  - **Set Goals**—Define retirement vision and financial targets.
  - **Assess Finances**—Calculate net worth and analyze income/expenses.
  - **Create a Budget**—Estimate future costs and adjust for inflation.
  - **Maximize Contributions**—Contribute max to 401(k)/IRA, use catch-up contributions if over 50.
  - **Have a Retirement Plan with Tax-Free Strategies**—Consider Life Insurance as a vehicle that can provide tax-free retirement when it is structured properly along with Living Benefits and create generational wealth.
  - **Estate Planning**—Update will, set up trusts, ensure beneficiaries are current, and designate power of attorney.
  - **Review Regularly**—Annual plan review, rebalance investments, adjust for life changes.
- Plan for retirement, remember and consider these key points:
  - Start Early and Save Consistently.
  - Understand Your Retirement Needs.
  - Diversify Investments.
  - Maximize Retirement Accounts.
  - Automate Savings.
  - Track Progress with Financial Tools.
  - Understand Social Security.
  - Plan for Healthcare Costs.
  - Create an Emergency Fund.

- Consider Inflation.
- Minimize Debt.
- Seek Professional Advice.
- Stay Informed on Tax Laws and Investments.

Dr. Shirley Luu
Financial Planner and Insurance Broker
Shirley Luu & Associates (SLA): Financial Services and Insurance
www.shirleyluuassociates.com
luushirley@gmail.com

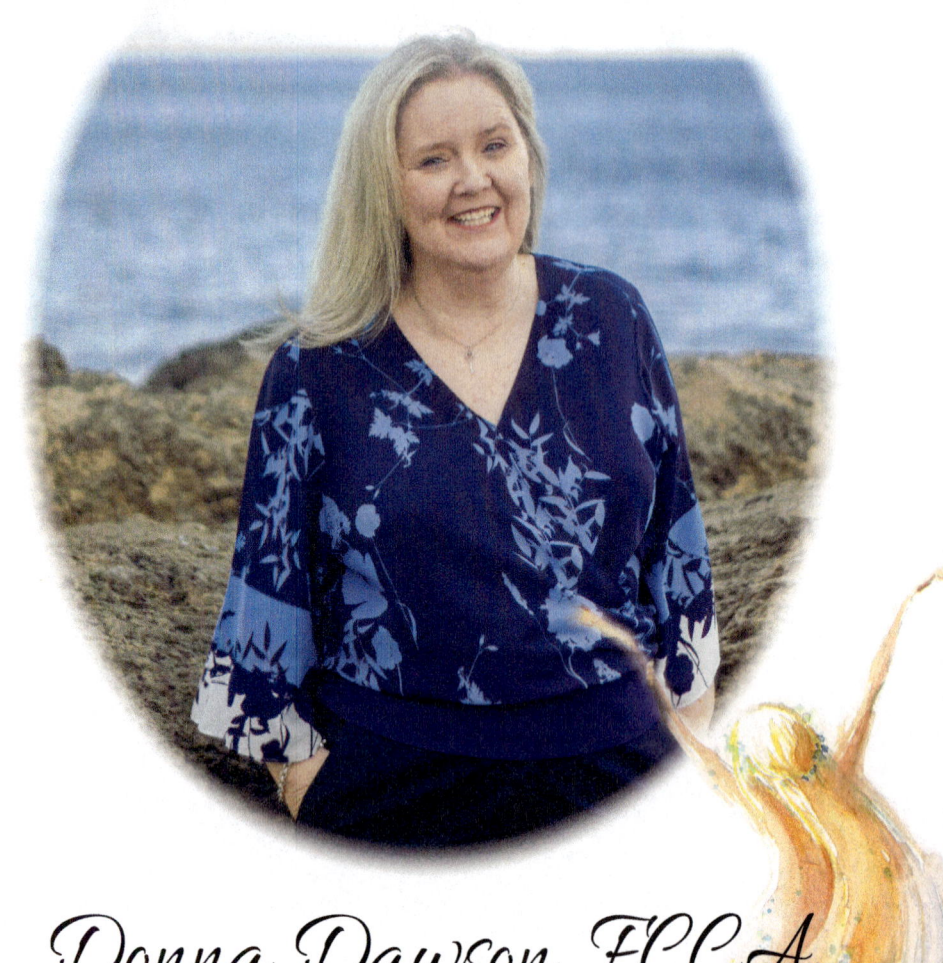

Donna Dawson, FCCA

Proverbs for the Soul: My Legacy

*"What's the worst-case scenario?
If you can live with that, you have already won!"*

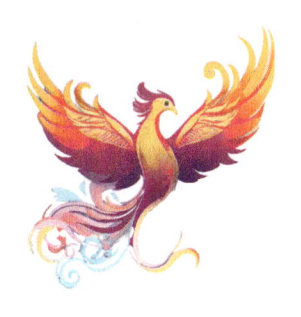

Intention:

The essence of a woman has been passed down through the generations through the incredibly strong Scottish women who walked their path before me. Their strength and courage to live fearlessly are etched into the rebirth of the next generation through their soul connection and the life lessons that they passed down through the proverbs of the ages.

I call these proverbs for the soul. I am not talking about the proverbs found in the Bible, which do have power, but the old wives' sayings that still resonate and are as pertinent today as they were generations ago. May these proverbs penetrate your soul as well.

Story:

I was born and raised in Scotland, a cross-section with a rich heritage of historical figures that bestowed significant breakthroughs to the world—the steam engine, penicillin, insulin, the telephone, and television. The greats that we know about were all men but dig a little deeper, and you will find very strong women who stood in their own greatness and had the courage to stand firm for their beliefs, self-educate themselves, and pave the way for generations of strong women who followed.

I was surrounded by these typically Scottish solid women who were the backbone of the family. My grandfather was a fisherman who braved the unforgiving North Sea to provide for his large family and due to his work, was absent for long periods of time. However, I never felt a void because it was my grandmother who was the golden thread that wove the family together. As a young child, I was not surrounded by material possessions as money was scarce, but love, laughter, and a powerful sense of family and community were abundant. Her wise words that made a lasting impression on me always came from these quick-witted, feisty women who could take the perceived pain of any life situation and turn it thoughtfully on its head.

Excelling in school initially was difficult for me, as I moved around to many different schools, and found it challenging to keep up with the variety of teaching styles. Equally challenging was the stability to socially fit in and build and sustain strong peer relationships with my fellow classmates. My one constant ebb and flow was always my grandmother who used to tell me "Whit's fur ye'll no go by ye!", now my life quote, which I did not appreciate until much later in life. During secondary school, I had a crushing dose of reality in a conversation with a career counselor. I knew deep down in my soul I wanted to be in finance, but economic circumstances did not afford me the opportunity to go to University. Instead, I commenced the trudging work from the bottom of the financial labor ladder and studied tirelessly during my off-time. When I saw a door slither open to the next step up, I grabbed that door handle and hung on, to progress—which moved slowly, relentlessly, but surely in the right direction.

Another of Grandmother's pearls of wisdom was "If you don't ask, you don't get!" I remember early in my career being brave enough to ask my then boss if I could be on the same pay and conditions as other team members because I was performing the same role. I was abruptly admonished that I was not the same level because I did not possess that magic piece of educational paper. Again, I asked for a pay raise, to which he replied I would always be stuck at this level. I heard the proverb resounding in my soul again: "If you can live with that, you have already won." I decided not to settle, and I felt that win when I departed the autocratic environment seeking opportunities where they appeared. I studied and eventually became a qualified accountant. Years later, I had elevated to a corporate position for a major global company, when my old boss came up to me. He was still with the company that provided the accounting support to my company. He looked down his nose at me and said: "So you have returned to the fold?" To which I replied, "No I work for the company!"

That fateful and victorious day, I heard my grandmother's voice resounding in my heart and mind as she kept telling me to leave the small town behind, go out into the world, and have a full, blessed, and abundant life. She was my everything and we had the strongest bond. I was with her when she was diagnosed with stage 4 lung cancer and her words still ring into my soul that day and continue through today. She looked directly into the consultant's eyes with dismay and said: "But I am a good person. I can't have cancer."

Our family proverbs of the soul collectively made a promise as a family, whereby she would not enter hospice. I too took my turn staying over to nurse and care for her as she had cared for me throughout my early childhood. Witnessing and loving her even to her last breath, was the most beautiful and the most heart-wrenching life moment I have ever experienced! Calm and peace washed over me that day of her transitioning, knowing that all the wisdom from her soul would continue through me and always live.

I wrote a poem for her that I read at her funeral. That day is still a blur to me, but speaks to a woman's life of legacy:

Goodbye

Goodbye is not a word I ever thought I'd say,
I thought that you'd be with me forever and a day.

But as the days go by, each day you grow weaker,
I pray each day don't take her yet, she's not ready to meet her maker.

Her blue eyes still sparkle, her smile still shines,
Still sharp as a pin that Grandma of mine!

I must be brave and shed no tears, for you have been so strong,
You were the one throughout my life that taught me right from wrong.

Just know that I love you, I'm fighting for you too,
But if it is your time to go, I understand that too.

We've made a promise that when you go, your presence will always be around,
For your soul will shine so bright, as you are heaven-bound.

So goodbye Grandma, I love you, more than you'll ever know,
As time heals, I'll understand just why you had to go.

To this day, I still hear her voice reverberate when I am at a crossroads in my life. She assists me even then to bring me back to listen to my soul.

Even though we had deep conversations about 'making something of yourself' and not settling, I stayed stuck in my grief for a few years. It wasn't until the birth of my first baby girl that those words resonated within my soul. I gazed into my daughter's eyes, illuminated with the pure essence of the female soul—now passed down through the generations. What a formidable force we are when we connect with the divine feminine essence.

"Going out into the world' manifested itself when my hubby and I took an around-the-world trip that included Australia. There was something that drew me to the world *'down under'* and we decided to immigrate with our young daughter and start a new life: just the three of us. Our family of three grew to four—but one of the challenges has been the void of the extended family support that I grew up with in Scotland. My husband and I dig deep into our generational Scottish heritage, make it work, and fill life with great memories. We both know that this move was propelled to build on the legacy and to give our daughters enhanced opportunities and choices. My girls are my everything! I am determined to ensure their essence in confidence, independence, and individuality: individual—strong and capable women who can be, do, and have all that they desire in life—just by applying the proverbs of the soul.

Throughout my life and career, I have made a conscious choice not to be a "show pony." There is a stoic strength in staying away from the spotlight and preferring to be the quiet achiever. The proverbs have built my personal fortress to be strong enough in my own skin to not be intimidated by the opinions of others. My preference is to be the cheerleader at the back of the room, allowing others to shine and step into their brilliance. I stand strong within this inner knowing of who I am as I shine in my own *essence* to shine and radiate no matter what! A brilliant piece of wisdom that has resonated with me throughout the years is to *'walk away'* from any situation that goes against my soul. I encourage you to do the same: live in your soul. Do not live in the opinions of others.

I am writing the 'Proverbs of the Soul' series to pass down the legacy not only for my daughters but for all the daughters around the world. These global women can choose to be, do, and have all that they desire if they apply the powerful messages of wisdom that have been passed down from the generations from the strong Celtic women who came before me. The time is now to unleash their feminine souls into the true essence of their womanhood.

Belief:

The proverbs have stood me in good stead in their wisdom and strength within the mire and wonderment of my life. The following are a few 'rock solid' examples:

"Better to ask the way than go astray"—This is *not* about asking directions, so you don't get lost—although a woman I would instead ask, then wait for a man to admit they need to ask for directions. Rather ask the question and see if the answer resonates with your soul. The answer's essence lies within the quality of the question we pose. If our question is poorly worded, how can we expect to navigate through life with meaning and grace? For example, if you are in what seems to be a heated debate with someone, and you ask them "Why are you so angry?"...this will only provoke a very emotional response which can escalate quicker than you can blink an eye. Try a reframe along the lines of "I can see this is upsetting for you. How can we work through this together?" A reframe can save relationships along with your sanity!

"Whit's fur ye'll no go by ye!" (What's meant to happen will happen.) When that one thing that you were chasing doesn't come to fruition, it was not meant to be yours. Sit with that disappointment for as long as you need, but while you are there, ponder and glean what lesson you need to learn. The lesson is there. If you dig deep and apply the lesson, next time you will win. Without this analysis, the lesson's voice will get louder and louder until the Universe forces you to listen to your own soul.

"Seeing is believing"—If you visualize the ultimate outcome, that is where the magic starts. That vision will be the driving force to get the results, but only if the action steps are applied to make the vision a reality. Only visualizing and wishing for something without engaging with the universe through your actions—will lend you a long wait! Gear into action, even if steps and course corrections change along the way. What you learn through those lessons will guide you toward that end goal that you visualized at the beginning.

"The eyes are the window of the soul"—One of the greatest gifts given to me as a child was being told if someone can't look you in the eye, they don't belong in your inner circle. If you really look into the energy and frequency of someone, look deep into their eyes—to read their true essence. Women are intuitively wired to pick up on the energy emanating from the soul—a true gift that has been passed down through the generations.

"Real friendship doesn't freeze in winter"—My grandmother used to tell me that true friendship will see you through your winter. Every woman has been left disappointed throughout my life by so-called friends who vanished into thin air as soon as they experienced a bit of a temporary 'situation.' Most of us are blessed when we can count our true friends on one hand. Those are the ones that you cherish for life and support you through all of life's seasons. Celebrate your friends and reciprocate 'in kind' when they encounter their version of winter.

"It will all come right in the wash"—This proverb reveals multiple meanings. Repeatedly resonated as I was growing up, and one of my favorites I've shared with my family as well. I will always be found out—maybe not today, but eventually the lie and the liar will be exposed. If life has taken an uncertain and stressful turn, or more importantly you feel like you have hit the wall, breathe and remember everything has a way of working out. The outcome may not be as you imagined, so next time you feel that stress enveloping you, visualize cleansing the issue first and hand it off to the Universe.

"Because is a woman's reason"—Certainly the Universal Woman response whether with a child, sibling, or significant other. We enter a discussion that goes round and round in circles and then utter the magic words "because I said so." The resultant sound is silence. Only a woman's conviction can carry this off. Not bombastic nor clever, but always achieving the desired results.

"Home is where the heart is"—I internalized the literal meaning while growing up. Moving often as a child could've been unsettling, but a constant and stable home was my grandmother's home. Realizing later as a young woman that her stability wasn't the brick and mortar of her home, but the beating pulse of her heart and unconditional love. When a woman is one with her own soul, she is truly living her essence and is truly home.

Take time to nurture yourself and your soul today and every day. Be grateful for all that is in the present, and all that was in your past as you step into the future. Know that you have a strong foundation if you follow the path of your soul. My life has been an evolving revelation of what has been *'fur me'*, and proverbs can resound in your heart for your legacy and the essence of your womanhood.

Action Steps to Soothe Your Soul:
- **Focus on Family**—family is also the extension of friendships. Build that wall so high that nothing else matters—Your cup will be full.
- **Deal with Disappointment**—A reminder it's time to course correct—the real reason, and the next step will follow.
- **Health above Wealth**—Healthy boundaries foster physical health and will keep you on track to build lasting wealth.
- **Mentorship provides Growth**—Whether a physical or virtual mentor, maximum growth evolved through adversity. Push completely through with another and watch the magic happen.

- **Embrace Challenges**—The Universe will never give you challenges that you can't handle—Its way of affirming you to push through and win.

Donna Dawson, FCCA
Certified Accountant
www.proverbsforthesoul.com
donna@proverbsforthesoul.com

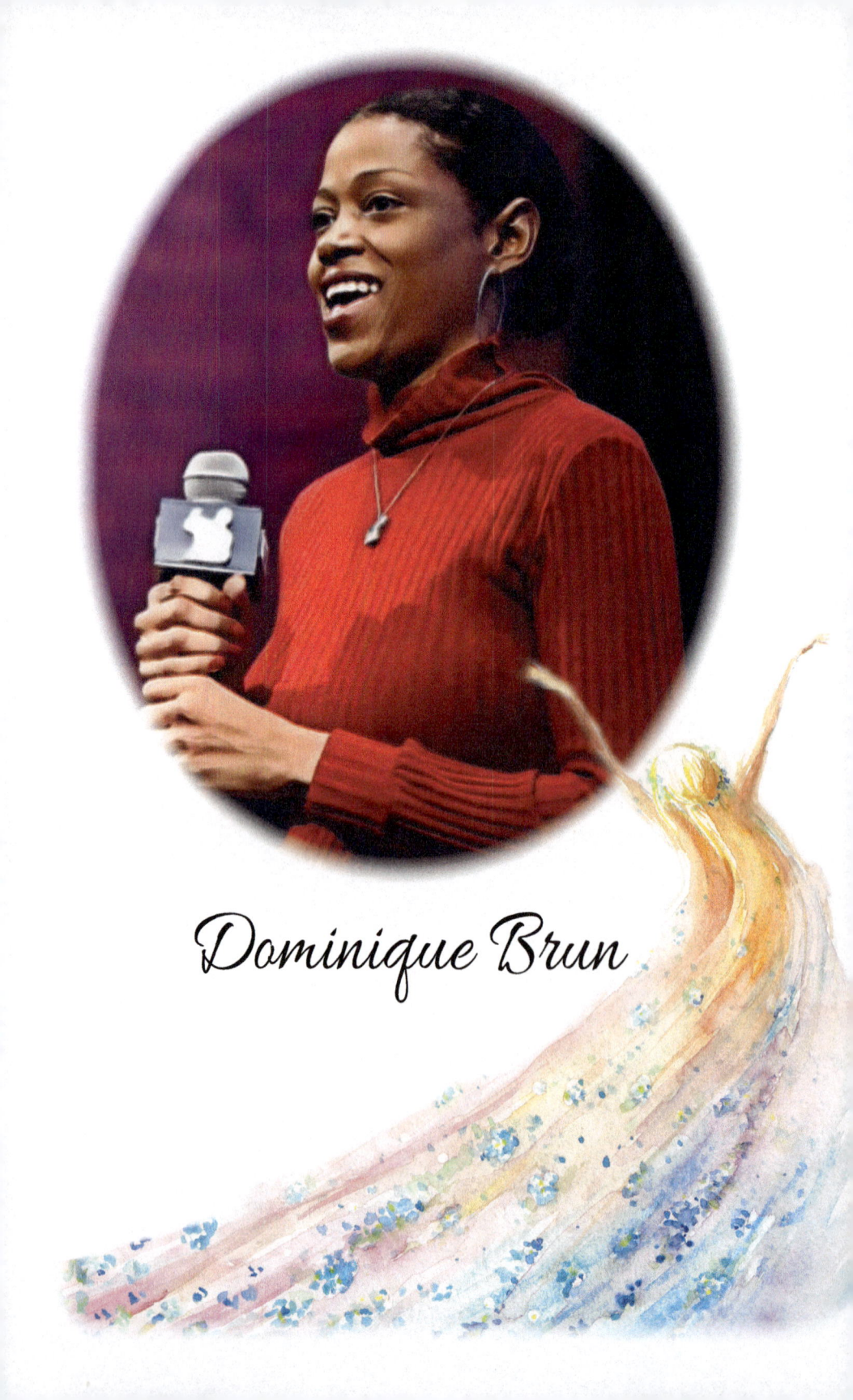

Dominique Brun

The Turning Point: Embracing the Domino Effect

"Stand tall—Create a 'domino' ripple effect of resilience. Turn your obstacles into opportunities."

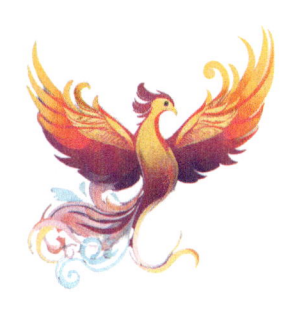

Intention:

"I'm not just surviving; I'm thriving. The dominoes in your game of life can either fall down or go up. Make sure yours go up." Staying in your divine feminine creates stability, power, and resilience. May you find your domino sequence fall into play while standing strong in your life's purpose.

Story:

Life has a funny way of throwing curveballs at you, and I've seen my fair share. My name is Dominique, and I'm here to share my journey from the depths of despair to the heights of empowerment.

Grab a seat, get comfy, and let's dive into the story of a black female founder who turned her life around with grit, humor, and a whole lot of *'Domino Effect'* determination.

Growing up, I had a childhood many would envy. I was blessed with a loving mom and dad, a great stepfather, and the opportunity to travel the world. From Germany to Hawaii, and eventually to locating my permanent home in Sacramento, California, I experienced different cultures and saw the beauty of diversity. My childhood was filled with fun and adventure, but life took a dramatic turn when I first met 'him.'

He seemed charming at first, but that charm quickly turned into a nightmare. I found myself trapped in a toxic and dangerous relationship, becoming a statistic where one in three women experience domestic violence. It was a domino that didn't have to fall, but it did. I felt isolated and alone, a stark contrast to the vibrant and supportive upbringing I had known. It was naivete and a lack of awareness of the neon red flags that landed me in my situation.

One night, he threatened to kill my dog because I was trying to leave him. My parents were out of town, and I was held hostage in my own home! I waited until he fell asleep and called my parents, who, thankfully, drove down from Los Angeles to rescue me. That was the last time I was ever with him, but the torment was just beginning. He stalked us, and the fear and isolation I felt were emotionally and mentally crippling. I turned to alcohol as a coping mechanism, making poor decisions that led to a few DUIs (Driving Under the Influence). It was a dark, hopeless time, and I was at war personally, professionally, and with the legal family court system, which seemed indifferent to my plight.

Finally, the district attorney in Sacramento picked up my case, deeming it serious enough to place a permanent criminal protective order against him. With this layer of support, I entered therapy, faced my trauma head-on, and started to reclaim my life. It was a long road with many detours, but I began to find myself again as a loving mother and a determined soul. Like Shakespeare's Macbeth, this was my dark night. But it was also the beginning of my total transformation.

As I rebuilt my life, I realized the power of the domino effect: one piece upon another. Negative actions and experiences had set off a chain reaction, but so could positive ones. I chose the latter for my life. I embraced entrepreneurship with renewed vigor, driven by a desire to create impact and help others. I wanted to empower women, to show them that they could rebuild their dominoes and rise above their circumstances, just as I was beginning to.

My <u>DominoFX Group</u> was born out of necessity and my unbridled passion to be and do more for myself and, consequently, other women. Small business, finance, and entrepreneurship changed my life, giving me confidence and power. I faced this daunting challenge *head-on*! I found my purpose in helping others navigate the often intimidating world of finance, especially the need and skill to access a variety of necessary capital. As I broke these personal barriers, I desired to create the next generation that would access new avenues of finance—a haven and space where women could feel supported and empowered.

If this is resonating with you and you are feeling like you're in a similar abyss, know that you're not alone.

Belief:

The domino effect guides everything I do personally and professionally. It's about recognizing the interconnectedness of our actions and understanding that we can rebuild no matter how many times we fall. The Ancient Chinese Proverb says:

> *"Fall down five, get up Six."*

There are naysayers and negative people out there who want to keep you stuck. Identifying them and removing them from your life is crucial. Rebuild with a supportive inner circle and watch your life and dominoes rise.

Today, I'm surrounded by world changers, people who inspire me to keep pushing boundaries to unleash my feminine soul. My journey from despair to peace and gratitude is proof that you can transform your life. These are no longer tears of terror but tears of joy and gratitude, the cleansing of a transcendental and healthy soul.

In the words of Maya Angelou:

> *"Nothing can dim the light which shines from within."*
>
> —Maya Angelou

Now, time to talk real and raw about finance, honey. Because the truth is, finance isn't just about numbers; it's about freedom, security, and empowerment—your true essence of a woman. When I first dipped my toes into the world of finance, I felt like a fish out of water, unable to swim, but I just kept dog paddling. There were so many terms, rules, and strategies that seemed like they were designed to confuse the hell out of you. But here's the thing: once you break it down, it's not rocket science. It's all about understanding how to make your money work for you and, most importantly, using your voice to *'ask for help!'*

I began with a simple question for financial health: How can I make my money work for me instead of the other way around? I read books, attended seminars, and surrounded myself with people who knew more than I did. The learning curve was as steep as Mt. Everest, but the rewards were and still are worth it.

Finance became my passion because I saw it as a tool to help people like me—women who felt stuck, overwhelmed, and powerless. I saw it working for my mentors, my clients, and my role models. I wanted to demystify it, make it accessible, and, dare I say, accelerate the domino build so that it could even be fun. I mean, who said talking about money had to be boring?

One of the first things I learned was the importance of budgeting. I know it sounds basic, but trust me, it's the foundation of financial health. Budgeting isn't just about restricting yourself; it's about understanding where your money goes and making it work for you. Think of it as giving every dollar a job. That dollar is employed by you, the owner. Once you know where your money is going, you can start making informed decisions about where you want it to go. In business, this is doing all the 'unsexy' work—gathering financial documents, putting your P&Ls together, and getting with your accountant. However, working the numbers to make sure you're going to profit is very sexy. When I first started my business, I knew nothing of the importance of this first step. Now, this is where everyone starts.

I also embraced the theory of the importance of credit. In this uncertain financial climate, there's often a lot of mistrust around credit, and for good reason. But when used wisely, credit can be a bridge, a powerful tool, and a successful means to an end. Especially business credit. Did you know that the biggest companies in the world utilize business credit to maximize profits and cash flow? I'm talking about Google, Facebook, Walmart, and Target, right down to HD Supply and Lowes. Once I discovered this concept, I was able to help multiple businesses and entrepreneurs change their lives. I have focused on women who were heading back out into the workforce after staying home with their families and living on their husband's credit. Others were ready to be poised to start businesses and needed assistance with where and how to embark on their business foundation responsibly and successfully. It's not about getting into debt; it's about leveraging your credit to create opportunities! Whether it's buying a home, starting a business, or investing in critical-mission-driven education and mentorship, good credit can open doors that would otherwise be closed.

Next up in the financial arsenal—investing—a true personal game-changer. The idea that my money could make money while I slept was revolutionary. My present goal unfolds within philanthropy through leverage: to invest in small businesses, create opportunities through communities, and drive equity back into those neighborhoods. As my confidence grew, so did my network and my capacity to one day go out there and purchase a business—my next goal within the year. Through education, finance, and mentorship, I unearthed the value of patience and the power of compound interest. Like planting a tree, you put the seed in the ground, water it, and watch it grow, knowing that one day, it will bear fruit.

The ultimate fruit-bearing tree for me is that business unfolds with entrepreneurship. Starting my own business was both the scariest and most rewarding undertaking in my life. It was a leap of faith, a test of my resilience and determination. Similar to the legal advocate I attracted into my personal life, entrepreneurship has been a professional confidence-building process. Being a business owner avails me the opportunity to create something meaningful, give back, and make a difference in the world. Not solely about making money; I am allowed to solve complex problems, create value, and as Les Brown says:

"Build a legacy that will outlive you."

Similar to Motherhood, entrepreneurship was like raising my daughters. It requires daily nurturing, patience, focused intention, and plain work. There were sleepless nights, moments of doubt, and times when I wanted to give up. However, the moments of triumph, joy, and immense pride made it *all* worth it! Every milestone, every success, was a testament to my tenacity, resilience, vision, and determination.

Networking in business is truly the art of focus, communication, and connection. *Who* you know can be just as important as *what* you know. Building a network of supportive, like-minded individuals continues to be crucial for success. This collective were professionals who believed in me, supported me, and helped me blossom and grow. I believe I was their tree! They remain my best cheerleaders, mentors, and partners.

Financial health begins, however, with daily self-care. As women, we're often taught to put others first, to sacrifice our own needs for the sake of others. A valid constant: 'You can't pour from an empty cup.' Taking care of yourself isn't selfish; it's necessary. Whether it's taking time to relax, pursuing a hobby, or simply taking a moment for breath work, daily self-care is essential to your well-being and overflows to personal success.

I've evolved to embrace my strengths and examine my weaknesses, finding humor in my mistakes and celebrating my victories. Just like the call and cry for help to my parents that fateful night, it's okay to ask for help and lean on others when you need it. Most importantly, I've embraced the concept that I am enough. Just as I am, with all my flaws and imperfections, I am a whole human being—a woman of essence. I am enough.

The great news is that *you* are enough, too! If I can rise up and do it, you can do it too! Be the first domino that topples the chain in a positive direction. Create impact, seek help, and never, ever settle. The possibilities are endless, and that first empowerment step starts now.

Break down the barriers, shatter the stereotypes, and we will all rise together. We are creating a world where every woman, no matter her background or circumstances, can thrive, thereby benefiting communities and empowering the world.

As you embark at the starting gate for your financial health and success, you are powerful, you are resilient, and you are capable of achieving greatness. The road may be long, with life's twists and turns, but every step you take brings you closer to your dreams. Keep moving forward, keep pushing boundaries, and always focus on your unique worth. Your ultimate financial health and abundance await.

Action Steps for Financial Health:

- **Acknowledge Your Situation:** Admit that you're struggling: the first step towards healing.
- **Seek Help:** Regardless of the word "no," persist until someone listens.

- **Don't Settle:** If something feels off, trust your gut and intuition. You deserve the best.

- **Believe in Abundance:** Something better is on the horizon. Stay consistent with your purpose.

- **Embrace the Light:** After darkness, there's a dawn. Keep pushing forward to 'fresh air' and clarity—vision to fruition.

Dominique Brun
CEO, Founder, Coach
DominoFX Group
www.dominofxgroup.com
dominique@dominofxgroup.com
linktr.ee/dominofxgroup.com

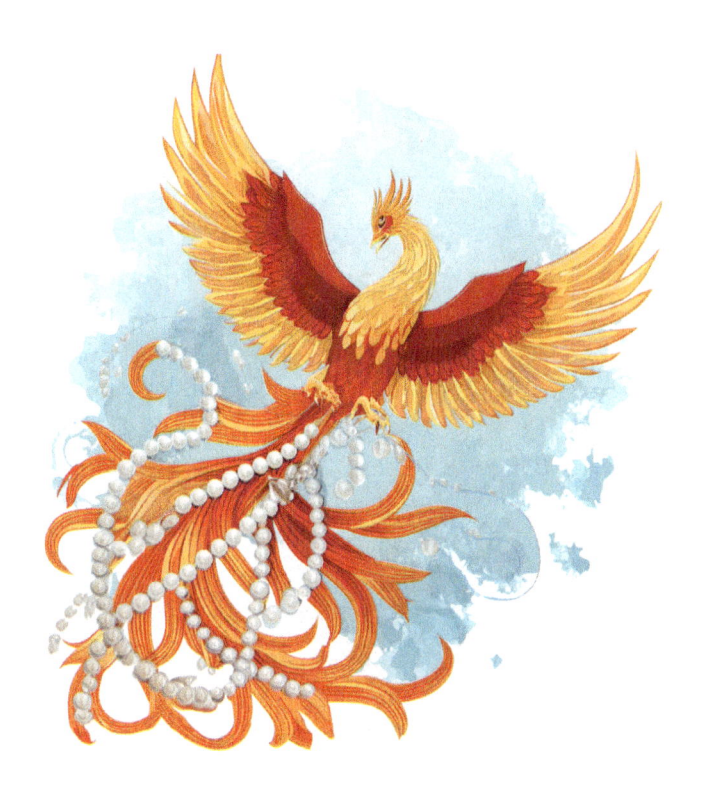

Dominique Brun | 317

Laura Ibarra, AbD

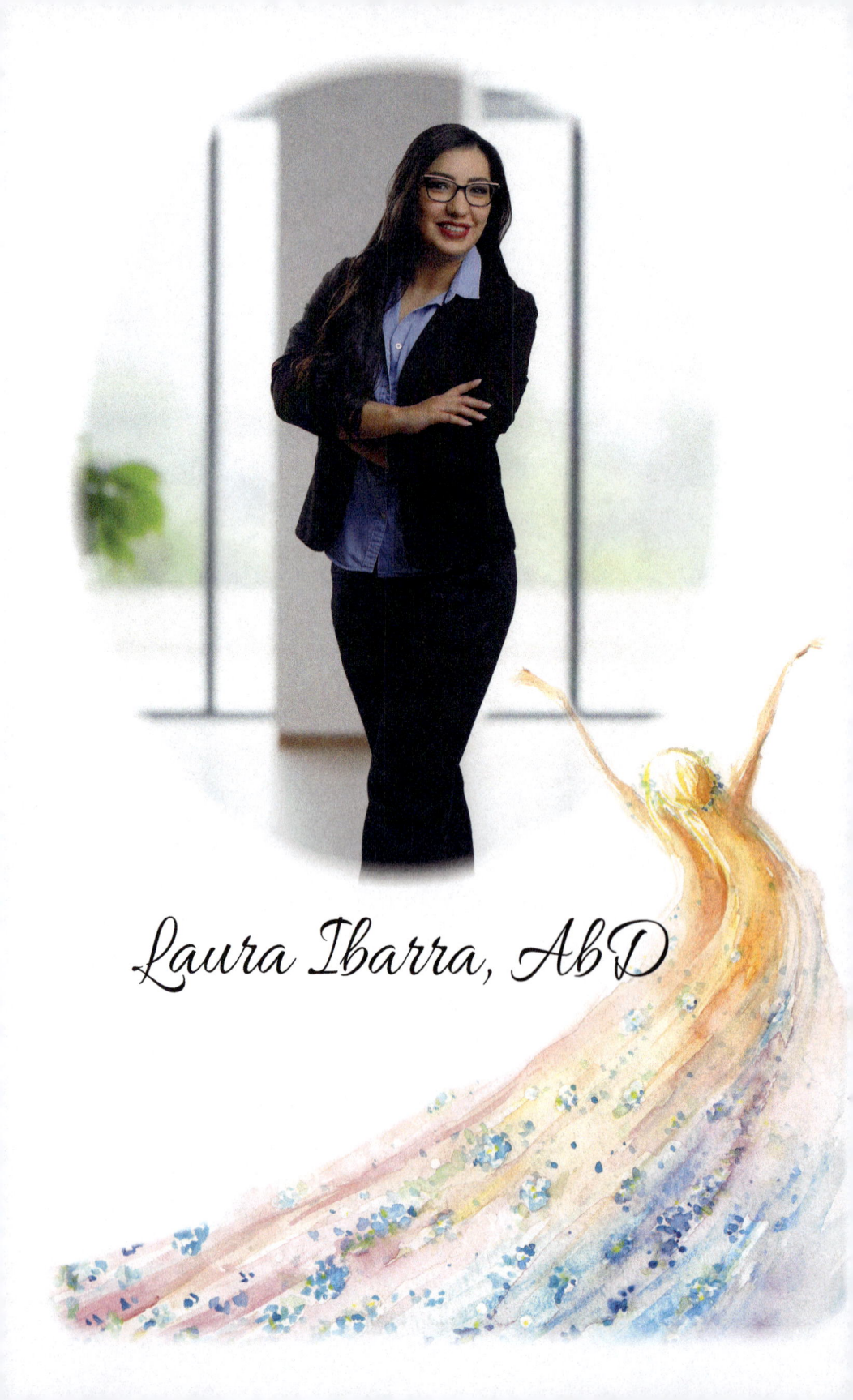

Healthy Mindset: Game, Set, and Match!

"The essence of winning lies in giving yourself permission to play with your mindset."

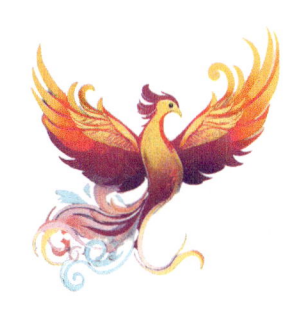

Intention:

Explore with me the transformative power of overcoming fear and cultivating a positive mindset to win in life. May all women be inspired to embrace challenges, seek mentorship, and unlock their full potential.

Story:

Fear is more than an interesting feeling. It's debilitating. Rather than suppressing it, I have always had the tendency and been aware to check in with my body: Is my belly aching? Is my blood pressure rising? Is my vision becoming more focused and clear? All of these changes are so important: they are detectable, we can feel them, and we can sense them. I love how these feelings allow me to recognize my next move.

Am I safe? Should I hide or run? Should I confront this situation? Do I feel strong enough? All of these questions happen in the amazing human mind—within a fraction of a second. Our mind is such a powerful, beautiful guidance system, and we are blessed to have it throughout our lives.

I believe some of us cannot recall when we realized we had this system activated. Do you remember when you finally said, "Yes, I need to start using my mind wisely?" Me neither. What I feel like saying is that it often happens near the point where we had some significant experiences, for example:

> *"Would you marry me?"* he asked me.
> *"Yes,"* I said, *"but I am afraid."*

Usually, the more impactful the experience, the more quickly we tend to recall it. When I was a child playing the popular plumber Mario's video game and couldn't defeat the Crazy Badass Sun in World 2, I soon realized that if I kept doing the same moves, I would continue to get the same results over and over again. So, what did I do? I managed to change the strategy! I was able to solve it by creating new moves, going further, and seemingly inadvertently, I finally won the game, becoming a master of it.

Mind and emotions are perfectly intertwined. The way Mother Nature intended it is so marvelous and at the same time a mystery with so many layers. Human beings love certainty and clarity because they give us peace of mind, one of the most precious things to have. Whether it's a simple decision about what to eat for lunch or whether to marry someone, as my personal example above, having clarity, with both mind and emotions, on these questions makes life a joyful place to live in. On the other hand, when our minds are overthinking, driving us down many a treacherous road, we will be stepping into a downward spiral of anxiety, which unfortunately is the anteroom to depression, anger, and hatred.

As a young girl growing up in Torreón, Coahuila, México, I had the privilege of having a beautiful home with my mom, dad, and my beloved brother. Both of my parents were professors, so reading, learning, and teaching became integral parts of my youth. It was fascinating to have access to a continuous menu and vista of so many ideas about human development and self-development at a young age. Both of my parents were passionately working in the field of human development. I can joyously recall afternoons at home, making packages and organizing copies for their courses, creating massive binders with all the information from the Masters. Carl Jung, Erich Fromm, Daniel Goleman, and Edward de Bono are a slice of some of the authors I remember from those Xerox photocopy days.

I'm clear that at such a young age, I couldn't understand or grasp the real use of those theories or have clarity about the meaning of human development. However, one thing I'm certain of is that I was absorbing the essence of their work in both my mind and soul. Now, as a mature woman, thirty-nine years old, I can finally feel that I'm starting to internalize and master more about why both of my parents were so passionate about teaching those principles for the betterment of people's lives, which thankfully included my brother and me.

Now, as a young adult woman, I have had the opportunity to be on stages, speaking about mastery, and being in rooms where great mentors have shared their knowledge. I have had the opportunity to be a professor at different universities in my hometown, and I can proudly say that I have been a professor at my favorite university in Mexico: Ibero Torreón, my alma mater. I can recall the feeling of excitement when I see in the faces of my students, as I teach them something new, an aura of a light switch that beams with an 'on' button. I can actually see the moment when participants' brains receive that new information and say, "Hey! I have never thought about that!" The process doesn't stop there. Once they get a new idea, they need to start using and implementing it. Great ideas without action will vanish. As the saying goes: A mind is like a parachute. Both work best when opened.

It seems super easy, but we always have some extra homework to do. Personal development, like housework, is never-ending. Sometimes we are able to receive a new idea—something that sounds exciting—but at the same time, we are so afraid of following up on our dreams. The key is to be willing to do the work. As my mentor, master coach with the Napoleon Hill Institute, Luis Jimenez says, "Many people don't achieve their goals simply because they don't fully commit."

Let me share another example. When I got married almost six years ago, I moved to the United States. I felt happy to have found a great man with whom to share my life. When I said yes to his proposal to leave my country, I was afraid, yet I was willing to commit. However, as with everything in life, this came with a cost. One thing I hadn't anticipated was losing my economic freedom. The immigration process is very complicated.

For those unfamiliar, a TN visa allows immigrant professionals from Canada and Mexico to work in the United States without intending to stay permanently. Dependents of TN visa holders, such as spouses and children, receive TD visas, which allow them to live in the U.S. but not to work. Later, if the TN visa holder's employment situation changes, it may be possible to switch to an H-1B visa, which is for specialty occupations. In such cases, dependents receive H-4 visas, which also allow them to live in the U.S. but generally do not permit them to work.

My husband, also from Mexico, was working in the U.S. for an international automotive company on a TN visa. I entered the country with a TD visa, which later changed to an H-1B visa for him and an H-4 visa for me. We knew if we wanted to stay permanently, we would need to obtain a Permanent Resident Card, also known as a Green Card!

While this might seem like a good deal, what many people don't know is that the spouse who receives a dependent visa loses their economic freedom, relying entirely on their partner's income. In my personal experience, I've been blessed with a husband who has taken care of my economic needs. But what about my profession, my self-esteem, my sufficiency, my identity? This can be a scary conundrum, not allowing for a playful life.

Living this experience day by day, year after year, can be incredibly discouraging. I felt like I was just waiting in the sports locker room, waiting to play in the game. My life was essentially put on hold due to an immigration status.

One day, I came across an article titled "Life Inside the Golden Cage: The spouses of workers with H-1B visas come to the United States and find themselves trapped at home." I saw myself reflected in the stories of professional and successful men and women who came here seeking a better life in the U.S., only to suffer from anxiety, depression, and various mental issues. It was clear to me that this environment is perfect for violence to arise, whether physical or psychological. While I've been blessed with an amazing husband, I can't help but think about how many people are trapped in this situation, unable to legally earn money and stuck in a violent environment.

This is when I realized how crucial it is to seek help and find a mentor to navigate such challenging situations. In 2021, I received a scholarship from the Hispanic-American Women's Association to be part of the Fearless Leader Program led by Kathy McAfee, who gave me one of the greatest gifts anyone can receive: the freedom of a creative mindset. During one of our calls, I shared my situation, struggles, and desires with her. She listened attentively and offered me a suggestion that changed everything.

"Laura," she said, "if you're willing to move forward in developing your strategic design skills and accept that, for now, you won't receive any payment for your services, would you be willing to invest your time serving pro bono on projects? These projects could help you keep your portfolio growing, meet new people, and improve your English skills, which will benefit your future business endeavors. Are you willing to let go of your frustration and put yourself in positive service, upward momentum, and advancement?"

That was Kathy's big question. I couldn't help but embrace the idea. I needed to move forward in my profession, even if my reward wouldn't come in the form of cash. Instead, it would succeed in relationships, language improvement, future business opportunities, and most importantly, lasting collaboration and relationships with so many people who now feel like family.

Abundance is a mindset, and I somehow managed to flip the switch and light beam to sufficiency. It wasn't easy for me to see it at first, but once a mentor pointed out that roadblock in my mental programming, I was able to clear it, break through it, and make anything possible!

Working on my personal development and mindset has made me stronger. Each step of this journey has been transformative, teaching me invaluable lessons about resilience, growth, and endless possibilities. Now, I know that if I give myself permission to play and explore, I discover an inner strength that helps me overcome any obstacle and allows me to experience victory.

The more I allowed myself to embrace new experiences and challenges, the more I realized how powerful a positive mindset can be. It truly unleashed my hidden potential, and propelled me forward, no matter the difficulties I face. The shift in my mindset didn't just change my perspective; it changed my entire life.

I learned that embracing abundance isn't just about material wealth. It's about feeling rich in love, opportunities, and personal growth. It's about understanding that there's enough out there for everyone.

To give you a glimpse of the future, after an almost six-year journey, I am currently the holder of a Permanent Resident Card, AKA Green Card! Now I am legally allowed to work in the U.S. and, even more, I am the CEO of my third and newest business, "3 Wins International LLC," which came as a result of my patience, resilience, and mindset. This has allowed me to support conscious entrepreneurs in expressing alignment between their products and services and their visual identity and brand message through our custom-made design processes. By helping others and contributing positively to the world, you too can create a cycle of abundance that benefits all.

It's truly magical when you start seeing results manifesting in your life. There's a tingling sensation that fills me with accomplishment and joy, making me feel like a real Wonder Woman!

This profound realization has become the cornerstone of my life philosophy. Now, every challenge is an opportunity to grow, every setback a chance to learn, and every success a testament to the power of a well-nurtured mindset. By giving myself permission to engage fully with life, I have unlocked a world of possibilities and endless potential.

Belief:

Our precious mind is always trying to avoid pain, making sure that we survive in this world. When we receive an idea that includes some kind of risk, we start evaluating what the iconic author Napoleon Hill of "Think and Grow Rich" calls the "What ifs." See yourself in these situations:

- What if you marry him/her and he/she cheats on you?
- What if you take the job and fail miserably?
- What if you tell a joke and nobody laughs?
- What if, what if, what if…

This is a real never-ending story, and at the same time, a gift of opportunity. However, this can be ignored or fearfully paralyzing, just as the bride in the proposal above. What stops us from growing is always some kind of fear.

Referring again to Napoleon Hill, who addressed these key six fears in his Masterpiece. He actually uses the term "ghost." His choice of the word 'ghost' is far more accurate because it feels just like that—they are chasing and scaring you all the time and must be avoided at all costs. These fears are:

- Fear of poverty
- Fear of criticism
- Fear of ill-health
- Fear of loss of love of someone
- Fear of old age
- Fear of death

Address these fears 'head on' at the onset of every undertaking. Once you deeply understand these fears and go through a process of identifying and introspection, you will surely find the root cause that paralyzes you. Sometimes, it's not an easy process, which is why it's said that we all need a mentor to guide us to our greatness—someone who has already walked the path we want to take. They are truly the bridge and pathway to legacy work and living. It won't always be your parents or your friends, but instead, someone with more experience who can show you the way to work on and develop your inner power.

Eventually, your daily work in self-development will gradually grow and transform you into that person who guides others. There comes a moment when you look back and see individuals with the same desire as you, following in your footsteps to be guided, leaning on your shoulder to be mentored, and walking by your side in collaboration. Life is truly a gift and becomes the ultimate opportunity when you live within that frequency of knowing, volleying the ball of life: The art in the game of a victor: Mindset, Game, Set, and Match!

Action Steps—Mindset:

- Be able to receive a new idea.
- Test it! You need to start using it. Take action.
- If you're still struggling, deep dive into your fears and go through a process of introspection to find another way.
- For total success in life, get a Mentor!

Laura Ibarra, AbD
PhD Student Social Research
www.3winsinternational.com
laura@3winsinternational.com

Gloria Kurz, JD, SRS

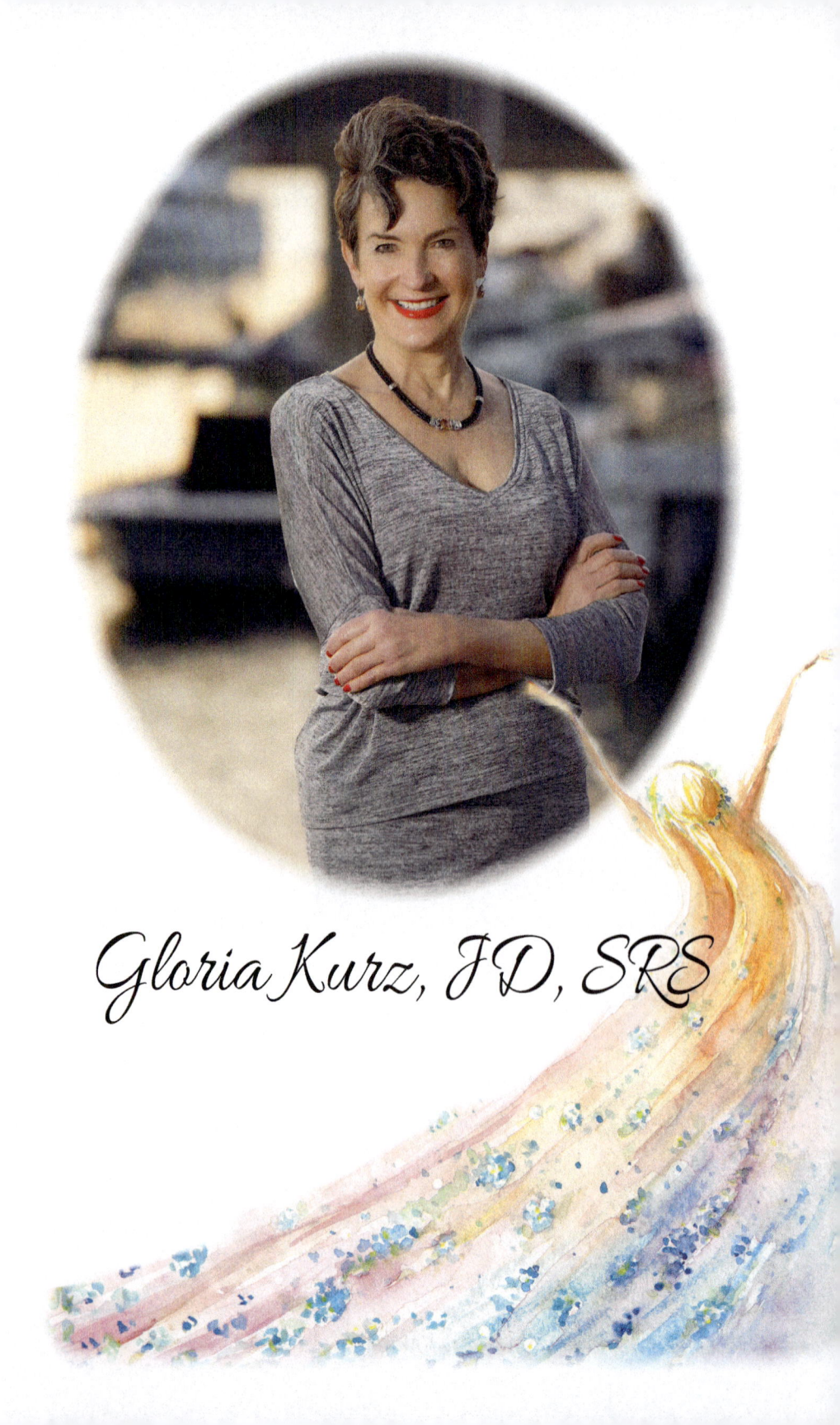

Pursuing My American Dream

"Passion and purpose power your dream."

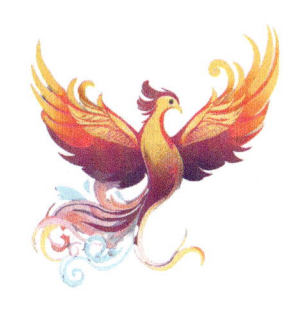

Intention:

Amelia Earhart said:

"The most difficult thing is the decision to act, the rest is merely tenacity. The fears are paper tigers. You can do anything you decide to do. You can act to change and control your life; and the procedure, the process is its own reward."

May pursuing your dreams lead to a healthy, balanced, successful, and financially independent life, not defined by the circumstances of your birth but created through your growth, patience, and perseverance.

Story:

I was the third of eight children in a military Air Force family. While still a toddler, we moved to Fürstenfeldbruck Air Base in Germany, west of Munich. My earliest memories were of a lakefront restaurant and our German Shepherds, Blondie and Dagwood. It was the beginning of a lifelong love of food, open water, and big dogs. As our family traveled back and forth across the Atlantic, it grew. My younger brother was born in Germany before we moved to Riverside, California—March Air Force Base. Three more of my siblings were born before we transferred to Seville, Spain—Moron Air Force Base, where my youngest sister made her entrance.

Money was always in short supply. It was impossible to support our growing family on just my father's military income. Early on, my mother inventively pawned her wedding rings between paychecks to make ends meet. My paternal grandfather loaned her money to buy our home in Riverside, providing stability and rental income when we were stationed elsewhere. As we got older, Mom worked part-time and then full-time.

While at Vandenburg, my father added a paper route for extra money. My sister, brother, and I helped. At age 8, I sold newspapers for tips in 'mess halls'—my first taste of having my 'own business.' In just a month, my reward from my business was an English-racer 3-speed bicycle—an exhilarating, empowering experience that began my quest for self-sufficiency. Over the next eight years, I branched out and other jobs included mowing lawns, babysitting, lifeguarding, and teaching swimming.

My parents were instrumental in us being independent and self-motivated. My Mom was born in Lvov, Poland (now Lviv, Ukraine) and was the pinnacle of strength, determination, and resilience, with a unique ability to overcome adversity. We lived below the poverty line but never knew it—she was adept at providing on limited means. Dad was a meteorologist in the Air Force, a fitness fanatic, and a semi-pro boxer. He bicycled 15 miles to work. Health conscious back then, neither of my parents smoked or drank—true role models of health.

Selected to attend college at the University of California, Riverside as part of an advanced high school/university program, I started UCR as a high school senior. After graduation, I began UCR full-time with the assistance of a Federally Insured Student Loan, an Economic Opportunity Grant, and a 20-hour/week work study program. When my work-study program was reduced to 5 hours/week, I supplemented as a waitress, restaurant hostess, and jewelry store salesperson.

Ironically, my future purpose unfolded when my older brother and roommate were arrested in Alameda County for underage drinking. I drove overnight to attend his arraignment, a stark eye-opener. Nearly sent to prison with adult offenders as he couldn't make bail, grace and justice prevailed. He was released on his own recognizance after the judge involved the Public Defender. It was a pivotal, life-changing moment for me. I saw firsthand how easily economic disparity influences outcomes in the judicial system and the importance of having a competent advocate. After watching the Public Defender, my inner voice clearly said: "*I can do better than that.*" My personal commitment to and passion for advocacy was born and my goal of being financially independent cemented.

My sister and I bonded closely growing up and became roommates in Riverside, then Balboa Island and Corona del Mar after we both transferred to UC Irvine, where I changed my major to Social Ecology, specializing in Criminal Justice and Environmental Health and Sciences. UCI's Social Ecology program was the first college program to require real work experience related to one's field and remains at the forefront of developing interdisciplinary approaches to social problems.

As part of the field study program, I volunteered as Project Director and Grant Coordinator for the new Human Relations Commission. I worked on a grant for a Pre-Trial Release Program through the Law Enforcement Administrative Agency. This program was designed to ensure individuals, like my brother, without economic resources, arrested for non-violent crimes and posing a low flight risk, could be released on their own recognizance pending trial. I was later hired as a Vocational Counselor with the Opportunities Industrialization Center, a federally funded program.

Subsequently, I became an Employee Development Specialist with Orange County's CETA Title 1 program and was then promoted to Personnel Specialist and Administrative Manager. My passion for advocacy was nourished as I helped individuals who met the program's affirmative action criteria get into interim jobs, and then into permanent positions. I confronted discriminatory attitudes across the board and learned some lifelong lessons. I was proud to be a change agent breaking down barriers to entry and becoming a more effective voice for clients.

I began at Western State University Law School to hone my advocacy skills. Since I had to work to afford law school, I attended classes evenings, weekends, and summers while working a 40-hour week. Passion and perseverance prevailed and I received my Juris Doctorate degree in 3½ years.

During this time, I rented homes in locations on or close to the water in Newport Beach, Balboa Island, Corona del Mar, and Laguna Beach. I spent more income than prudent but loved the locations and fell in love with real estate. Serendipitously, I received an American Jurisprudence award in my real estate law class.

Exhilarated to pass the California Bar on my first try, I interviewed for jobs in Public Defender and District Attorney's offices and accepted an offer from the Stanislaus County DA's office as a Deputy District Attorney. I was elated—particularly when I found out their first choice had accepted a different position. The DA is the ultimate advocate, representing the collective interests of *'We the People'* in court and I was determined to prove myself worthy. I was young, idealistic, motivated, with high aspirations, and even took a pay cut to accept the position.

A majority of our cases were driving under the influence, mostly alcohol. I was a liaison with the Battered Women's program, which opened my eyes to another underserved demographic. I was asked to manage a satellite office, a real accomplishment since professional women were still very much a minority.

As my legal career started to take off, my personal life was unexpectedly upended in another life-changing moment. This time, by a man. His name was Rick. He was mature, handsome, stylish, sophisticated, successful, and drove a 280Z. He relocated to Modesto from Manhattan. I had finally met my match and it was a whirlwind romance. Just months later, I was previewing apartments in Manhattan after Rick accepted an offer with Singer Corporation and asked me to join him. The 'Big Apple' was an adventure for this small-town California girl. We leased a 900 sq. ft. penthouse on 35th Street in Murray Hill with a wraparound terrace overlooking the East River, Empire State Building, and World Trade Centers.

My job search commenced with an interview at the Bronx DA's office. It wasn't a fit, so Rick's professional network kicked in. I was introduced to a Park Avenue law firm, where I became a Litigation Associate and was assigned to the Lachman estate litigation. Charles Lachman, the co-founder and "L" in Revlon died at 81, leaving a $30,000,000 estate ($129,000,000 today). Our firm represented his daughter who challenged whether his fourth, 39-year-old wife should inherit half his estate. At issue was the construction and interpretation of a will provision requiring she "shall have been married to me and living with me as my wife at the date of my death." The Judge eventually ruled for the wife, who was awarded almost $15,000,000, about $1,000,000 for every month of marriage. It was a jaw-dropping moment.

About that time, a major issue was raised with my status at the firm as the New York Bar refused to recognize my law school, which wasn't yet nationally accredited. Although I passed the California bar, the most difficult in the country, I wasn't allowed to sit for the New York Bar. I unsuccessfully petitioned for an exception. I refused to go back to law school, so consulted with a friend who left a successful legal career to open a boutique fashion business. I subsequently interviewed for positions in the cosmetics, fragrance, and wine industries before settling on a position with the Brazilian marketing department of Avon International.

After Avon, I teamed up with a talented sales executive who had purchased Sonya Rykiel's perfume *'Septieme Sens'* from Parfum Rochas and started a fragrance company, just as I was diagnosed with a potentially life-threatening tumor and had surgery. I powered through the surgery and embraced entrepreneurship. We introduced the first color cosmetic 'gift with purchase' tied to fragrance in the industry. The partnership was short-lived but I had a blast and became hooked on being my own boss (years later, he founded an extremely successful PR firm representing high profile fashion, beauty, and wellness brands). Rick and I then relocated to New Canaan, CT., after he left the helm as President of Somerset Wine Company and joined Marketing Corporation of America in Westport as a Senior Consultant.

At that point, I was figuring out what I wanted to be "when I grew up." While interviewing for a corporate marketing position in real estate, I was introduced to Tamar Lurie, an extraordinary woman and real estate professional married to Ranan Lurie, a world-renowned political cartoonist. It marked the beginning of my real estate career. I obtained my sales license, thrilled with this new venture. My diverse experiences in human resources, law, and corporate marketing all came together!

Coincidentally, my former senior law partner had clients who owned the last waterfront subdivision on Cos Cob Harbor in Greenwich. These 10 lots, priced from $595,000 to $1,595,000 became my first listing—a great kickstart to my career. I had numerous lots under contract when 'Black Monday' hit on October 19, 1987, causing a severe market downturn and global financial crisis. As a new realtor, it was baptism by fire—a lesson on how to focus in a volatile market, be flexible, have the ability to pivot, persevere, and 'stay the course.' Thankfully, Greenwich was a 'recession resistant' oasis. It recovered quickly and I soon represented buyers there in one of the first $3,000,000 transactions.

While I built up my real estate practice, Rick shifted careers and accepted a position outside of Hartford. We relocated and I changed my business focus to Jamestown, RI, where we had a second home. It was my third foray into the world of entrepreneurship. Mansions & Manors® was born.

At that time, a luxury sale in Rhode Island was anything over $500,000. In May 1995, my first sale was $855,000, a big deal. Earlier in 1995, I published an overview of the 1994 market in "Real Estate Views"©—the first real estate newsletter. It was before computerized statistics, so I'd have writer's cramp from generating everything by hand. I introduced corporate practices to our area, originated print invitations for broker open houses, and placed whole-page ads and center spreads. I was an early adopter and innovator of best practices, marketing techniques, and technology and had the first computerized window display. Advocating strongly for clients, I became known as a problem-solver.

We set records for sales and became adept at competing with larger local, regional, and national firms. Using skills learned practicing law and in corporate marketing, I focused on the quality of our representation, productivity, client service, and retention—creating and serving 'customers for life.'

I incorporated another lifelong love and created one of the first dog-friendly offices. We once had golden retriever puppies in our window with a sign that said *"Dog House $75, Puppies Priceless."* People weren't sure if we were a pet store or a real estate office. We're now on our fifth golden greeter, Cotton, who is a beloved team member and people magnet.

Federally registered, Mansions & Manors® was and remains a brilliant brand—instantly recognizable in the luxury market. With over $250,000,000 in sales and counting, I remain passionate about supporting my clients in RI and SC, where I'm also licensed. Sitting in the courtyard of our historic Beaufort home where Clara Barton, Founder of the American Red Cross and *'Angel of the Battlefield,'* lived while directing relief and recovery efforts after the Hurricane of 1893, I reflect on recent changes in my life. I think of Clara and the challenges she faced as I consider my next move.

Where do I go from here? With decades of practice, how do I best leverage my experience and give more back to the community? I want to channel Clara's essence and energy and be an equally effective *'angel advocate'* for clients in the 'brokerage battlefield.' Contemplating the future, I think about the past, my life-long dreams, and what I've accomplished. I'm proud that I've lived and worked with passion and purpose and grateful to have done so with patience and perseverance.

Belief:

Success is less about a specific job and more about creating financial health by following your passion and purpose. As a consummate career woman, I have been self-sufficient and entrepreneurial since I bought my first bicycle at age 8. I know we can unlock our potential at any age/stage of our life. Clara Barton was 72 when she challenged governmental indifference and managed the aftermath of the devastating 1893 Hurricane.

As women, we must advocate for our own health and financial well-being while balancing our personal, family, and/or marital lives as the support of partners, spouses, family, and friends is critical to our success. It often feels like we're walking a tightrope but the ability to remain whole, healthy, strong, and balanced when being pulled in multiple directions is unique to women and part of our essence.

Making mistakes and losing business opportunities is natural. It comes with the territory. Retrench and keep going. Ensure you infuse your business with passion so that it survives, thrives, and inspires. Success is measured by the strength of your convictions, adaptability, willingness to change, and ability to endure. These principles aren't static and will morph over time. They're powerful, persuasive attributes for your business and a healthy, balanced life. Do what you love, love what you do, be successful and the dollars will follow.

Action Steps for Financial Health:

- Find a job you love. If you find passion in your career choice—you will succeed.

- Embrace change. Cycle through until you identify a career path that maximizes your talents and skills.

- Be thoughtful. It's easier to get a job when you have one.
- Practice mindful spending. Spend less than you earn.
- Achieve financial security. Create a safety net to achieve financial freedom.

Gloria Kurz, JD, SRS
Principle, Real Estate Broker
www.mansionsandmanors.com
gloria@mansionsandmanors.com

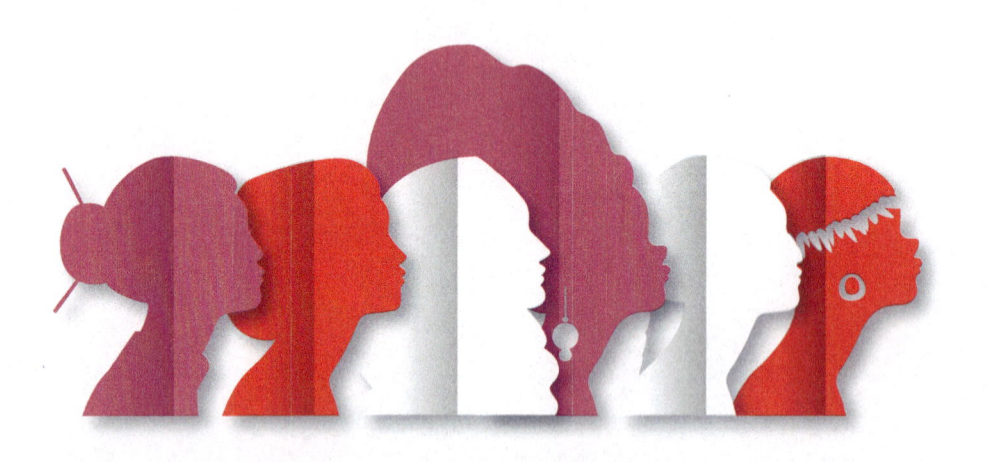

CHAPTER SIX

Social Pillar

"Beauty isn't about having a pretty face it's about having a pretty mind, a pretty heart, and a pretty soul."

—Drake

"Outer Beauty Attracts, but Inner Beauty Captivates."

—Kate Angell

"Beauty is about enhancing what you have. Let yourself shine through."

—Janelle Monáe

"True beauty is not related to what color your hair is or what color your eyes are. True beauty is about who you are as a human being, your principles, your moral compass."

—Ellen DeGeneres

"There's nothing more inspiring than the complexity and beauty of the human heart for humanity."

—Cynthia Hand

"Beauty, to me, is about being comfortable in your own skin. That, or a kick-ass red lipstick."

—Gwyneth Paltrow

"You cannot change a person. Let them be. Let them be the way they are."

—Melania Trump

"You should never view your challenges as a disadvantage. Instead, it's important for you to understand that your experience facing and overcoming adversity is actually one of your biggest advantages."

—Michelle Obama

Tiffany Haddish

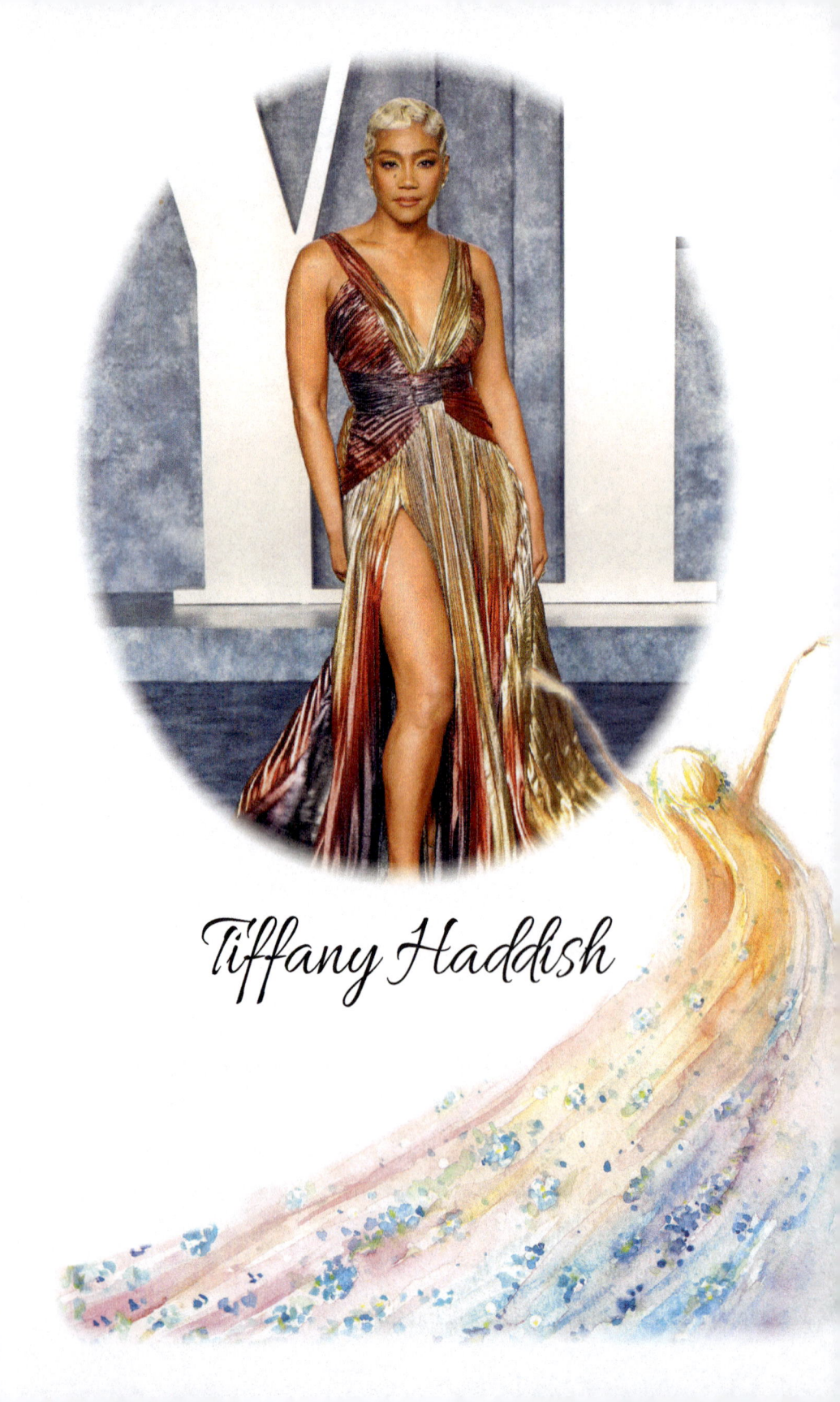

Woman Up!

*"Life's Lesson: Be Authentic, Be Resilient,
Be Love—Be 'SHE Ready."*

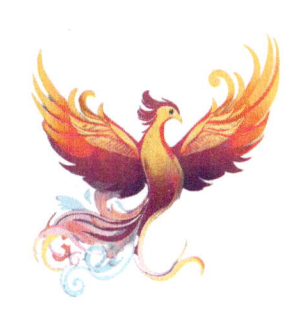

Intention:

May your authentic essence of a woman be found in your personal resilience, tenacity, strength, vulnerability, and spirituality—all wrapped in your heart filled with joy and love.

Story:

What's the essence of a woman? Now, that's a deep question, and if you know anything about me, you know I'm not afraid to dive deep. The essence of a woman isn't just one thing, and it's not something you can sum up in a few words. It's a whole lot of things mixed together—strength, love, humor, resilience, spirituality, and above all, authenticity. It's about taking whatever life throws at you, whether it's roses or rotten tomatoes, and turning it into something beautiful. Baby, let me break it down for you, Tiffany Haddish style. You see, the essence of a woman ain't just one thing—it's like trying to describe the taste of gumbo. You got all these flavors in the pot—strength, love, humor, resilience, spirituality, and a whole lotta "I ain't got time for your nonsense!" And honey, that's just the appetizer!

For me, beyond an appetizer, the essence of a woman is about survival. It's about finding the light even when you're surrounded by darkness. It's about loving fiercely, laughing loudly, and never, ever letting anyone dim your shine. I've been through a lot, but every experience, heartbreak, and struggle has only made me stronger. And that, my friends, is what the essence of a woman is all about.

This essence appears as bright as finding the light when all you've got is a busted flashlight and you've found some duct tape. It's about loving so hard that even heartbreak gets tired of trying to bring you down. And don't get it twisted—I've been through enough to know that when life throws you rotten tomatoes, you don't just make ketchup, you open a damn restaurant!

Resilience: The Foundation of a Woman's Strength

Speaking of resilience, let me take y'all back. *Picture* lil' Tiffany, 13 years old, living with a foster family that treated me like I was just another piece of furniture. They were more interested in the check they got from the state than making sure I was okay. I was hungry and lonely, and the only thing in my corner was my stubborn will to survive. But did I let it break me? Heck no! I looked life dead in the eye and said, "You better ask somebody! I'm Tiffany Haddish, and I'm not just gonna survive—I'm gonna *thrive*!" I didn't know how, but I knew I had to.

Let me take you back to where it all started. Growing up wasn't easy for me. My childhood was a whirlwind of uncertainty, bouncing from one foster home to another, never really knowing where I belonged. But in those tough times, I learned what it meant to be resilient. You see, when life tries to break you, you discover just how strong you really are.

That's where the essence of a woman starts—with resilience. It's that inner strength that keeps you going, even when everything around you is falling apart. It's that voice inside that says, "You got this, girl," even when the world is telling you otherwise. For me, resilience has always been about survival. It's about getting up every time you get knocked down, about finding a way to keep moving forward no matter how many obstacles are in your way.

Resilience is like wearing high heels on a bumpy road—you might wobble, but you ain't gonna fall! And let me tell you, that's where the essence of a woman starts—with the ability to get knocked down and bounce back up like a damn basketball!

Humor as Survival: Finding Light in Dark Places

Now, humor? Oh, that's my jam! Comedy was my escape plan when life tried to hand me lemons, but I turned those suckers into lemonade so sweet, it gave diabetes a run for its money! When you're in foster care, and everything feels heavy, you either laugh or cry. And you best believe I chose laughter every time. That's what women do—we find the light in the darkest places and then crack a joke about it to make it just a little bit brighter.

In my New York Times best-selling book, *The Last Black Unicorn*, I talk about how I used comedy to survive those tough times. Humor was my escape, my way of coping with the pain and the loneliness. I'd crack jokes to make people laugh, but really, I was just trying to keep myself from crying. That's the thing about women—we find a way to survive, no matter what. We find a way to turn our pain into power, to take the things meant to break us and use them to build ourselves up.

If you've read any of my books or seen me on stage, you know that humor is a big part of who I am. But what you might not know is that comedy was my lifeline. When you're a kid going through the kind of stuff I went through, you either laugh or you cry. And I made a decision early on that I was going to *laugh*.

One of the first times I realized the power of humor was when I was still in foster care. I was in a group home, and it was one of those days when everything just felt heavy. You know what I mean? The kind of day where you just want to crawl into a hole and disappear. But instead of doing that, I started telling jokes. I started making the other kids laugh, and you know what? It made me feel better too.

That's when I learned that humor wasn't just about making people laugh—it's about survival. It's about finding the light even when everything around you is dark. It's about taking control of your narrative, about me saying,

"Yeah, life is tough, but I'm tougher."

And that is a big part of the essence of a woman.

When I started doing stand-up comedy, it was my way of taking all the pain, all the struggles, all the heartbreak, and turning them into something positive. I'd talk about the craziest things—my mom's mental illness, my time in foster care, my failed relationships—and people would laugh. But what they didn't know was that every joke I told was a way of healing myself.

In my best-selling book, *I Curse You With Joy*, I talk about how humor became my shield, my armor. It was what protected me from the world, what kept me going even when things got tough. And that's the thing about women—we find a way to laugh through the pain. We find a way to turn our struggles into stories that make people smile. Because at the end of the day, that's what the essence of a woman is all about—finding the light, no matter how dark it gets.

Love: The Heartbeat of a Woman

Now, let's talk about love. Love is at the core of everything a woman does. Whether it's the love we have for our families, our friends, our partners, or ourselves—love is what drives all of us—what keeps us going. But here's the thing about love—it's not always easy. Sometimes, love hurts. Sometimes, love requires you to give more than you get. But we love anyway because that's who we are.

Love is the engine that keeps this woman-powered train running. But let me tell you, love ain't always a fairy tale. Sometimes it's a horror movie where you're the only one who brought popcorn. I've loved hard and lost harder, but every heartbreak was like a dress rehearsal for the woman I was becoming. And honey, when you learn to love yourself first, you become unstoppable.

I've had my fair share of love and heartbreak in my life. I've been in relationships where I gave everything only to end up with nothing. But you know what? I wouldn't change any of it. Because every time I loved deeply, I learned something new about myself. I learned about my strength, resilience, and capacity to forgive.

In my New York Times best-selling book, *The Last Black Unicorn*, I discuss my first marriage. Now, that was a roller coaster. I was so focused on being the perfect wife and on making him happy that I lost myself in the process. I forgot about my dreams, my goals, and my happiness. But when that marriage ended, I found something even more important—I found myself.

That's the thing about love. It's not just about loving someone else; it's about loving yourself. It's about knowing your worth, about not settling for anything less than you deserve. And that's a big part of the essence of a woman—loving fiercely but never losing sight of who you are.

Self-love is something I had to learn the hard way. I spent many years looking for validation from others, trying to prove that I was worthy of love. But then I realized that the only validation I needed was my own. I had to learn to love myself, to accept myself—flaws and all. And once I did that, everything else fell into place.

Love is powerful. It's what connects us, what binds us together. But it's also what makes us strong. Nothing can break you when you love yourself and truly embrace who you are. And that, my friends and sisters, is the heartbeat of a woman.

Turning Pain into Power: A Woman's Superpower

One of the most powerful things a woman can do is turn her pain into power. We've all been through things that could have broken us, that could have left us bitter and defeated. But instead of letting it define us, we rise! We take that pain and use it as fuel to propel us forward. That's a woman's superpower right there! Life tried to knock me out with a whole lot of hurt, but instead of tapping out, I turned that pain into the punchline. And that's the beauty of being a woman—when life hands us pain, we don't just take it. We remix it, flip it, and turn it into something that lifts us up, and leaves the world in awe.

I've been through a lot of pain in my life—abuse, homelessness, rejection. But instead of letting it break me, I let it build me. I took all that pain and turned it into something positive. I turned it into comedy, into storytelling, into motivation. And that's what the essence of a woman is—taking the worst that life throws at you and turning it into something beautiful.

In *I Curse You With Joy*, I talk about how I've used my platform to speak out about what I've been through and let other women know that they're not alone—that their pain is valid—but it doesn't have to define them. We have the power to change our narrative, take control of our story, and turn our pain into something that empowers us and others.

Pain is inevitable. We're all going to go through things that hurt, make us question our worth, and inspire us to give up. But it's how we respond to that pain that defines us. Do we let it break us, or do we let it build us? Do we let it defeat us, or do we let it drive us? The essence of a woman is about turning pain into power, about using our experiences to become stronger, wiser, and more compassionate.

I've learned that pain is a part of life, but it doesn't have to be the end of your story. It can be the beginning of something beautiful. It can be the spark that ignites your passion, the push that gets you out of your comfort zone, and the motivation that keeps you going when you want to quit. That's the essence and power of a woman—the ability to take her pain and turn it into something powerful, something meaningful, something that can change the world.

Embracing Authenticity: The Freedom to Be Unapologetically Yourself

There's nothing more freeing than being unapologetically yourself. For too long I tried to fit into a mold that wasn't made for me. I tried to be what other people wanted me to be, to say what they wanted me to say, to do what they wanted me to do. But you know what? That's not living! That's just existing. And the essence of a woman is about living your life to the fullest, being true to yourself, and not apologizing for it.

I've always been a little different. I've always had a big personality, a loud laugh, and a unique way of looking at the world. And for a long time, I tried to tone it down, fit in, and be "normal." But then, I realized that being normal is overrated! Being normal is boring. And more importantly, it's not who *I am*.

In *The Last Black Unicorn*, I talk about how I was always the odd one who didn't quite fit in. But instead of trying to change who I was, I embraced it. I embraced my uniqueness, my quirks, my flaws. And that's what made me who I am today. That's what makes all of us who we are—our ability to embrace our true selves, to stand tall in our truth, and to shine our light for the world to see.

Being unapologetically yourself means not shrinking yourself to make others comfortable. It means taking up space, using your voice, and standing in your power. It means knowing who you are, loving who you are, and not letting anyone take that away from you.

The essence of a woman is authenticity. It's about being real, being honest, being true to yourself. It's about not letting society's expectations dictate how you live your life. It's about embracing who you are, flaws and all, and loving yourself for it. Because when you're true to yourself and live your life authentically, that's when you're truly free!

Spirituality and Inner Strength

Let's talk about spirituality. Alright, let's get real! Now, I'm not saying I got a hotline to the Big Guy upstairs, but I've butt-dialed Him a few times! Spirituality is like that one friend who never lets you down, even when everyone else flakes. That inner GPS keeps you from getting lost in the chaos, even when you swear you're driving in a circle. For me, spirituality has always been a source of strength, a guiding light that's helped me navigate the ups and downs of life. I'm not talking about religion—though that's important to a lot of people—I'm talking about that deep, inner connection to something greater than yourself. That sense of purpose, belonging, and knowing that no matter what happens, you're not alone.

Growing up, I didn't have a lot of stability in my life. But one thing I always had was my faith. I believed that there was something bigger than me out there, something that was looking out for me, guiding me, protecting me. And that belief gave me strength. It gave me the courage to keep going, even when things were tough.

In *I Curse You With Joy*, I talk about how I've always had this inner voice, this intuition that's guided me through life. Some people might call it a gut feeling, others might call it a connection to God, but whatever it is, it's always been there for me. It's that *voice* that tells you to keep going, to keep fighting, to keep believing even when things seem impossible.

Spirituality is a big part of the essence of a woman. It's that inner strength, that connection to something greater, that keeps us grounded, that gives us the courage to face whatever life throws our way. It's about knowing that you're not alone, that there's a purpose to your life, that you're part of something bigger than yourself.

I've learned that spirituality isn't just about believing in something—it's about living it. It's about letting that belief guide your actions, your decisions, your life. It's about finding strength in your connection to the universe, God, and whatever it is that you believe in. And that, my friends, is a big part of the essence of a woman.

Community and Sisterhood: The Collective Power of Women`

One of the most beautiful things about being a woman is the sense of community, of sisterhood, that we share. There's something powerful about women coming together, supporting each other, lifting each other up. It's like we have this unspoken bond, this understanding that we're all in this together.

I've been blessed to have some amazing women in my life—women who have supported me, encouraged me, and helped me become the person I am today. And I've always tried to do the same for others. Because that's what community is all about—being there for each other, lifting each other up, and helping each other shine.

In *The Last Black Unicorn*, I discuss the importance of mentorship—having someone in your corner who believes in you and sees your potential even when you don't see it yourself. I've had a few mentors, and they've made all the difference. They've helped me navigate the challenges, overcome the obstacles, and find my way.

But mentorship isn't just about having someone to guide you—it's about giving back. It's about using your experiences, your knowledge, your wisdom to help others. It's about being there for the next generation of women, about helping them find their way, about lifting them up and helping them shine.

Sisterhood is powerful. When women come together, when we support each other, when we lift each other up, there's nothing we can't do. That's the essence of a woman—being there for each other, supporting each other, and lifting each other up.

Belief:

Listen, I've had my moments where I was like, "God, if you're listening, can you send me a sign? Maybe a winning lottery ticket? Or at least a decent parking spot?" But here's the thing—spirituality isn't about getting everything you want, it's about trusting that when you don't, you still got this! It's knowing that even when life feels like a bad reality show, there's something bigger out there, making sure you don't get voted off the island. So, yeah, spirituality is real, and it keeps me grounded—well, that and a good wig on a windy day!

So, what is a woman's essence? I sang about it in my video: "Woman Up"! It's resilience, humor, love, the ability to turn pain into power, and being unapologetically yourself. It's about standing strong in adversity, laughing through the tears, loving fiercely and deeply, and owning your truth. It's about knowing your worth, embracing your uniqueness, and shining your light for the world to see.

The essence of a woman is complex, multifaceted, and ever-evolving. It's a beautiful mix of strength, vulnerability, power, and grace. And it's something every woman carries within her, whether she realizes it or not.

I've been through a lot, but I wouldn't change any of it. Because every experience, every challenge, every heartache has contributed to the woman I am today. And I'm proud of that woman. I'm proud of my resilience, my humor, my love, my power, and my authenticity. That, my fellow women, is the essence of a woman—being *'SHE Ready'* for whatever life brings you. This *SHE Ready essence* is standing tall when life throws shade, cracking jokes when you'd rather cry, and loving yourself so fiercely that even heartbreak gets scared to mess with you. It's about being unapologetically you, trusting that there's something bigger guiding you—even if you can't always see the map. The essence of a woman is knowing your worth, shining your light, and turning every challenge into your next success story. And baby, that's not just the essence of a woman—that's the essence of Tiffany Haddish and you, too!

Action Steps: *'She Ready'*:
- Find resilience to go from surviving to thriving
- Find humor in the dark places
- Find spirituality inside of you

- Find your authenticity in being you
- Find community in sisterhood
- Find your heartbeat in love

Tiffany Haddish
Comedian, Actress, Author
Instagram:@tiffanyhaddish
YouTube: @thaddish
#icurseyouwithjoy
https://shop.tiffanyhaddish.com/collections/shop-all

Dr. Jo Dee Baer, PhD

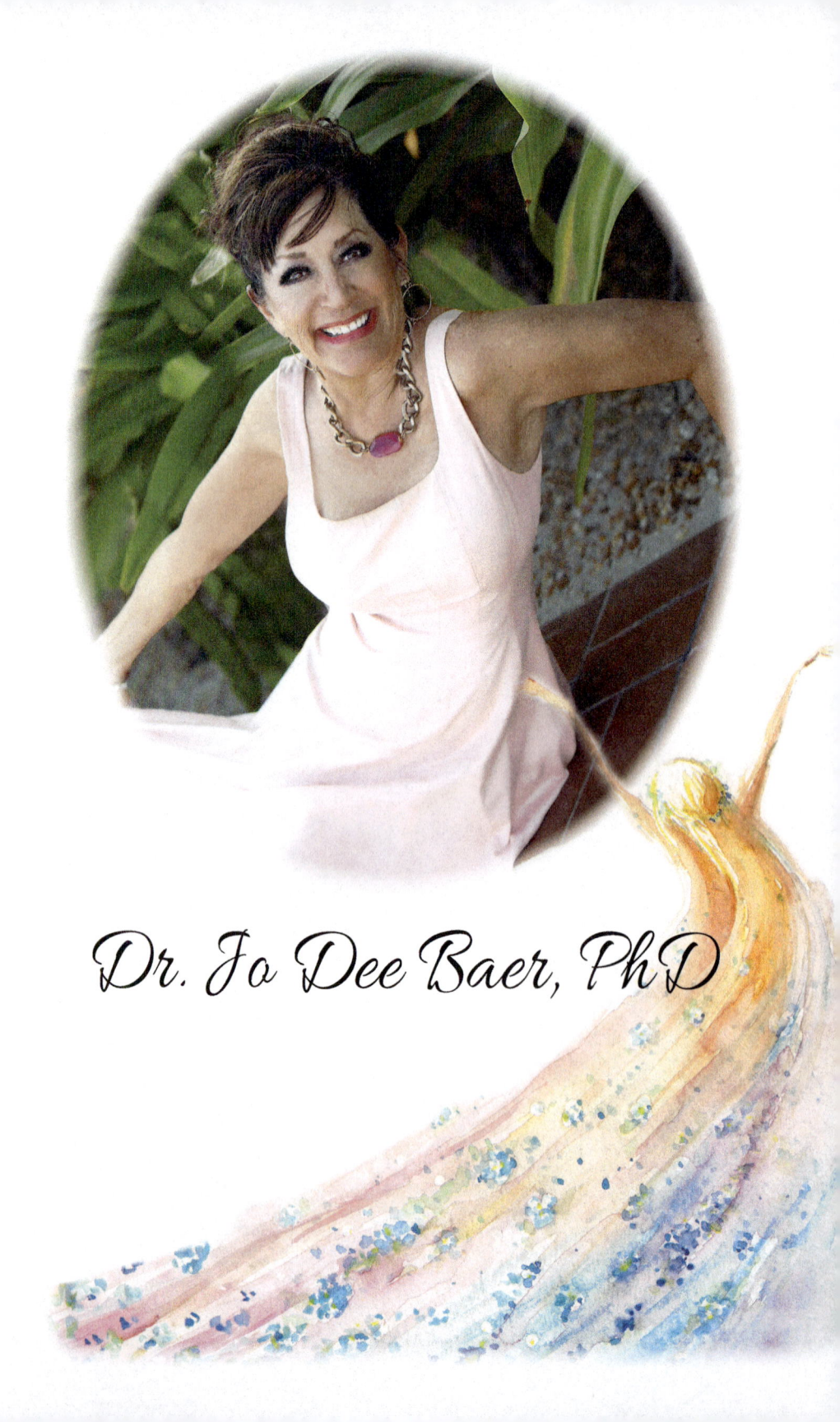

The Woman in a White Robe

*"Immerse in the flow of who you are—
and how you are becoming."*

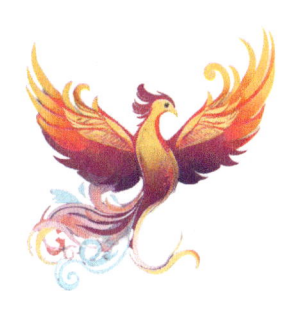

Intention:

With a personal and 'recognizable and achieved' bond that goes deep, high, and wide within yourself—security, community, and legacy emerge like the Phoenix within each of us. Each woman has been in the deep and dark recesses of her inner and undiscovered soul. Acknowledging and subsequently embracing the personal darkness within, she transversely will accept the present within the beauty of the ***now***. She then naturally celebrates in perpetual gratitude the heights in this bright abundance of personal awareness that transcends into a passion and the ecstasy of becoming, which is truly living.

Story:

My earliest childhood memory was one of my three-year-old plaintive cries as I was awakened from a restive sleep: "Mommy, my tummy hurts; I, I can't go potty." My Mother assured me that it would all get better, caressed the tresses of my brown hair, and sang a lullaby until I once again returned to sleep. However, more often than not, every week, I found myself on my knees, posed in an embryo position as my Mother administered an enema to me to mitigate my constipation and subside my constant tummy pains. My chronic *tummy* condition was one of constipation, an emotional outcome of the sadness I subconsciously buried inside of me. Still, one day, this little toddler made the connection and tearfully bellowed out: "Mommy, did I make Daddy die?" My Mother lovingly held me as she reassured me I had nothing to do with daddy passing." I believed her and was consoled and temporarily appeased whilst we were both coping with catastrophic and gut-wrenching grief: the sudden passing of my father. For much of my childhood, I assimilated these pains as part of my daily M.O. Still, later in life, I unleashed the link between physical constipation, my gut pain, and the grief of my emotions, resulting in manifesting into chronic sub-optimal health conditions, until as a young novice and curious health coach, I attracted the Iconic Dr. Hulda Clark, N.D., into my life.

While still a preschooler and in the Beta Stage of development, I discovered that the pain in my tummy and my emotional pain were often automatically expelled and dispelled each time I sang or played my piano. Later on, I discovered, after two college degrees in Psychology, Neurolinguistics, and Psycholinguistics, that this entire physical and emotional malady was indeed bound up in the Electra Phase and Beta Stage of my innocence at age three. I had unconsciously fallen in love with the first man in my life, my Father. His life was needlessly snuffed out at the young age of 44, and my resultant abandonment cascaded like Niagara Falls into my subsequent adult life, fittingly summarized into the epitome of Dr. Seuss's book title: *Will You Be My Friend?* This childhood story is an analogy centered around an animal adventure that symbolizes kindness overshadowed by the constant yearning for acceptance, inclusion, and friendship. Coco, the Orphaned Rooster, faces continual rejection and sadness. But Coco continued with his perpetual co-co-doodle doo, never losing his faith and hope.

Assimilating Coco, everything I accomplished as a child into my teenage and adulthood was a continuing hopeful cascade of over-achieving, striving, and excelling at every personal and professional endeavor. The personal acceptance I continually longed for, personally and professionally, became a circle from where the transcendence of a weakness finally transformed into strength. This emotional and physiological roller coaster of constant achievement developed into my emergence as being commonly known as America's Top Foundation Health Coach and Holistic Nutritionist. It has been a four-decade road—dirt road or expressway—of guiding multitudes and supporting my clients/patients to their healing and wholeness—and ultimately to myself as well.

Philosophy:

Listening to and becoming their professional coach, confidant, counselor, and eventually professional friend, like Coco, has been gratifying and cathartic. This noble journey and pathway first arose, like a Phoenix at the height of my marathoning days, in my late 30s, when I first observed a class of yoga students in Savasana and post-practice meditation. I sarcastically called their experience '*adult naptime*.' My sharp and unfounded opinion, a mere expression of my personal and childhood unresolved anger, turned inward. This same '*adult naptime*,' after my epiphany and awakening to this essential component for health and abundance, became one I soon embraced as an anchor of personal healing for my emotional health.

During the devastating loss of my marriage and yet another intimate love, I turned my abandonment into the love of achieving optimal health for others. I immersed myself in my two loves of life, my practice/clients and my young sons, to the extent that I lost my personal perspective, which resulted in 'overachieving and over-giving.' One morning, that orphan woman collapsed onto the floor while making breakfast for my two sons. My legs folded like a paper airplane, and the next thing I knew, I woke up in the ambulance, still in my white fleece bathrobe. I was shivering to almost near convulsions, not because the ambulance temperature was quite cool, but because I was consumed by sheer fear and terror! The frantic question reverberating inside of me: "How did I lose myself in the midst of my life?"

Once again, Dr. Hulda Clark, ND, my esteemed mentor, came to my rescue and lovingly taught me the art of meditation. This meditation miracle saved me, restoring my health, my vitality, and my zest for life itself. It is a practice I still do daily to revive and rejuvenate the essence of me. Dr. Clark's sage words still resound in my soul 35 years later,

"Meditation is for your soul, your true essence of who you are."

Whether I consult my clients/patients with Complementary Alternative or Energy Medicine, each receives the keys to my 'Daily Meditation'—my personal 'routine' so I can be the best part of myself to those who seek personal and professional guidance. www.drjodee.com/blog/10-rituals-for-10-am-n38ba. Years later, the empowered flip side of this white robe unveiled itself again to me in a profound group mediation.

The first meditation I collectively participated in after becoming a single parent and empty nester was one at the Women's Personal Development Retreat. With my two sons launched successfully into College and Collegiate Swimming Careers, I gravitated to anything and any answers that could quell this resurfacing loneliness again, the despair of abandonment. I was ripe and longing for a self-revelation to break this life pattern. On the second day, the facilitator asked probing questions focusing on a personal life's higher purpose. He simply stated the following probing questions: "If you had a billion dollars in the bank:

- What would you do?
- Where would you go?
- Who would you be with?
- How would your life be?"

We all collectively closed our eyes, and instantaneously, a woman personally appeared to me full-frontal, serene, and lips pursed with a sliver of a Mona Lisa smile in a white circular flowing robe, with dolman sleeves and white chiffon cascading down to her knees. This brunette had tresses of long flowing hair billowing and succumbing into the rhythm of each movement like a ballerina performing the ballet of "Swan Lake." Just at sunset, her grace and gazelle-like movement skipped effortlessly across the smooth rocks and sand on the beach.

This woman, peaceful and secure in herself, her brown eyes sparkling and fully immersed in her glistening mission and vision in a panoramic view, was me, Health Coach Jo Dee, taking her passion and mission into the world of healing and hope—like Coco, but my Soul was *unleashed* from within. Now, looking back 24 years later, this was my first portent of things to come of what has now become *Health-a-Pedia*. At the time of this neon Fifth Dimension revelation in a futuristic meditation, I was merely practicing within the brick-and-mortar as a health practitioner and holistic nutritionist. The Universe and Creator of All, originally named "Yahuah," pre-ordained this vision into my personal life. This precursor life force knew I would first retire and then unretire after six weeks to develop what has presently emerged as the Global Expanse of Health-a-Pedia. The Mission and Vision to Fruition: A transcendent process, 'without walls,' whereby all who choose to 'be attracted' through the *Law of Attraction* can find transformative healing and hope. All these Six Pillars of Health:

Spiritual, Mental, Physical, Emotional, Financial, and Social are now in full all-embracing view. Within this meditative state lies the essence of pure and unbridled joy. True joy is the consummate prerequisite for hope.

Like Coco, hope reigns eternally in the soul and is constantly rejuvenating. The regenerative/degenerative apex turns as a result of either confidence or fear. Degenerative disease begets fear, which spirals downward to anger, hatred, disease, and regenerative life force unveils the Soul, transforming self from confidence to gratitude, joy, hope, passion, and ultimately ecstasy. The woman who collapsed in the white fleece bathrobe was the epitome of this degenerative cycle. However, like the flip of a coin toss, the regenerative white-robed woman conjoined as the Firebird (feminine) and Phoenix (masculine) in the Regenerative Circle of Life—can and will always appear. The self-actualization of a mindful daily, moment-by-moment personal decision for personal evolution in self-care begins with you—to center, feed, and thereby take care of and elevate the frequency of the world around you. Birthed within your divine soul, the Social Pillar of Health and the wider net of the world outwardly transcends from family to community, country, the World, and the Universe. The first cornerstone lies in your personal epi-center: the epitome of peace and self-love.

This Six Pillar Philosophy of Foundational Health reveals to all who inwardly seek this constant: that *transformation* is truly an inside job! I have built my personal and professional life around these Six Pillars of Health in coordination with the Quintessential *Five Elements of Traditional Chinese Medicine*: Supplementation, Sleep, Exercise, Prayer and Meditation, and lastly Physiotherapy. A simple daily self-care accountability in mindfulness for mastery is to look at your hand. The fourth component of Traditional Chinese Medicine is indicated with the fourth finger, the ring finger. In meditation, the primary tenant is that one is 'married' to oneself: masculine—mercy—and feminine—stability. Integrate them both into the essence of Y-O-U, and you are never alone. You are the only person that will never leave you. Husbands may. My Father did in an untimely and sudden manner, and children in some stage of life better! The acrostic of Y-O-U stands for:

Y-es,

O-pportunity of

U-niqueness."

Celebrate Y-O-U every day in every way. One way is to celebrate Y-O-U in meditation, which I genuinely espouse consistently. I end my meditation with all or some of these parts daily. I enjoy the energy of a meditational Symphonic 'finale' and encourage my client/patients to engage in it as well. Merely finish your meditation with a toe-to-head Visual Meditation—a 'Celebration SCAN.' This energetic focus is aimed at each organ and body part, which goes as follows: "I love my feet; love my pinky toe (mention each one)." Include a perceived flaw as you ascend, for example: "I love my bunions. I truly love their character and remember all the miles they have run." As you go up your ankles, calves, and thighs, remind **you** of the varicose veins. Have a sense of humor because most of these varicose veins have been 'very close' to an accomplishment, a personal event of some sort! Then, the fun begins with celebrating each female body part, your vagina and labia, whether you have birthed your children through this birth canal or by Caesarian. Now is the time to celebrate each birth and child you have brought forth on Planet Earth.

Continue with each organ: your colon, large and small; uterus; ovaries; pancreas; liver, stomach; gallbladder; breasts; lungs; sternum; thyroid; neck; throat; vocal cords; ears; lips; nose; eyes; and brain. Stop at any time and take a focused detour, whereby this is, as I prefer to call it, rather than a disease, a temporary 'situation' within any organ. Focus and speak vitality, healing, and wholeness. Any personal health 'situation' can be mitigated because the body is a miracle-making machine. It can and will heal itself. For example, if you find out that your liver function is less than optimal, call to your liver at the end of your meditation, saying something like this: "Liver, I love you. Move and release! My liver is subtle, alive, and toxicity-free." Call and command wellness and wholeness into every organ of your body. An energetic release will abound and rebound, akin to the connection of fear, stress, depression, and disease. With this meditative self-care love **scan**, you emerge as **the** triumphal woman in your own white robe, shedding your 'Coco' tendency and immersing in the flow as the ***phoenix*** ballerina of your life and purpose—for you and humanity. Transcendently, this energetic frequency release expands and resounds into true passion and peace within this meditative celebration of Y-O-U. This celebration truly evolves to what the Scriptures say:

> *"The Peace Passeth all Understanding"*
> —Philippians 4:7

That Peace is the regenerative and upward flow of accurate transcend health.

The Woman in the White Robe IS the healing flow of all who chose this healing path of expansive abundance, gracefully skipping across the rocks of life in genuine knowingness. Glinda, the Good Witch in *The Wizard of OZ,* told Dorothy: You have always had the Power within you. That power begins with grasping and owning your personal deserve level. That deserve level is embodied in Rex Sikes renowned NLP/Mentalist, whose poignant two-word quote from his book, *Life on Your Terms*:

> *"Celebrate Everything."*

When you c*elebrate everything* in the social pillar of foundational health, transformation expansively elevates to the essence of the world. One of my favorite personal quotes is:

> *"Life is like a Milkshake. Choose your ingredients wisely."*

That first ingredient in life's milkshake unleashes your personal deserve, the level of your inner soul. Loving yourself to and through self-acceptance **IS** the greatest love and feeling of all. You, too, can be the woman in a white robe. That Phoenix will unleash to arise within each woman who diligently searches for her white robe of serenity, tranquility, love, and joy. Hope is the outgrowth of your inner work. Deserve it first. Build your personal life's milkshake, and then your life will savor the sweetness of life's dessert!!

The Three Action Steps to *'SEE'*—Simple, Easy, and Effective–Yourself:

- **SEE** yourself daily as a whole human being: Stare into the depths of your eyes in the mirror daily.

- **SEE** yourself as 'body beautiful:' Scan your body in a full-length mirror and celebrate it all!

- **SEE** your body at the end of your meditation as 100% whole, abundant, and if applicable, pain-free.

Dr. Jo Dee Baer, PhD
Certified Health Coach; Holistic Nutritionist
Board Certified NLP Trainer
Foundational Health
and Health-a-Pedia
www.drjodee.com
www.healthapedia365.com
jodee@healthcoachjodee.com

Kim Jacobs, MBA, BD

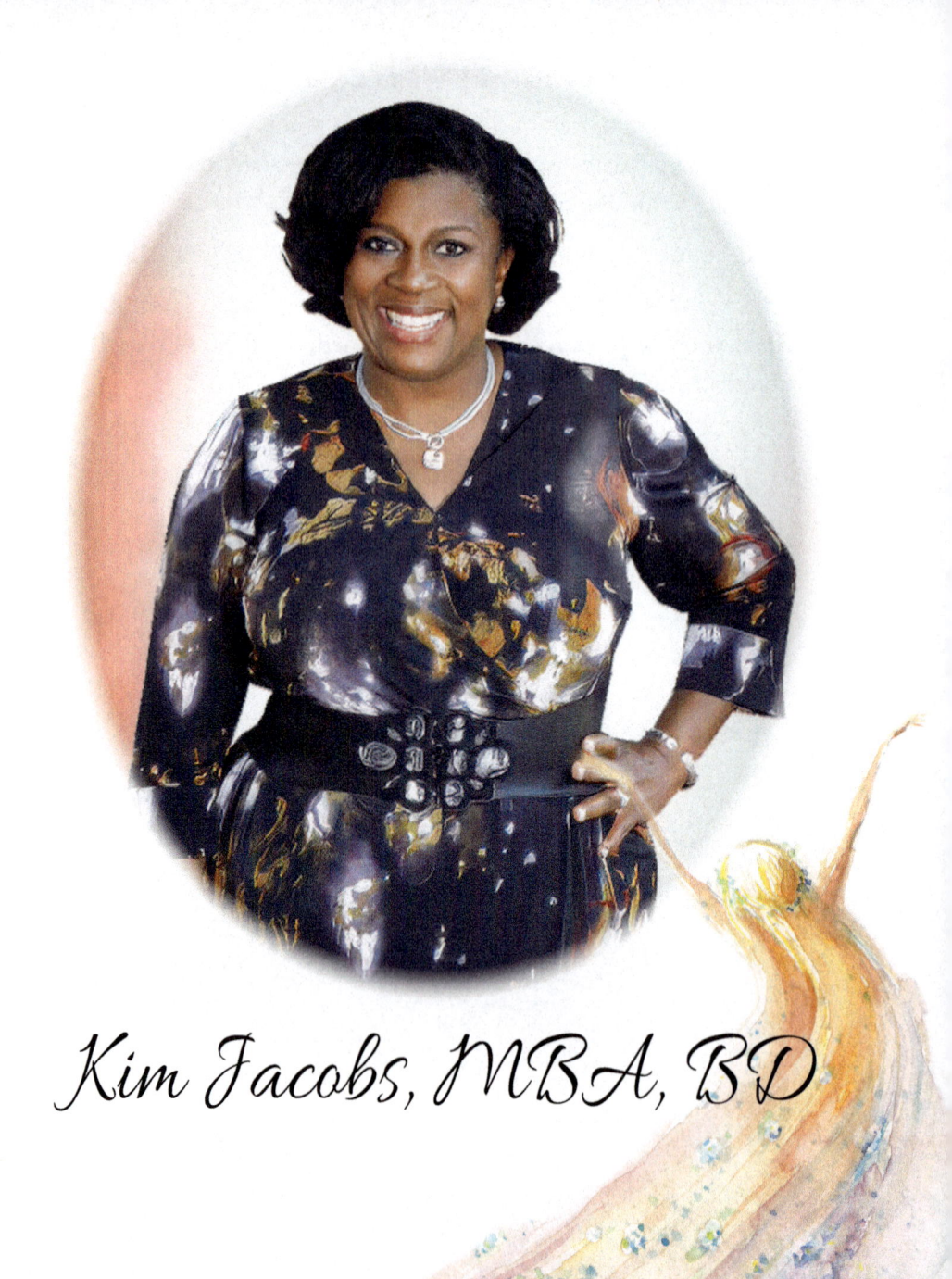

Who Knew? God Knew!

"Use every gift God has trusted you with to salt this Earth."

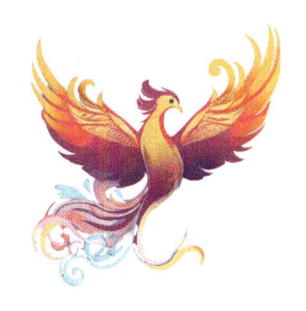

Intention:

Be your purpose and leave no stone unturned by using each gift in part and collectively. May that same God who leads me, lead you to your miracles of life: Salting the Earth with your personal 'essence of a woman.'

Story:

I was celebrating the island atmosphere as a newlywed in the Bahamas for my honeymoon, relishing in the love of my new marriage; suddenly, on my way back home, I experienced excruciating stomach pain and was rushed to the hospital. I was told that I had an ovarian cyst the size of an orange that would rupture if I didn't have immediate emergency surgery! During the procedure, my family was notified that the cyst was wrapped around my ovary and that the doctor would have to take a significant portion of my ovary, possibly preventing me from having children. The decision was made on my behalf, and I would face my life as a married woman with no childbearing possibilities.

Who knew I would give birth to my first son five years later and four more children following him? *Who knew?* God Knew! Motherhood became my greatest gift, and I cherish it deeply! There is nothing compared to my unconditional love and bond with these five human beings that God entrusted me to oversee, lead, and guide them to their destinies! This assignment is my life's mantle because I have birthed messengers of hope. Everything we do collectively and individually will impact many people's lives worldwide. *Nothing happens by chance.* God ordains or authorizes things to happen in our lives for a specific purpose. I truly believe God has a pre-ordained plan for my life, and these five miracle children formed in my womb.

> *"Before I formed thee in the belly, I knew thee, and before thou camest forth out of the womb I sanctified thee, and I ordained thee, and I ordained thee a prophet unto the nations."*
>
> —Jeremiah 1:5 (KJV)

No matter what your diagnosis, remember God has the final say in your miracle.

My five miracle children now are 27, 23, 19, 16, and 12 forever. My oldest son, Frank Jr. (27), graduated with a Computer Science degree from UNC Chapel Hill and is one of the most brilliant men I know. I learn so much from his wisdom. He has always been an avid reader since his childhood. Once, he entered an accelerated reading contest and needed one last book to win the competition. We rushed to the library to get the treasured book, where the person in front of us turned around and said, "Frankie, are you looking for this?" His name was Pradeep! Frankie came in second place to that young man that year but won the reading contest for years to follow. Seeing this giftedness and insatiable thirst for knowledge, I vowed always to have access to any book he needed, and now he has cultivated a brilliant mastermind.

My son Ivan (23), who battles Cystic Fibrosis—a chronic lung disease that fills the lining of the lungs with mucus, making it more difficult to breathe, is a student at UNC Charlotte, a Cystic Fibrosis Student Ambassador with Boomer Esiason Foundation, a National Association of Sports Medicine Certified Personal Trainer, and a Cystic Fibrosis Foundation Ambassador. He has lost over 100 pounds on his own personal natural weight loss journey and created his own brand to teach his program to others, outlined on www.majorpt.com. My son Jeremiah (19) recently graduated high school. An avid fisherman, actor, and working presently in roofing. With an innate sense of finance, Jeremiah will be the billionaire in our family. He also lives with Cystic Fibrosis and serves as a Cystic Fibrosis Foundation Ambassador, as an advocate and liaison before Congress to present bills to be considered to assist CF Patients with quality of of life.

My daughter Jayla (16) is an "A/B" honor roll student and National Art Honor Society Member who works at Chick-fil-A. She draws animations on a professional level. Jayla also kicks Cystic Fibrosis in the head. She also serves as a Cystic Fibrosis Foundation Ambassador with her brother and speaks before Congress to have them consider particular bills.

According to the National Institute of Health, 1 in 17,000 are African American. Therefore, it is rare for three African American children to be diagnosed with Cystic Fibrosis in the same family. Jayla and her two brothers, Ivan and Jeremiah, are three of those individuals, and they are anomalies who live in the same household. *Who knew? God Knew!* God knew these warriors would inspire other young people battling life-altering diagnoses and encourage them to pursue their dreams and goals. This CF Family Trio recently helped raise $2.2 Million with the Cystic Fibrosis Foundation. I was just in awe, watching these miracles create a miracle for others.

I referred to my last child as 12 forever. My son Gabe is 12 years old, and he is 5'10' and a gentle giant. We call him "Diesel!" He loves football but loves humans so much more that he stopped the football game to ensure that the person he tackled was OK! Gabe gets excellent grades in school and treats everyone as if they are his best friend. His middle school principal spoke about Gabe in a documentary where she told her staff, "If you all treat the students like this child, Gabe, treats everyone, then you are doing a wonderful job as staff."

Gabe serves as the anti-bullying mediator at his school in the 6th grade, and his peers call him "Guardian Gabe!" Gabe is considered Deacon Gabe in our Church and wants everyone to know Christ as their personal Savior. He prays and raises his hands high during service. Living his higher calling, Gabe was named after two angels, Gabriel and Michael.

However, on April 9, 2015, Gabe, his siblings, and his Dad were playing a family game of basketball on a newly installed Basketball hoop. Suddenly, Gabe looked up to the sky as if someone was calling him by Name, and lay down on the ground peacefully, and was no longer with us. Heaven became his home that day! *Who Knew? God knew!* God knew that over one hundred children would accept Christ as their personal Savior at Gabriel Michael Jacobs's funeral—a miracle home-going Celebration of Life. Gabe's heart still *'Just Keeps Beating'* through www.Gabesheartfoundation.org where we spread awareness of sudden cardiac death and raise funds to place defibrillators in public spaces where youth congregate. Gabriel would be 21 years old today as I write this chapter, but to me, he will be 12 forever and always be my son.

I take my role of encouraging and understanding my children to know that they can be and do *anything* they choose. There are no limits to what they can do! God gave me the Mother he did for me to become the mom I am today. My legacy was ordained by my Mother, Ella Mae, who raised me as a single parent in a low-income housing project called *'The Bottom.'* My mom had a tremendous support system with my Great-Grandmother Vater Perkins and Grandmother Mary Liza Kee, who, together, instinctively created a nurturing family and faith-filled ecosystem for me and my siblings. At the same time, she worked to provide for all of us. She was the most loyal and compassionate woman I know; she was dedicated and had worked the same job for 40 years. She was living proof that circumstances never dictate the outcome of one's destiny! She encouraged me to participate in pageants and serve as President of my class in both high school and college. She instilled in me that I could be anything I wanted to become, which truly shaped who I am today. When it was time for me to get married, my Uncle James walked me down the aisle. Although my mom and dad divorced when I was young, God interceded through my Grandmother Tomcena Clark, Aunt Erma, and Aunt Sadie to eventually reunite me with my dad—witnessing the miracle of him becoming a Bishop. I was afforded the gift by God to hold his hand on the day he transitioned from this earth. His final loving words to me were, "You will always be my daughter!"

My professional destiny became first as a teen, where I would emulate Oprah Winfrey and Phil Donahue. I would sit in front of the television and read the closed captioning out loud. Everything that Oprah Winfrey would say, I would say it as if I was *literally* her. I was just playfully acting out in jest; I had no idea that as time progressed, I would become an actual Talk Show Host! My first audition was at the former Praise the Lord Studio of Jim and Tammy Faye Bakker. It was called 'Daily Balance' with Kim Jacobs and aired on PBS™ and on The Word Network™. So honored to interview household names as guests like Dr. Les Brown, Dominique Wilkins, Emmitt Smith, Pat Smith, George Fraser, Mother Love, Ralph Sampson, Humpy Wheeler, and many names we may not know, but they too are everyday heroes. The Balance Doctor™ became 'my brand' as I helped countless people find harmony in their own lives. Part of my gifting expanded to formally teach business owners, motivational speakers, authors, and entrepreneurs. It was called 'How to Start a Show from Scratch' www.Kimjacobsconsulting.com.

I meet with them one-on-one virtually and help them create an actual show from ground zero. They own their own content and rights, and I get the uplighting and continuous reward. *Who knew? God knew!*

Who knew that I would be God's vehicle to inspire mothers? Someone who was told I couldn't bear children is now the founder of 'The Mother Dreamer Movement'™ www.Motherdreamer.com/join. What a blessing to encourage, and inspire Mothers to dust off their dreams and goals that are sitting on the back burner and make those dreams a reality! Some members are not physical Mothers but are birthing their dreams to share in the connected thread of love and vision by joining the movement.

Who knew that I would be appointed as the Managing Director for a 500,000-member women business entrepreneur group called eWomen Network? The founder, Sandra Yancey, is a CNN Hero and a masterful business leader. I had been a member for over 15 years and didn't even know I could be considered for this special role. *Who knew? God knew!*

Who knew I would lead God's people for over 20 years in a leadership role? I don't take for granted that I am assigned to lead people to Christ and help them decide where they will spend eternity. Me, an ambassador for Christ! A little girl from the projects that many people didn't believe would achieve much based on my circumstances. *Who knew? God knew!*

> *"For I know the thoughts that I think toward you, saith the Lord, thoughts of peace, and not evil, to give you an expected end."*
>
> —Jeremiah 29: 11 (KJV)

I am so grateful that God trusts me enough to possibly be the only Bible that some people may ever read. I am humbled and honored to be bestowed with this mantle.

From the T.V. impersonation, I was confident that I would impact the masses, but I was surprised to find out which vehicle it would take place in.

While in my twenties, with a budding career in pharmaceutical sales, I heard one of the most profound speakers I've ever encountered in my entire life, Les Brown. This Icon commanded the stage, and he talked about how: "*I* was necessary, how *I* was possible, how *I* was going to make a difference on this earth. I felt like he was presenting to an audience of **one—me**! I waited patiently backstage after that presentation and conversed with this gentleman only to learn that he was about to embark on a National Tour teaching people 'How to Start a Seminar Business.' His mission would focus on pulling out the greatness in people by teaching them how to share their stories to earn money. He allowed me to spend the entire day with him and his team to learn more about his vision. From the one-day encounter, I was allowed to be mentored by *THE Dr. Les Brown*! I traveled the Country with him and spoke before thousands of people, teaching them his famous quote: 'You've Got to be Hungry!" We literally impacted the Masses! *Who knew? God knew!*

I have experienced tragedies in life that I wouldn't wish on anyone else. I couldn't predict some of those outcomes: I *never* saw it coming until it happened. Some things could have ended horribly for me and would have changed everything for my family. I am thankful that God spared me and allowed me to continue and always has gone before me on this journey called life.

My personal essence of a woman's testimony is that I have decided that nothing will separate me from the love of Christ! Romans 8:38–39 sums it up best for me:

"For I am persuaded, that neither death, nor life, nor angels, nor principalities, nor powers, nor things present, nor things to come, Nor height, nor depth, nor any other creature shall be able to separate us from the love of God, which is in Christ Jesus our Lord."

Just as we all do, you will experience trials and tribulations; don't get discouraged to the point where you give up or quit on life. God needs you to use your gifts and talents to salt His Creation Earth. If you haven't heard these words recently, experience my family's mantra for yourself now:

'You are valuable! You are needed! The world is a better place because you are in it! No one else can do what you are assigned to do! You are important. You are fearfully and wonderfully made by God. You are somebody in Christ. The Whole World will miss out if you don't use your gift!'

Even when you don't know, your doctor doesn't know, your family or friends don't know! God knows all! He loves you, and He wants the very best for you! *Don't give up on Him because he will never give up on you!*

God has special blessings in store for you. Hold on and hold fast so they become a reality.

In fact, it is clear what you can expect:

> *"Yes indeed, it won't be long now."*
>
> —Amos 9:13–15

Belief:

This is God's Decree. Things are going to happen so fast your head will swim, one thing fast on the heels of the other. You won't be able to keep up! Everything will snowball all at once—and *everywhere* you look, blessings! Blessings like wine pouring off the mountains and hills. I'll make everything right again for my people, Israel:

> *"They'll rebuild their ruined cities.*
> *They'll plant vineyards and drink good wine.*
> *They'll work in their gardens and eat fresh vegetables.*
> *And I'll plant them, plant them on their own land.*
> *They'll never again be uprooted from the land I've given them."*
>
> —Amos 9:13–15

Why? Because God, your God, says so.

Get your mind right to be the vessel, and know that it won't be long now; your blessings are right around the corner.

Who knew? God Knew! He *knows* for each of us.

Action Steps from the Balance Doctor:
- Keep your eye on your Eternal Prize of Salvation.
- Look for the blessing in every adversity.
- Remain a humble servant with your giftedness.

Kim Jacobs, MBA, BD (Balance Doctor)
Host of The Kim Jacobs Show
Founder, Gabe's Heart Foundation
www.kimjacobsconsulting.com
www.gabesheartfoundation.org
kimjacobs@ewomennetwork.com

Deborah Dennis

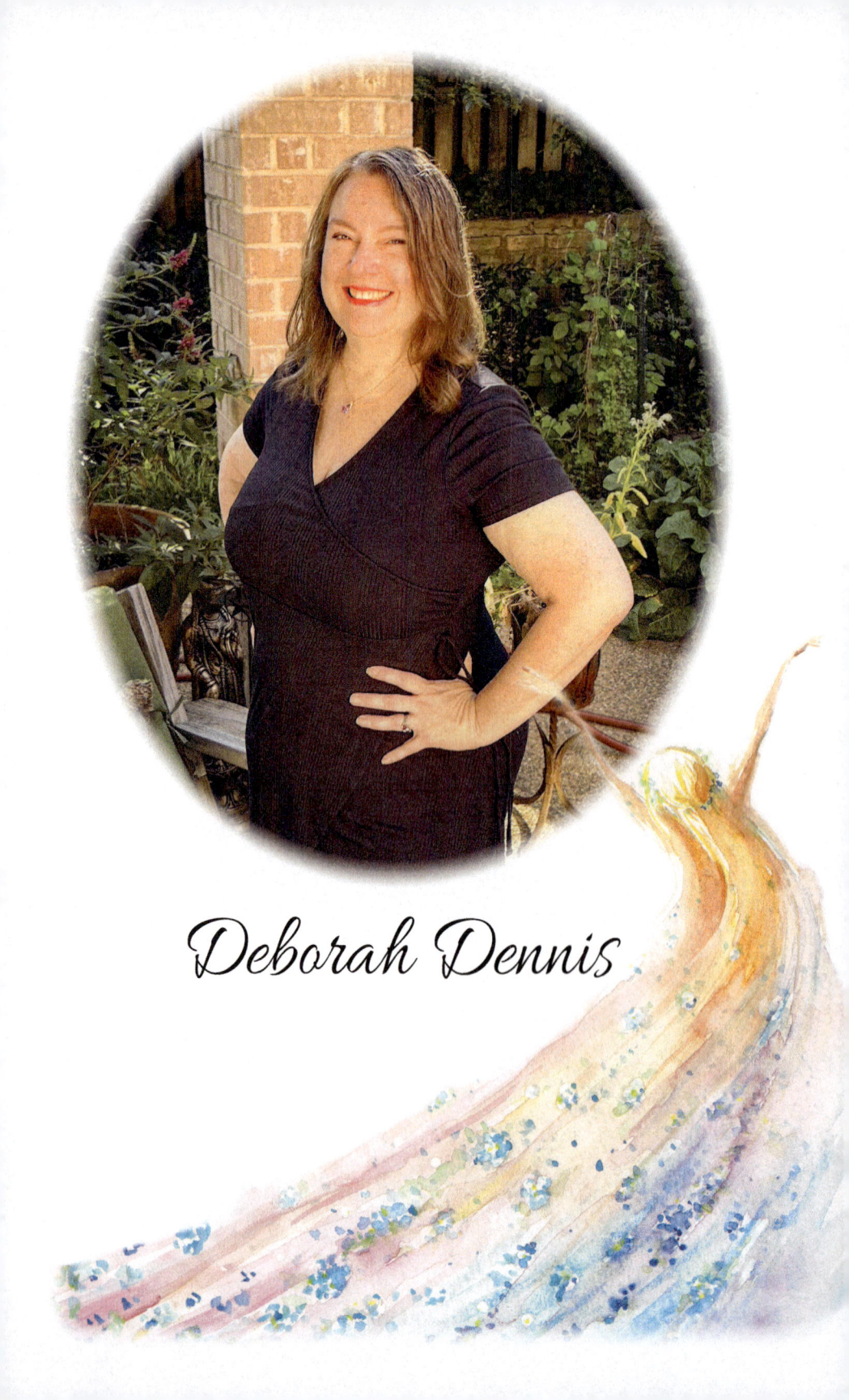

Parenting Xtra-Growth Families

"The artful expression of love is a human life."

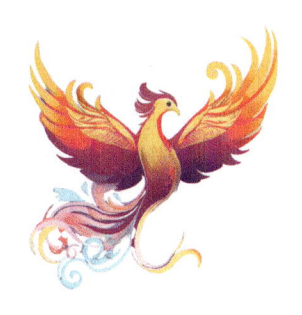

Intention:

Parenting, mothering, is an artful expression. When a child is born, divine purposes collide. The uniqueness of the disposition of each child is a reflection of their soulful desire. Recognizing and harmonizing with each child's individuality can guide a parent's choices.

Story:

On the North Sea of Scotland, my parents had me. Romantic stories of castles, lavender fields, sheep, and quaint bungalows in the distance as you gaze almost anywhere, all that amazing history is where I started. They love telling me about it. We moved to Rochester, New York when I was two. At age nine we moved to Orlando, Florida enjoying all the visitors that naturally came. Eventually, I settled in Texas at age 15. We followed my patent-laden father's illustrious career in the telecommunications industry. My mom was by his side. I love to say that I come from a long line of mothers who have had little girls. It makes me think of just how special life is, and how we take turns being so innocent and then so responsible.

I met David at the University of North Texas. I graduated and started my career in Technical Recruiting in 1990. By December that year we were married. We told everyone, as they were asking, that we planned to wait 10 years to have kids. We did! We welcomed our Year 2000 Golden Dragon Baby, a beautiful girl, and the three of us started off on the most magnificent odyssey.

Oh boy did this dragon baby roar!! As I was pregnant with her, I drove to work with the top down, music blaring. We did not realize, then, how easy it is for a developing baby to hear. As we gained so much more knowledge than we knew was possible to apply, it dawned on us how successful we were when we noticed and played along with what each baby was observing moment by moment.

I am so excited to introduce the unique individuals that came to David and me. Yes, they chose us. They knew our personalities and what they would face from us and our bloodline, so naturally, I have confidence they are strong enough to handle whatever comes their way as they mature.

First came the forward-facing "Swivel Head" Baby that demanded to be held in front of your body facing out, and her head steadily went right to left, right to left. When she was hungry and when she wanted anything at all we were met with a huge intake of air. The air was sucked in with as many breaths as needed, up to seven inhales without exhaling. The air was to develop a scream that could rattle glass! We accommodated this baby, an enormously powerful creature.

Today, she continues to command respect. She was a 10 out of 10 in every way. We met her with love, thus allowing her to soften. We were amused. Everyone was. She had 20 lemon wedges brought to her by waiters happy to do so, and she had command of even the colors she wore. Pink was a no, the inhales started if I went for any pink outfit. She recently married her high school orchestra stand partner. She graduated from SMU and is solid in the medical industry. We are immensely proud parents watching her move from our odyssey into a new one with her husband, Joshua.

Next came the "Seagull Crier" Baby, a glowing bright happy all the time serene baby. She was both aloof and easygoing with a cry that sounded like a seagull flying over the ocean docks. No surprise, I listened to ocean sounds to soothe my morning sickness. This baby did not have all the blaring music because the louder baby was sleeping.

A huge inner world with characters developed for these two babies. Two years apart, together they found an imaginary friend, a bear named Farrar, at the Peabody Hotel in Memphis. Farrar stayed with them for three years; I read to him too. Fairy wands, still to this day, come from magnolia tree blooms. Everything spoke to these two—trees, clouds, flowers, especially snapdragons. They are responsible for the branding of snapdragons on our XtraGrow product.

The Seagull Crier Baby was found to have a speech delay that we vanquished just in time to see dyslexia keep her on the same reading level for years. With much work, she adapted to complete advanced placement classes and got into college. She did not want to stay there. She left after the first year to our surprise and concern. Within a short time, she became a full-time artist with her own distinctive wow factor. I do believe she is going to be famous—she sort of already is in Denton! She personifies the most chaos that I have ever known. Even with this, she is a gifted visionary conscious of even the most minute components of what she sees as if she has a thousand eyes herself. Her following is joyfully taking her work in and sharing it as a part of themselves.

Our third baby is the "Pure Love" Baby. He is everything Corinthians 13 commands of what love is and is not. He could patiently smile at the grouchiest person in the room until they smiled back. A playground bully hit him in the head with one of those old birdhouses on a pole when he was five years old. Tragically, he was not his normal self afterward. He was under disciplinary circumstances every day at school and the topic of many families' dinner conversations. As we chased down possible therapies and guidance for his traumatic brain injury, nothing official could be determined. They said possible ADHD and put in accommodations for that at school. By 6th grade, he was still enigmatic to teachers. Resisting advice to drug him, we were steadfast in our determination to do our best for him when he discovered his athletic body and musical ear. Success became his as he lovingly shares his gifts with others. He plays piano as if the famous Rachmaninoff is under his hat. He sings and plays the guitar. He did not want lessons, he wanted to teach himself. We also watch him smile and be friendly during wrestling matches. His coach said that he could make a more menacing facial expression, but like the rest of us, Coach must sit back and watch this boy be his charming self.

This brings me to the quintessential tiny baby, the "Hide Me" baby. She was deeply and fully fine until someone outside the immediate family approached. As this often happened, she would attempt to go down my shirt or squish into my shoulder or leg with all her mighty strength. Very introverted, she found it easy to charm others and have a small circle of friends once she started kindergarten. Always on the underdog cheering team, she is also an artist and excellent writer. Her own world developed fast as she spent hours reading and drawing, refusing ballet and swim team, and doing everything with the older kids and their friends. It was as if she preferred mature company, but silly antics are her favorite. She gets every joke.

She was diagnosed with Juvenile Diabetes, also known as Type One Diabetes, at 18 months of age. Every day we manage her blood sugar, one meal and one snack at a time. We do not panic. Early on, I decided to join a support group. I was given much sympathy. This showed me that I could not allow this disease to become an identity for us, we are not victims of it, we are managing it. It is something to manage just as many other things are managed. She is so much more than all the extra details that go into her care. As a new teenager, she is committed to healing herself. We are incredibly proud of her as she takes the reins more and more. She will change the world! She is there for any child that needs a hand. She is so kind, so fair, and unafraid to bring things up that are on her mind or could benefit another person.

Belief:

XtraGrow is one of the companies our kids participated in. They witnessed experiments, helped with packaging, listened to thousands and thousands of phone calls, and grabbed faxed-in lab reports from the plant in Nebraska. They watched us speak to groups about regenerative agriculture. People would visit our home, even live with us for a time. They have met the most interesting people and have been told how our product helps the world in richly fundamental ways, ways that fit into what they really care about.

As these cool people were around my kids, they said my kids were fortunate to have parents like us. People respect others by the value they have. If you are authentic, your value is obvious, and people treat you in the way they see you. It is validation and a happy way of being in this world that fosters creativity. Others like you see you and bond with you in a safe way. Loneliness is not even something that makes sense as a concept to you. This alone hedges off some of the main challenges of modern parenting.

The boundaries you set in caution and love and how you move within your world gift your children their values. Never take the word of an authority figure over your child; this is not wise under any circumstance. As you take personal responsibility and are accountable for your choices as a parent, you thrive as a parent!

Have your home be the social go-to haven. Volunteer where they participate, read what they read, shop and cook together, share in mundane chores together, and try new adventures. Be involved in letting them have their own time by simply knowing where they are and who they are with.

Bad influencers are something that can be misconstrued. The most challenging thing that ever happened to us as parents was when a family member told their kids that ours were the bad influencers. So ashamed, one of our kids subsequently ran away. Their note said we would be better off without them. In shock, David and I eventually called the police; it was getting dark, thank goodness they found our child! Asking for help is okay, even if there are consequences. It took us a while to piece everything together. It is so very important not to judge or hold a grudge that divides. All is merely unfolding in front of you for a reason. When parents try to be good parents, they often put a lot of weight on what they don't want. Some parents lose confidence because of an ex-spouse, drugs, drinking, mental issues, infighting, self-harm, or mistakes made. The list is a long one, but whatever the story, it is a story. When a parent repeats the story of "why we do not" it goes on forever until you stand up to it in love. Sounds like parents are being called to be Christ-like. Or, what would Jesus do? He did talk about other people, but He forgave them. He warned and allowed some things to happen for the sake of what the people are learning.

Every one of us has ancestors with every behavior and communication style that ever was. If we can identify what we don't want, we can identify what we do want. A startling story happened when I was a baby. My mother's older sister attempted to get a divorce in "the old days." My grandparents were having a New Year's Eve party back in New York. My aunt attended with her two sons and her violent husband appeared. She managed to shove their kids into a closet, and they survived, but several people did not. This man who was so consistently a threat to those around him arrived intent on killing my Aunt, and he did. My mom lived with survivor's guilt and needed much comfort. I was a small baby when this tragedy occurred, and it really did affect our relationship and how I became the woman I am today.

The venues of energy around the positive are vast. A lot can get done when you do what you want to do. You don't get stuck in quicksand, like you would if you were actively avoiding or allowing interference to dominate over what is coming into your life; especially in the parental role where it is not just you that such choices affect. What is intended for you is to be happy and able to create a true home.

Kids are innocent even if they look guilty. They are confident looking because youth is beautiful. They do not know what they do not know, and you might not want to tell them yet as you stand between them and harm, until they are ready. Deciding what is harmful is part of the wisdom you gain. Say "no" on matters that could affect their future readiness to do what they love. There is no need to ensure that they intellectually understand everything, we want them to figure stuff out for themselves in their own time. Provide the tools, resources, and a well-balanced presence in their lives.

Remember the relationship between me and my mother? One of the most poignant things I recall is how incredibly protective she was regarding dating and being around guys in general. It is not that she was strict, she was reliving the tragedy of my Aunt when I was a baby. I still hear her words resonating as she warned about how easy it is to attract and how hard it could be to get out of a relationship. Being a force for good and positive global change, Hermine Tobolowsky, the mother of the Texas Equal Rights Amendment, lived and worked in Dallas. I was honored to work by her side, in her home even, on anti-stalking legislation that would have helped my Aunt. Women's rights was her child, and the dream was for all of us to have the ability to care for ourselves as empowered and capable individuals. This became a pivotal archetype for me as a mother and in business. People must realize that they are their own highest connection, free to choose everyday for their own good and well being.

Everyone is a genius at something. It is safe to be around someone who has more skill than you. Celebrate their art: you will get prolific kids! And by all means, be mindful of music; it could set the whole tone for their adorable baby personality and their future greatness!

Action Steps:
- *Be truly yourself:* kids can tell.
- *Be firm:* so they trust you.
- *Be involved:* for an amazing relationship.
- *Protect them:* for their future.
- *Include them:* so they are competent.

Deborah Dennis
XtraGrow, LLC
Deborah@XtraGrow.com
Deborah@XtraGrowFoundation.org

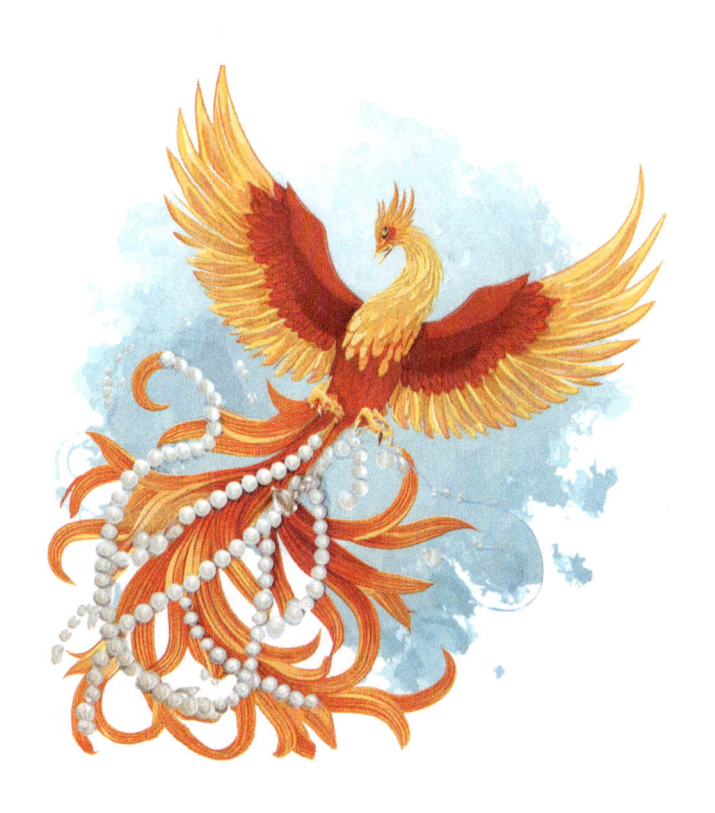

Cristina Candullo-Dody

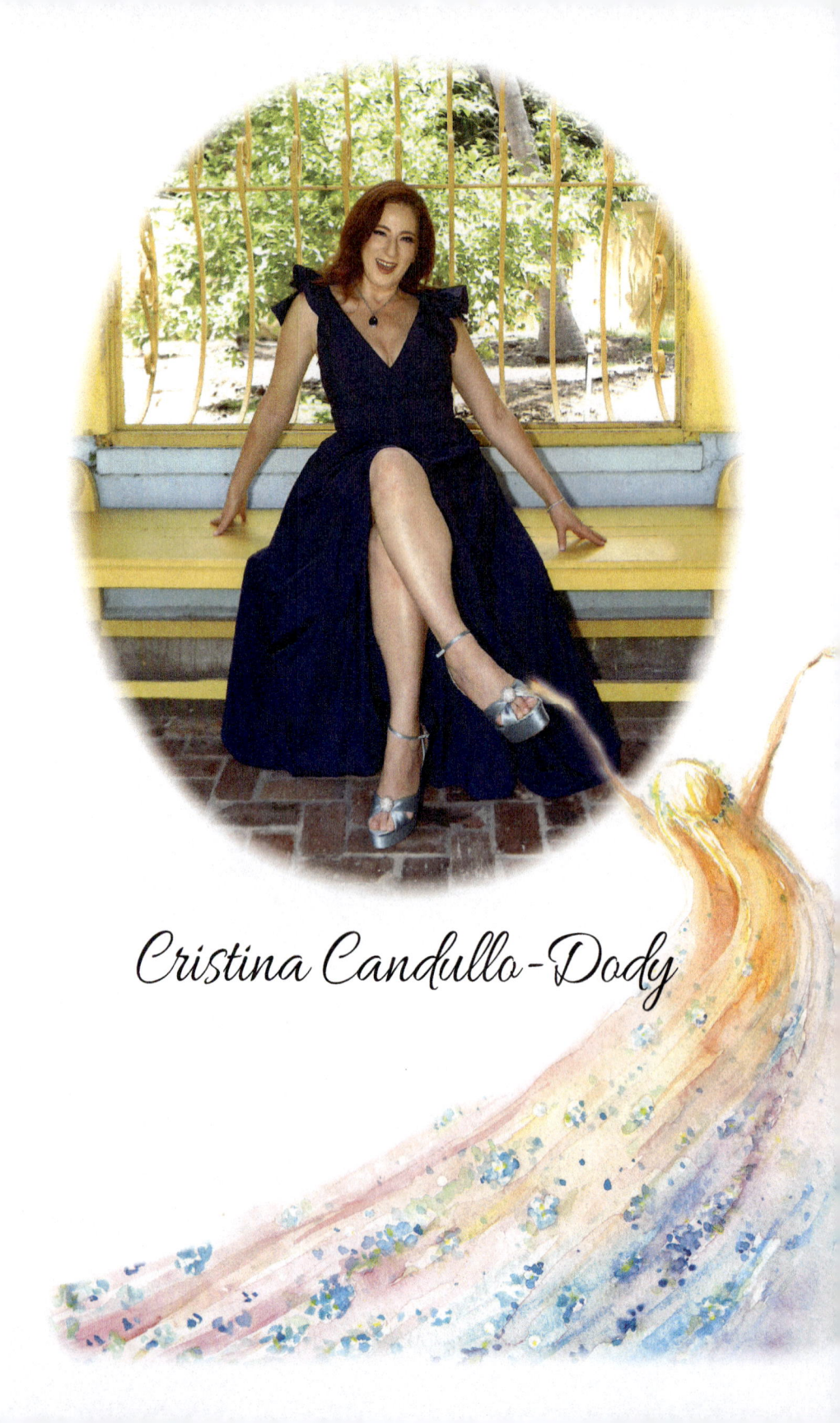

The Loyalty of Love

*"Love: A manifestation in your mind—
becomes your reality."*

Intention:

Know that hope is eternal and in every situation in life it is only temporary. The true essence of a woman is someone who reaches out for help and support. It is crucial to true empowerment. From being socially awkward to becoming a social butterfly—was a choice. In the same way, may you experience this testament of manifestation in the power of resilience and love.

Story:

Born into a large traditional Italian family, it's no wonder they call me *"Momma Tina"* when I make a vat of sauce to feed an army when I cook! I am the oldest of seven siblings, born in Brooklyn and raised in Staten Island, New York. I never remember a time when my mother wasn't pregnant, and I spent the majority of my childhood babysitting siblings.

We moved from Brooklyn to Staten Island when I was two, but we visited Brooklyn every weekend for Sunday dinner to be a part of our larger family, which included my grandparents. A Quintessential Tradition was an Italian Dinner complete with mouthwatering marinara sauce on Sunday with the whole family. I can still smell that sauce! Sunday was considered our family day.

I was a bright student academically but socially awkward. With six brothers and sisters of various ages, I was forced to be responsible, and quiet, forced to quickly mature. Despite the close-knit nature of my family, unfortunately, we weren't shown a lot of affection as children—which left me feeling somewhat internally troubled, shy, and silent—often feeling alone and by myself. I was the victim of fellow student abuse and bullied badly because of my social awkwardness, always yearning for my voice to be heard. In a big family, it was easy to feel overlooked, and I developed a habit of repeating myself until someone finally responded, thinking they just must *not* have heard me the first time. The bullying was so vicious and cruel, that it made me believe that I was unattractive, annoying, and disposable socially.

I remember sitting with my head down, my arms crossed, and my hair hiding my face—pretty much all the time. Why? Because I felt ugly, and invisible, and wanted to hide. Ugly was not something I was born with—it was something I learned from the words that were said and reverberated to me over and over again. Despite that horrible bullying, I still excelled in school. I was the brainy girl, a science nerd who wanted to be an astronomer, actually attending two schools at once. My high school specialized in accelerated learning whereby I was able to even begin college while still in high school. When we moved to New Jersey, things changed dramatically. I was awarded a reprieve from my previous peer labeling and reputation, for a fresh *new* start! Late in my junior year, I moved to a new school where nobody knew me. I wanted to make friends, something I struggled with in Staten Island, only being accepted by a few close friends. Now I could manifest more in my social circle—something very sweet for this 16-year-old young girl.

In my new school, I hid my intelligence to fit in, putting more emphasis on my social life, which had me neglecting my academics a bit. I played with make-up and began feeling pretty at last. And it was *fun*! My new persona even manifested something new in my academic vista. I started an astronomy club, carving out a new academic comfort zone. I expanded my social horizons by joining the color guard and getting a summer job while school was out. The wings of the new social butterfly fluttered around my work at a theme park. Who knew I'd spend my leisure time as an adult at Walt Disney World? This monumental move helped me become more confident and proficient. I was happy to have a new beginning and learned important social skills—navigating teenage life.

Coincidentally, I saw a girl in my new high school, who I knew from Staten Island, who reconnected with me, becoming fast best friends. We planned to go to the Prom together that spring because my strict parents wouldn't let me go with a boy. My friend convinced my parents with the ultimate sales pitch that there was nothing to fear or worry about, assuring them we'd just have a good time, and come home safely.

However, she ended up canceling with me to go with a boy at the last minute, leaving me heartbroken and feeling ditched again. Little did I know that Anthony, who would become my future husband, was at that Prom that night. Ironically, The Prom was the catalyst that brought us together—even though I wasn't even there. He ended up being a blind date for his friend's friend. I didn't even know the girl that he went with: true unconscious manifestation in action! With another twist of fate, I ended up becoming friends with Anthony's date, after we graduated, through our mutual job.

Years later, I was out with my sisters and girlfriends, including this work friend, who had been Anthony's Prom date. As silly girls can sometimes do, on a whim, she began to call people she hadn't spoken to in a long time, including *that guy* who was her Prom date. I attracted my husband through a prank call orchestrated by a mutual friend and a one-time Prom date. After he finally figured out who was calling him, he was eventually put on the phone with one of my many sisters, then me. However, I, the eldest sister, commanded the cell phone waves on this destined night. It was funny—when it was my turn to talk to him, magic happened as if we had known each other for years. We talked incessantly! We had so much in common that we finally exchanged numbers. I never thought he would actually ever call me, though. In those days, not everyone had a cell phone, and he was one of those who didn't. So, he wrote my number on a piece of scrap paper. It was a miracle he still had it weeks later when he called me.

Just a typical Saturday work day, I experienced one of the most harrowing and traumatic days of my life—I got *Held Up*—at gunpoint working at my bank! I spent the entire day being interviewed by the FBI and went home exhausted, collapsing in bed. Wouldn't you know it! That was the day and time Anthony decided to call. I calmly told him about the events of the day. It was the first time he called me, and naturally, he thought I was blowing him off, where he must have pondered to himself, "Was that *the* best blow-me-off excuse ever?" Saying to himself, "Now I've heard it all." Despite that, he hesitantly called me again two weeks later. Once again, he found that same scrap of paper where he wrote my number. That fateful get reacquainted call was where we connected and lasted hours. Our destiny for 'our journey to forever' was etched in stone.

Anthony and I were an hour and a half apart during our early relationship. Those strict Italian parents who forbid me to go to the Prom with a boy were the incredibly fearful parents—especially my mother—who made us resort to hiding our relationship initially. Our time from '*like to love*' was our version of Romeo and Juliet. Despite the challenges, Anthony further helped me gain the confidence to grow socially and blossom as a woman. He was my first real boyfriend and made me feel like no one ever had, beautiful and confident. My true essence as a woman emerged and was born. With my newfound and empowered version of myself, I started my first company: The Shoe Society. I wanted to help other women feel as poised and beautiful as I did, since my transformation from nerd to social butterfly. My company ran events that felt more like parties, where I would have contestants walk a pink carpet for 'Best in Shoe.' It was so exhilarating because our events almost always benefited a non-profit—backing a good cause. This is where I got my start planning events, which I put to instant use when we got engaged.

Manifestation to Reality 1.0! Everything I had planned for my wedding as a teenager came true, from the dress to the horse and carriage. I planned it all myself and just about everything I had on my wedding vision board came to reality, down to the location. I even got to meet my dream wedding dress designer. I discovered when I have a vision that I want to create, I cannot and will not settle. Everything I wanted was brought forth to reality. It was a bride's dream come true—such a wonderful day in our lives. Manifestation and my marri*age have created our own Disney "Magic Kingdom."*

Life was Wonderful! We faced the usual newlywed couple getting to know each other while adapting to everyday life and acclimation. Until one fateful day, Anthony got in a car accident at work. He was rear-ended hard. The woman driving wasn't paying attention and hit him while he was waiting at a light. The impact was so intense, that she took off the entire driver's side back corner of the car. She was in a big SUV and he was in a tiny little compact car the company had given him. When I got the news that my dearest husband was in a car wreck, I broke into a million pieces as well. Unfortunately, that was just the tip of the iceberg. What should have been a quick recovery turned into a long-term severe ordeal.

Anthony was diagnosed with a concussion, which we were told should get better on its own. Unfortunately, it did not and the doctor that he was assigned to was devoid of answers. Two weeks after the accident, we were playing miniature golf with the family and Anthony went to the public restroom. A stranger who was in there as well sought us out and admonished us to get him help. His father attended to him whereby Anthony began to projectile vomit everywhere. We called an ambulance, and from the very beginning, the treatment he received was deplorable. Due to mistakes by the hospitals, incorrect notes, tainted opinions, and just outright lying, the medical system could not help my husband. In fact, they made him worse. Through our own trials and struggles, we were forced to look outside the traditional medical system for answers. I continued to work, and at the same time thrust into being a caretaker.

I lived the purest form of loyalty in love as I circumvented the myriad challenges that occurred from Anthony's injuries. A concussion turned into what is called "Post Concussion Syndrome"—something hard to diagnose and something many doctors don't understand. It changed his personality. Many other obstacles and health challenges mounted and continued to arise from just a minor car accident. Luckily during this time my job, in the telecommunications industry, was stable and my bosses were understanding. I continued working at the same company, eventually earning a promotion that allowed us to move to Florida, which we both concluded would be better for the medical challenges he faced.

If that plate wasn't full enough, it grew to the size of a Turkey Platter, when I decided to go back to school. I knew that if I wanted to be a good candidate for a promotion, I had to go back to college. I chose Penn State for its clout, prestige, and quality education. Looking for support, this now adept professional communicator and manager in a tele-communications company, realized there were no sororities for online students. Always desiring a better way, I was inspired by my previous experience starting an astronomy club. I pondered, "Why not create a virtual sorority?" This was a unique and novel social experiment. Coincidentally, in 2019 a girl named Jona Hall reached out to me via email about starting a virtual sorority with philanthropy to fight against human trafficking. I felt this Manifestation 2.0 was my calling. I was shocked at how quickly my thoughts became reality with my strong sense of justice through philanthropy in anti-human trafficking. We kicked into action and I became an officer—Zeta Mu Phi's first Treasure and Executive Board member to build the organization, and expand to multiple schools. We support women in love in multiple ways, and I treasure my contribution to making my mark on this sorority.

Belief:

We are all born with an innate ability to envision and execute a plan. For me, this was a gift that I was born with. In addition to my wedding and the sorority, I have witnessed knighting ceremonies three times, and I have had the knowing that I would one day have the opportunity to plan one myself. That opportunity came when I was asked to plan the first knighting ceremony in Florida—a huge privilege—Manifestation 3.0! This propelled me to start my next company, Cristina Candullo Events.

We have now recently expanded our first Zeta Mu Phi Gala in Las Vegas for our sorority, to support 'Illuminate,' a nonprofit to combat anti-trafficking. When we started our sorority, it was paramount to include the philanthropic focus. Throughout the challenges that Anthony and I have faced together, we have always believed that giving back is a constant for abundance and reciprocity. I am always thankful for my strong values of loyalty and justice, instilled by my parents, which drive me to help those in need.

You, as a woman, can create the life you want and whatever you visualize within your mind can turn dreams into reality. It is essential that when you get to a place of power it is your responsibility to empower others. No matter where you start, you can visualize and spread your wings of a Phoenix to fly where you want to go and be—and then help others do the same. Unleash your feminine soul and lead with love, even in the most challenging situations—it's only temporary. Have empathy within the loyalty of love.

Action Steps for Manifestation:
- Visualize what it is you want specifically.
- Write it down and create a vision board to visualize it.

- Feel the feeling you would feel as though it is already done.
- Take action steps to move toward the goal that you are trying to manifest.
- Step into opportunities—even when you don't feel confident.

Cristina Candullo-Dody
www.cristinacandulloevents.com
www.zetamuphi.com
www.illuminateltw.org

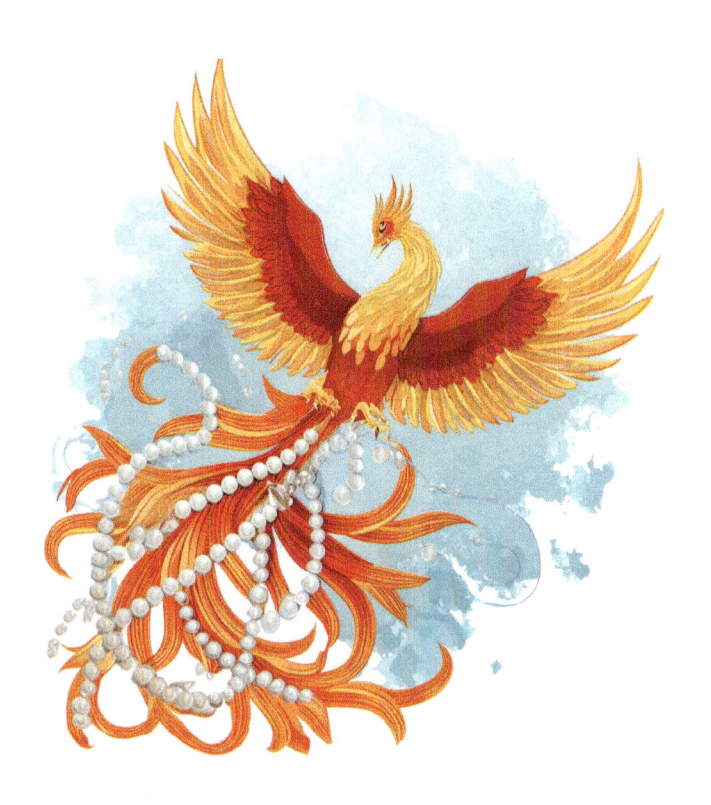

HRH Princess
Dr. Moradeun Ogunlana

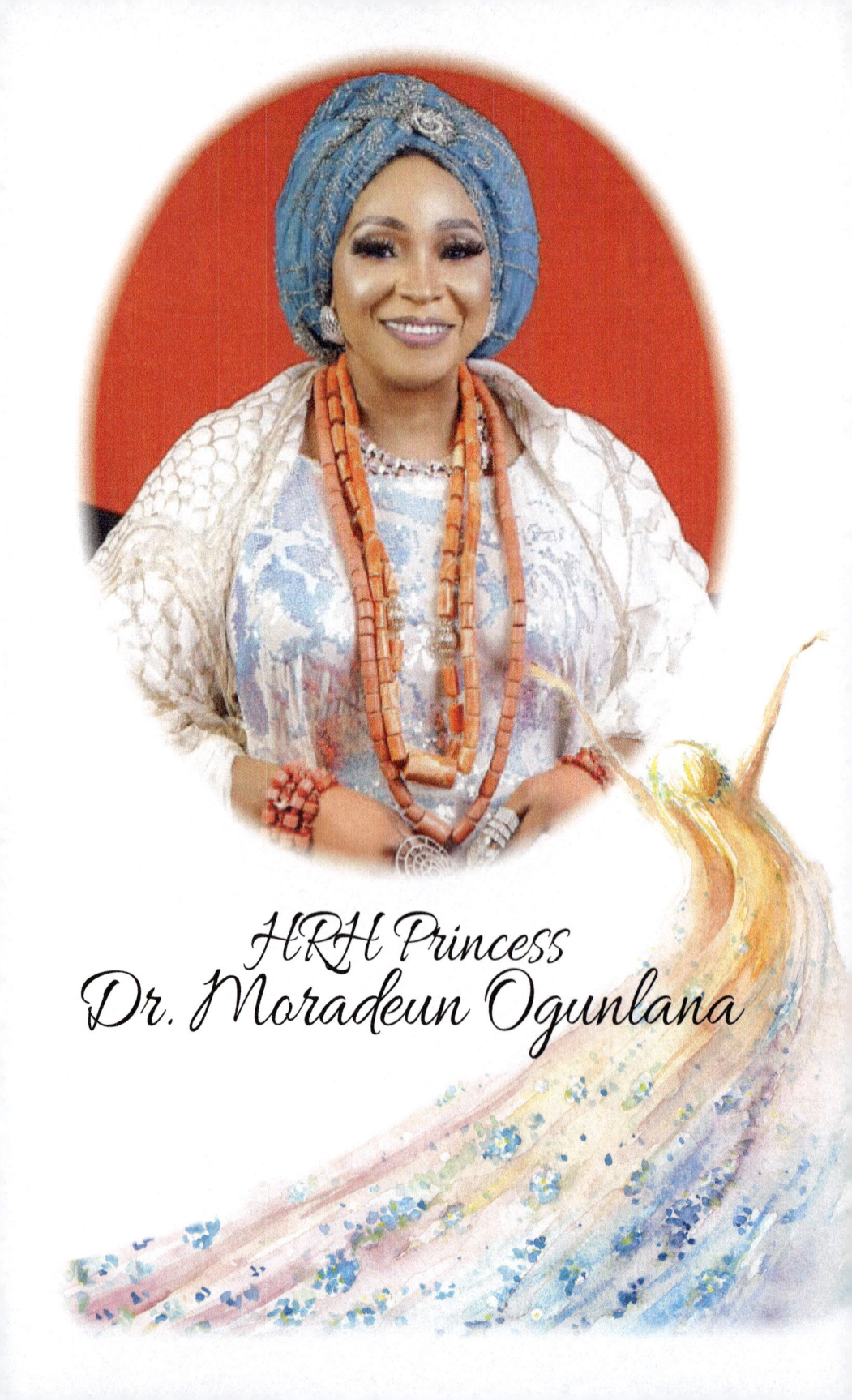

The All-Empowered Woman

*"A woman is not just the whispers of her soul,
but the elegant grace that echoes through eternity."*

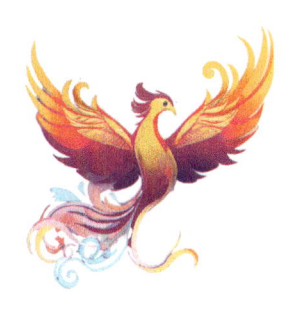

Intention:

The Essence of a Woman is a profound and intricate tapestry, woven from the threads of her power, voice, impact, and influence. It is the culmination of her experiences, values, strengths, and passions which converge to form a unique and dynamic force. This essence is not something external, but rather an inner radiance that illuminates her path, guides her decisions, and inspires her actions.

For centuries, women's essence has been shrouded in mystery, misconceptions, and societal expectations. Yet, as we embark on this journey of discovery, we find that the essence of a woman is not something to be defined by others, but rather something she must uncover for herself.

Through the exploration of her power, voice, impact, and influence, a woman comes to understand her true nature, her deepest desires, and her highest potential. She learns to embrace her authenticity, celebrate her individuality, and unleash her inner strength. In this journey of self-discovery, we invite you to join us as we delve into the essence of a woman. Let us uncover the hidden treasures, confront the challenges, and unleash the full potential of what it means to be a woman.

Story:

Even as a Royal, I remember the day I discovered my essence as a woman. I was in my early twenties, struggling to find my place in the world. I felt lost and uncertain, like a leaf blown about by the winds of expectation. But then something shifted. I began to explore my passions, my values, and my strengths. I started to listen to my own voice, to trust my own instincts.

And slowly but surely, I began to uncover my power. I realized that my essence as a woman was not about conforming to societal norms or meeting others' expectations. It was about embracing my uniqueness, my creativity, and my resilience. It was about finding my own voice and using it to make a difference.

As I continued this journey of self-discovery and personal unfolding as a woman, I encountered many challenges. I faced self-doubt, fear, and uncertainty. But I also discovered a deep well of strength, courage, and determination within myself.

Today, I know that my essence as a woman is not just about me. It's about the collective power of women everywhere—truly a global movement of embracing your heritage as much as positively projecting your future. As I humbly trace my lineage back to two esteemed Royal Families in West Africa—a noble heritage is rooted in the ancient Kingdom of Lagos, Nigeria, and the Royal House of the Republic of Benin. As the granddaughter of the revered His Royal Majesty, David Ajasa Ogunlana, the 10th Obanikoro of Lagos, their collective sovereignty expanded over six decades. Significant developments in infrastructure, education, and healthcare have imprinted a lasting legacy in Lagos. Further embracing my ancestry, I am the great-granddaughter of His Royal Majesty, King (Oba) Liyangu Owabagbe Adenuga, the ninth ruling Akarigbo of Remo Kingdom Sagamu in Ogun State, Nigeria. Remo land was initially settled, Oba Liyangu's leadership was marked by wisdom, courage, and a deep commitment to his people. In addition, my beloved uncle was the late King (Oba) Adeyinka Oyekan, the King of Lagos. He was also a respected leader and a symbol of unity and progress for the people of Lagos.

I transcended my global heritage with me across the Atlantic Ocean as a teenager, first to Chicago, Illinois. We finally made our American home in Little Rock, Arkansas where I attended college at the University of Arkansas. Presently, when I am in America, I volley between Houston, Texas and New York City. I am a woman of the World. I thankfully credit the empowered visionary men throughout my heritage that live through my genes and vision to this day. My Global Empowerment Mission has been manifested into the world by the ways to support, uplift, and empower each other. It's about the ways in which we challenge systems of oppression and create a more just and equitable world.

My essence as a woman is a work in progress—one of continuous growth, exploration, and transformation. As I elevate and continually evolve, I am at peace, knowing that I am not alone. I am part of a larger community of women who are discovering their own essence, their own power, and their own voice. Together, as a heart centered and mission driven collective, we are unstoppable.

There is a profound and empowering framework for women's personal and collective growth. It's a holistic and foundational approach that encompasses *four key* aspects:

- **Discovering Our Power:** Identifying sources of power, navigating fears and obstacles, and unlocking potential.
- **Discovering Our Voice:** Exploring voice from a feminist perspective, developing voice as a tool for communication and advocacy, and refining voice to reflect identity and personality.
- **Discovering Our Impact:** Defining impact, planning actions to achieve goals, and measuring positive difference made in the world.
- **Redefining Power and Influence:** Periodically reassessing and adapting power and voice to respond to changing needs, opportunities, and challenges.

This framework has encouraged me, even as a young girl growing up in Nigeria to this present day. When we ask women to embrace her strengths and passions, we develop our unique voice and communication giftedness. By unearthing our individual uniqueness, we can positively impact our social influence in our world to expand this relevance globally, adapt and pivot to new circumstances, and perpetually elevate our influence.

Belief:

The journey to uncovering the Essence of a Woman begins with a fundamental question: *What is my Power?* For too long, women's power has been defined by societal expectations, cultural norms, and patriarchal structures. But what if I told you that your true power lies within?

I would like for us to shatter the illusions of external validation and embrace the authentic, unbridled power that has been waiting to be unleashed by exploring and reevaluating what is truly the essence of the woman.

Discovering a Woman's Power

The essence of a woman lies in her power to discover her own power.

This journey of self-discovery is the foundation of personal growth, empowerment, and transformation. It involves identifying and embracing her sources of power, such as values, beliefs, strengths, passions, talents, skills, knowledge, experiences, relationships, and resources.

A woman's values are the core of her being, guiding her decisions and actions. Her strengths are the qualities that make her unique and capable. Her passions are the driving forces that fuel her creativity and motivation. Her talents and skills are the gifts that enable her to excel and make a meaningful impact. Her knowledge and experiences are the wisdom that informs her perspective and decision-making. Her relationships and resources are the networks and support systems that sustain and uplift her.

However, this journey of discovery is not without its challenges. Fears, doubts, insecurities, and obstacles may hinder her power, causing her to question her abilities and second-guess herself. These barriers can be varied, but all personally debilitating—internal self-doubt and fear of failure, or external barriers of societal expectations and gender biases.

To overcome these challenges, it's essential for a woman to develop resilience, courage, tenacity, and determination. She must learn to acknowledge, then navigate her fears and doubts, reframing them as opportunities for growth and personal development. She must cultivate self-awareness, recognizing her strengths and weaknesses, and develop strategies to build on her strengths and work on her weaknesses.

Moreover, she must surround herself with positive influences, supportive relationships, and empowering resources. She must seek out mentors, role models, and communities that uplift and inspire her. She must also be willing to take risks, step outside her comfort zone, and embrace new experiences and opportunities.

Through this journey of discovery, a woman comes to understand her true power and potential. She learns to harness her strengths, passions, intuition, and talents to achieve her goals and make a meaningful impact in the world. She embraces these gifts as confident, self-assured, and unapologetic about who she is and what she brings to the table.

In essence, a woman's power is not something external, but rather an inner force that drives her to grow, learn, and evolve with elegance and grace. Her soul sparks and ignites her passions, fuels her creativity, and inspires her to make a difference. By discovering her power, a woman unlocks her true potential, becoming a force to be reckoned with, a change-maker, and a leader in her own right.

Discovering Her Voice

The essence of a woman lies in her intuitive insight to discover her voice. From a feminist perspective, voice is not just a means of communication, but a tool for self-expression, empowerment, and social change. A woman's voice is a reflection of her identity, personality, style, and tone, and is shaped by her experiences, values, and beliefs.

Discovering one's voice involves exploring and embracing one's unique perspective, values, and passions. It demands the insightful criteria required to develop the confidence to be vulnerable, speak up, share one's thoughts and feelings, and assert oneself in various contexts. A woman's voice is not just about speaking, but also about being heard, listened to, and respected.

Through developing her voice, a woman can express herself authentically, advocate for herself and others, and influence positive change. Her voice becomes a powerful tool for communication, connection, and community-building. By defining and refining her voice, she can navigate different contexts and situations effectively, adapting her tone, language, and style to suit her goals and societal audience.

Moreover, discovering one's voice is a journey of self-discovery and growth. It involves confronting and overcoming internalized oppression, self-doubt, and fear of judgment. It requires releasing past failures with grace and embracing one's uniqueness, celebrating one's differences, and finding solidarity and community with others.

In a patriarchal society, women's voices have been historically silenced, marginalized, or distorted. Feminism seeks to reclaim and redefine women's voices, promoting a culture of inclusivity, diversity, and equity. By empowering women to find and use their voices, we can challenge dominant narratives, create alternative perspectives, and build a more just and equitable world.

The core component with the essence of a woman lies in her power to discover her voice. By exploring, developing, and refining her voice, she can express herself authentically, advocate for change, and influence positive outcomes. Her voice becomes an integral tool for personal growth, social change, and collective empowerment.

Discovering Her Impact

The essence of a woman lies in her power to discover her impact. From a feminist perspective, impact is not just about achieving success or recognition, but about creating positive change in the world. A woman's impact is the difference she hopes to make, the lives she touches, and the communities she transforms.

Discovering one's impact involves reflecting on values, passions, and strengths, and identifying the issues that matter most. It requires envisioning the kind of difference one wants to make, whether in personal relationships, professional pursuits, or social justice movements. A woman's impact is not necessarily tied to grandiose gestures and achievements, but can be seen in everyday actions, conversations, and choices.

Planning one's impact involves setting goals, identifying strategies, and taking deliberate actions. It requires considering the resources, networks, and support systems needed to achieve those goals. Measuring impact involves assessing progress, evaluating outcomes, and learning from successes and setbacks.

From a feminist perspective, impact is not just individual, but collective. Women's impact is often seen in the ways they support, uplift, and empower others. It is seen in the ways they challenge systems of oppression, advocate for justice, and create spaces for marginalized voices.

Moreover, discovering one's impact is a journey of self-discovery and growth. It involves confronting and overcoming internalized limitations, self-doubt, and fear of failure. It requires embracing one's agency, celebrating one's achievements, and finding solidarity with others.

In a world where women's contributions are often erased, undervalued, and diminished, discovering one's impact is a paramount and radical act of self-love and self-assertion. By claiming and celebrating your impact, women can challenge dominant narratives, create alternative perspectives, and build a more just and equitable world.

This layer of the essence of a woman lies in her power to discover her impact. By defining, planning, and measuring her impact, she can create positive change, challenge systems of oppression, and empower others. Her impact becomes a productive tool for personal growth, social change, and collective empowerment.

Redefining Her Power and Influence

The essence of a woman lies in her power to redefine her power and influence. From a feminist perspective, redefinition is a vital process of self-reflection, growth, and transformation. It involves periodically reassessing and reevaluating one's power and influence to ensure they remain relevant, effective, and authentic in the face of changing circumstances.

Redefinition is essential throughout life, because women's roles are constantly evolving. New experiences, challenges, and opportunities emerge, requiring adaptations in how we assert ourselves, express ourselves, and impact the world. By redefining her power and influence, a woman can:

- Refine goals and aspirations
- Update strategies and approaches
- Expand personal influence and reach
- Deepen self-awareness and understanding
- Enhance resilience and adaptability

This process of redefinition also involves embracing new dimensions or aspects of oneself, such as:

- Exploring new passions and interests
- Developing new skills and talents
- Forming new connections and relationships
- Embracing new identities and labels
- Challenging new systems and structures

From a feminist perspective, redefinition is a radical act of self-love and self-assertion. It challenges societal expectations and limitations, allowing women to reclaim and redefine their power and influence on their own terms. By doing so, women can:

- Break free from patriarchal constraints
- Challenge dominant narratives and stereotypes
- Create new spaces and opportunities for themselves and others
- Foster solidarity and community with other women
- Drive social change and transformation

Moreover, redefinition is not a solitary process, but a collective one fostered by community. Women's power and influence are often amplified when they work together, support each other, and lift each other up. By redefining their authority and influence, women can create a ripple effect of positive change, inspiring others to do the same.

By re-defining this power, the essence of a woman is cementing her influence within her legacy and history. By periodically reassessing and adapting her power and influence, she can stay true to herself, respond to changing circumstances, and expand her impact and influence. Redefinition is a powerful tool for personal growth, empowerment, and social change, allowing women to reclaim their agency, challenge the status quo, and create a more just and equitable world.

This essence of a woman is a multifaceted and dynamic force that encompasses her power to discover and re-discover her Power, Voice, Impact, and Influence. Through this journey of self-discovery, a woman uncovers her sources of power, develops her unique voice, defines her impact, and redefines her power and influence.

By discovering her Power, a woman identifies her values, strengths, passions, and talents, and learns to navigate obstacles that may hinder her growth. By discovering her Voice, she develops a tool for communication, expression, and advocacy, and refines it to reflect her identity and personality.

By discovering and unlocking her Impact, a woman defines the positive difference she hopes to make in the world and plans the actions needed to achieve her goals. She measures her impact and assesses her progress, adjusting as needed.

By continually evaluating and redefining her Power and Influence, a woman periodically reassesses her power and voice, adapting them to respond to new opportunities and challenges. She expands her power and voice to include new dimensions and aspects, ensuring that she remains authentic, effective, and influential.

As I reflect on the Essence of a Woman, I am reminded of the incredible tapestry of qualities that have been woven in me to create the unique masterpiece of who I am today. I have become strong and resilient, capable of weathering life's challenges with grace and determination. I thrive on being a nurturer, a caregiver, and a source of comfort to those around me. My empathy and compassion constantly allow me to connect with others on a deep level, and my creativity and innovation inspires me to imagine and dream big. I'm thankful that I've become a leader, a visionary, and a force for change. I gratefully embody grace and beauty, not just in my appearance, but moreover in my resilience, kindness, and authenticity. My intelligence and wisdom constantly guide me on my journey, and my courage and perseverance fuel my passions. Embracing the Essence of a Woman is not just about celebrating gender—it's about embracing my own humanity, with all its complexities and gifts. All these gifts and qualities enumerated in the adjectives above are within each woman's grasp—yours for the asking.

Belief:

The palatable Essence of a Woman is her power to create positive change in herself and the world around her. It is the ultimate journey of self-discovery, growth, and transformation, and one that requires courage, resilience, and determination. By embracing her Power, Voice, Impact, and Influence, a woman becomes a force to be reckoned with, a true agent of change and a testament to the boundless potential of women everywhere. Become that woman who listens to the whisper of your soul and takes your place in our Global Community with your footprint of elegant grace to the World: The Power of the Universe.

My *BELIEF* Action Steps:

Practice Princess Moradeun's beliefs on the *Essence of a Woman*:

- **Believe** in your inherent power and strength as a woman.
- **Believe** that you, as a woman, have a unique voice and perspective that deserves to be heard.
- **Believe** as a woman, you instinctively create positive change in yourself and the world around you.
- **Believe** in the importance of self-discovery and self-expression as a woman.
- **Believe** as a woman, you're empowered to make your own choices and decisions.
- **Believe** in the value of female relationships and community.
- **Believe** in your personal experiences and perspectives essential to creating a more just and equitable society.
- **Believe** in the power of our women's voices to challenge and transform systems of oppression.
- **Believe** that your true empowerment as a woman is essential to creating a more peaceful and prosperous world.
- **Believe** in the limitless—your essence as a woman to continually grow, learn, and evolve.

HRH Princess Dr. Moradeun Ogunlana
UN Ambassador Nigeria
Founder and CEO
African Women's Health Project International
AWHPI GLOBAL FOUNDATION
Africa 2-5-9 Project Initiative

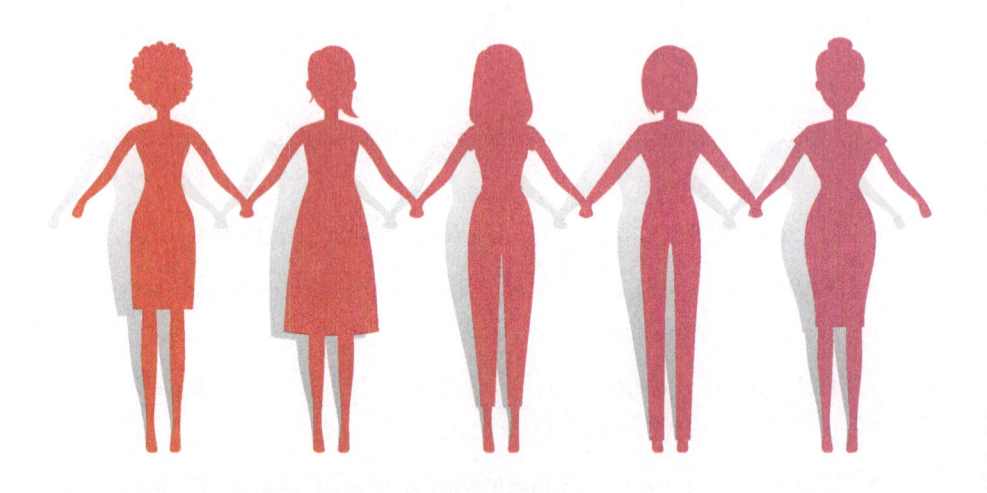

Author Testimonials

Being a part of a global community of amazing women has been an extraordinary experience. Bringing life, passion, and emotion to my story has been profound and transformational. The support of the team of women that have supported this book's compilation has been uplifting. The opportunity to contribute my story and message to the collection, each one of ours being as unique as we are, has been an honor. Dr. Jo Dee's love, leadership, and profound generosity in inviting us to contribute have made this possible. I am eternally grateful for her vision and trust in each of us and for providing the platform for us to contribute to *The Essence of a Woman* to the world.

—*Anne Borow-Lawrence, MEd*

Working alongside the caliber of women contributing to this project, with the unified focus of honoring the essence of a woman, has been an expansive experience. I have observed, learned from, and contributed toward an exceptional recount of the qualities we all illuminate when we align with the most significant outcome. I honor the spirit of collaboration present with women who have experienced great adversity, found exceptional depths of strength and courage for healing, and persevered in ways that many can only imagine. I am grateful for the opportunity to participate and walk this journey with each of you.

—*Anna M. McKee*

I truly thank God for calling me into the wellness ministry. Once I accepted the call, he led me to people and platforms I did not anticipate. This book project is another reminder that God is a promise keeper, especially when you are obedient to him. I have had the most fantastic experience with *The Essence of a Women* book team. The Pillars aligns with the message God gave me, so this opportunity to become one of the Authors in this book confirms that God is the controller of my vision.

I pray that every book team member, Author, and reader be mentally, physically, and spiritually blessed.

—*Dr. Annette Watson-Johnson*

Working with Dr. Jo Dee Baer and the other authors was a great experience. This book is my sixth compilation, and I'm already an international bestseller for all of them, but when Dr. Jo Dee asked me to write a chapter for this book, I jumped at the chance. It was the first time that I addressed my weight loss journey and how pernicious the topic is for women. I hope that my chapter will be inspirational to others, and I am proud and honored to be in this excellent book with epic women who took TLC to Betty Norlin's editing and Kathy Strauss' photography. I know this book will be a message for many!

—*Barbie Layton*

When Dr. Jo Dee reached out to me and asked me to be part of this book and the editing team, I immediately knew it was a big "YES," even though I was beyond busy!

This process has been fun, exciting, and humbling. I have had the opportunity to meet with almost every author on Zoom, learn about their stories, and guide them through the process. One of the things that has resonated the most for me is the power of each of these women, their stories, and the community and movement we are a part of.

I am grateful for this opportunity and for being part of a movement that will impact so many worldwide. Thank you, Dr. Jo Dee and your amazing team.

—*Betty Norlin*

Writing a book with multiple amazing women was a transformative experience. Collaborating with such talented individuals allowed me to learn about the diverse, intricate work that goes into crafting each story. The process required coordination and deep introspection to weave my insights into a cohesive narrative. It was a journey of discovery, understanding the writing process, and reflecting on my perspectives. This collective process showed me the tapestry of voices and experiences that resonate with authenticity and profound insight.

—Cathy Vergara, APRN

Writing the book under the direction of Dr. Jo Dee was incredible. I didn't have much of a story at the beginning of this project, but the total collaborative process drew my story out of me. This project has helped me realize my story and how important sharing our experiences with others is in life.

—Cristina Candullo-Dody

The sheer joy I have found in writing in *Health-a-Pedia* and *The Essence of a Woman* can be described as exhilarating! I've developed some lifelong friendships.

When we are open to possibilities, God, the Universe, sends them our way. I knew I wanted to write a book, and these two chapters have inspired me to write more. Dr. Jo Dee, Betty Norlin, and Renée Brown's coaching and editing were extremely beneficial to the messages in these books.

Thank you for the opportunity to tell a part of my story. I hope that the reader will be inspired to fulfill their own dreams and desires. May everyone find the love, friendship, and support I have seen on these unique expeditions—blessings and gratitude to all the authors and readers.

—Cynthia Hammel-Knipe C.P.E

What an honor to be invited to talk about my favorite projects—each of my amazing children! Thank you very much, Dr. Jo Dee Baer! This is my first-ever collaboration on a book. It has been a lot of fun reflecting on women's rights and just how passionate I am about having agency over relationships and choices about raising children in ways that are gentle yet highly effective at making a beautiful world!

—Deborah Dennis

It was challenging to start this adventure of writing my story, but as I started typing, the rays of light shone through the darkest area throughout my years of being in bondage. Taking this path showed me how broken I was. The turmoil of negative emotions seemed to rule my life as I fought to survive. I disliked myself and everyone around me, always acting as if everything was alright, but it was a tornado inside my soul.

It is always hard to look within ourselves to see the spectacle we carry; incredibly, the horror dissipates as the Holy Spirit reveals the truth. I was able to embrace my past and make peace with who I was. In my writing, it was another eye-opening experience of my new identity, as old things passed away. My heart was hardened by life and circumstances that overwhelmed me like waves crashing on the sea, and I was being pulled under and could not breathe. Then, as my heart softened, I saw the light that rescued me from myself. I was my abuser trying to protect myself but was continually dragging myself and others through the storm of my soul.

The revelation I got from sharing my story has transformed into healing, forgiveness, and love. All the pain and suffering I endured were for a better story, God's plan for me. My story is now part of a bigger story that will touch and bring others to know Jesus as their savior.

I am grateful I was asked to help unleash the feminine soul, as mine was a raging storm that is now calm. It is a joy to look back and see that my story has changed and is continuing to change as I embrace the future with strength and dignity!

—*Desiree Peacock*

I thrive by breaking barriers to capital, coaching women to access funds, and empowering them to grow and scale their businesses—each success lighting the path to limitless possibilities. This experience in writing my chapter has allowed me to do just that.

—*Dominique Brun*

The journey of collaboration and self-discovery has been incredible. I received amazing support and mentorship like no other. The energy transfer created within this inspiring group will resonate the world over for many generations to come.

—*Donna Dawson, FCCA*

As women, we are unique and uniquely empowered. Participating in *The Essence of a Woman* forced me to reflect on the twists and turns of the remarkable journey that is my life—a life that has experienced joy, sorrow, failure, and success—a life marked by constant change, growth, and the willingness to remain open. My life has epitomized the *American Dream*. I sincerely hope my experiences will encourage and inspire other women to tap into their underlying strength to live with passion and purpose unencumbered by sexism and ageism as they mature and achieve a sense of balance as they manage their multiple roles.

—Gloria Kurz, JD, SRS

I am honored to be one of these women who discovered her essence, wholeness, and mission on earth. Our stories are all connected. Finding authentic ways to collaborate is the next lesson that women today can model for the future. We are leading the way for all women to align their missions as we have done together in this book. Thank you, Dr. Jo Dee, for your willingness and courage to step forward and bring us together. I am grateful to be part of this anthology and to teach future women what is possible when we unite our heads, hearts, and hands.

—Dr. Golda Joseph, PhD

It has been a very interesting and inspiring process to work with these fantastic heart-centered women to weave our stories into a diverse yet unified story. It required me to focus on which of my experiences and the knowledge I've gained from them might be most relevant to our audience and most complementary to the contributions of the other authors in this collaboration. It was a challenge and a privilege to share in this process and in the final product.

—Dr. Hepsharat Amadi, MD, LAc

Writing this chapter on emotional intelligence has deepened my appreciation for its transformative power. It goes beyond managing emotions to enhancing self-awareness, empathy, and resilience. By offering practical strategies and biblical wisdom, I aim to guide you towards healing and growth. In writing this chapter, it's inspired me to use emotional intelligence to enrich both personal and professional relationships.

—Dr. Jacqueline Mohair, PhD

A Truly Inspiring Experience—Being asked to work on a project that elevates women's voices worldwide alongside a group of incredibly knowledgeable and inspiring women was a "pinch-me moment" in my life. Coming together beautiful, feminine minds for the world's greater good and collaborating on education to help other women make changes, no matter how small or big, for a better life is a beautiful spiritual journey of togetherness and enlightenment.

It was an exceptional, extraordinary, and exemplary experience witnessing our group shed layers of armor, be raw and vulnerable with each other, and indeed write from the heart. This project has not only empowered others but also deepened our connections and enriched our own lives. Dr. Jo Dee really understands how to bring a collective group of women together to gift something unique to the world.

—Jennifer Louise Kerr

Writing a chapter for the book *The Essence of a Woman* alongside so many incredible women has been a truly transformative experience. Collaborating with such talented individuals has opened my eyes to the diverse and intricate work that goes into crafting each story.

This journey required coordination and deep introspection to weave my insights into a cohesive narrative. Through this process, I discovered more about the writing journey, understood the various perspectives of my co-authors, and reflected on my own. My SOUL's Butterfly Journey!

This collective effort revealed a rich tapestry of voices and experiences, resonating with authenticity and profound insight.

—Karen Rudolf

My journey as a visual storyteller, turned creationeer, to now I'm known as a creative connector. It truly has been a long winding road. I'm passionate about creating memories and sharing that creativity which is something that every human being possesses. When asked to contribute to *The Essence of a Woman* to share my knowledge, experience, and creative eye, it tells me that I'm on the right path to a brighter and more colorful future! Thank you, Dr. Jo Dee Baer, my family and friends, for having faith in me and my message—that everyone is the artist of their lives!

–*Kathy Strauss, CCFC*

Being chosen to participate in this project has been a once-in-a-lifetime opportunity. It's not only because of the caliber of authors I am joining but also due to the challenge of writing my chapter in my second language—English. While technology aids us today, this endeavor showed me I can rise to the occasion. Collaborating with esteemed authors dedicated to this project's success is incredibly rewarding. My three wins were proving my capabilities, contributing to a collective effort, and learning leadership skills from Dr. Jo Dee Baer, PhD, and her team, in bringing this massive project to fruition. I am immensely grateful for this experience.

—*Laura Ibarra, AbD*

Becoming an author is something that I have always wanted to do. However, the magnitude of this experience has surpassed any dream I have ever had. Not only am I fortunate enough to be included in a book with other amazing women, but I can encourage, strengthen, and support every reader who comes across my story. Through this journey, I have learned that transparency and vulnerability are two things that we must sometimes embrace to make a true difference in other peoples' lives. The amount of reflection and prayer during this experience was transforming and healing. I hope to achieve this same revelation for each of you.

—*Lorina K. Sanchez, MSN, RN*

I am grateful beyond words for the experience of participating in *The Essence of a Woman*. Dr. Jo Dee and other authors' love, dedication, and sisterhood raise this experience to the top of the charts.

—*MarBeth Dunn, M.Ed. Somatic Healing Expert*
Energy Healer, Empath, and Intuitive

Upon taking on this assignment, I was unaware of all I would need to do and how intricately detailed it would be. After re-examining the instructions and thoroughly applying myself, I realized Dr. Jo Dee had laid the road map for the co-authors to follow. This realization brought relief and reassurance, knowing I was not alone in this journey. I was reluctant to start. It looked like too much, and my schedule was already full. I had to look again. At that moment, I realized I only needed to follow the path already laid. I feared taking the first step, something I rarely encounter. Despite everything, I wanted to keep my word and complete this chapter.

I want to express my heartfelt gratitude to Dr. Jo Dee Baer, Renée Brown, Kathy Strauss, and everyone who contributed to this project. Your guidance and support have been invaluable. I have genuinely enjoyed writing this chapter and am hopeful, anticipating its profound and positive impact on a global scale. As the saying goes, 'A journey of a thousand miles begins with the first step.'

—*Ambassador, Dr. Nephetina L. Serrano*

The coming together of us women in this extraordinary and influential way is a one-of-a-kind transformative experience I treasure. Thanks to Dr. Jo Dee, who created this epic book project to expand women's voices around the World. The opportunity to associate with such profoundly high-quality ladies is soulful and divine. We learn from one another, assist, and propel each other forward meaningfully. Each has a graceful intention to help other feminine beings on this beautiful path on planet Earth by crafting the inspiring message from our hearts and delivering their profound experiences authentically expressed, hoping to connect and uplift the vibrations for all. The process required heart opening and sharing the deepest parts of our souls in *oneness*, the Source of our true essence, **love**. I truly appreciate the unique conscious expansion lovingly shared to manifest the **heaven-on-earth** we all desire.

—*Dr. Nitikul Solomon, MD, MSHA, ABIHM*

I'm grateful to have experienced a life that has allowed me an array of opportunities and challenges. Struggles from my childhood have only made the rest of the moments in my life sweeter. It brings me joy to assist others to rise above their circumstances and feel connected and fulfilled. It's been a treat to have been in this book and to have met and bonded with some amazing and incredible women!

As a wife, mother, extended family member, and friend, I can easily say that nothing is more rewarding than the connections that give us more context as to who we really are in life. My relationships have inspired me to expand who I am and to serve.

—*Renée Brown, CEO, Next Level Recovery*

I am an accomplished, holistic provider and am grateful for the opportunity to collaborate with such an amazing group of individuals in creating this masterpiece! Together, we have created an educational resource to enlighten the reader regarding their physical, physiological, emotional, and spiritual well-being. I am blessed God chose me to be a contributor, and am thankful for this opportunity.

—*Shannon L. Roper, FNP-BC*

Being asked to contribute to *The Essence of a Woman* project initially left me perplexed and hesitant, and I questioned its significance. However, as I immersed myself in the writing process and learned about the diverse authors involved, my perspective shifted profoundly. Each author's story revealed layers of depth, resilience, and extraordinary impact on the world. It dawned on me that this book isn't just a collection of stories; it's a testament to the legacy each woman is creating.

Ultimately, I am thankful for being pushed to contribute, even when I hesitated. *The Essence of a Woman* project has not only enriched my life. Still, women have also underscored the transformative power of sharing stories and celebrating the diverse experiences that shape us all.

—*Dr. Shirley Luu*

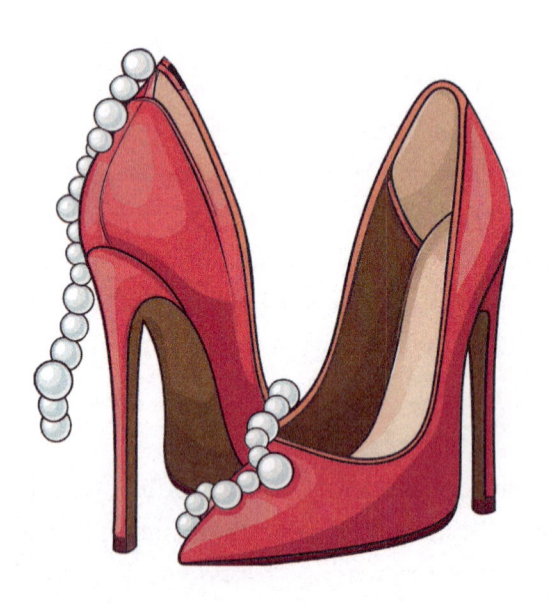

414 | The Essence of a Woman — High Heel Moment

High Heel Moment

"Pink, Pearls, Pumps, and Perfume"
—*All women identify with the Four-Feminine 'P's.*

Every woman has a time with these physical 'P's' inherently transmuted into a myriad of emotions when she felt the winning combination of Wonder Woman, Sheena: Queen of the Jungle, The Valkyrie Viking Princess, and could bellow the song lyrics to Helen Reddy's iconic women's empowerment song: "I am Woman."

"I am woman, hear me roar,
In numbers too big to ignore,
And I know too much to go back and pretend."

Slip into your own high heels to absorb and immerse yourself in the humor, emotion, passion, and triumph, in our following **SHE—*roe*** vignettes.

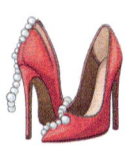

During the apex of my marathoning years, I was running approximately 80–100 miles a week and competed in a marathon a month for a year. Running was my consummate hobby and life. Frankly, the ego-driven personal applique insignia on the 'backside' of my running shorts said it all: "Of Course! I run like a girl! Try to catch up." Sporting a 7-minute mile—I was pretty fast.

One day, while running along the always-crowded Silver Comet Trail in Atlanta, Georgia, one of my fellow male runners approached me with the ultimate challenge. My personal pistons had indeed passed him on the trail, leaving his running ability a bit in question. So, if you think you're so fast, why don't you prove it and run in high heels?

The challenge was accepted, and the game was **on**! Purchasing a pair of 2-inch Mary Jane-style shoes, I showed up the next week at the Georgia Tech 5K Race, competed, completed, and placed first in my age group for that race! My calves, however, winched over that 2-inch elevation for over a week. I did see my fellow male running counterpart later on in the month and displayed the medal and picture with no words, just a smile.

—*Dr. Jo Dee Baer, PhD*

Nature's love: animals, plants, insects, and other creatures of nature live in a unique genus-specific communication. There is such an innocent and everyday communication between all creatures of Mother Earth. Becoming integrated in this process has had a significant impact on my life.

Three years apart, I became aware of this as an ongoing process thanks to my teacher, Dr. Jim Marinakis. Searching for help in a difficult situation in my personal life, I turned to the forest. I found peace and balance by walking through and leaning into the beautiful trees. Gratefully, I expressed my love and honor day by day, but the forest decided to help me further.

Shy animals, huge birds, and fish showed up surprisingly out of nowhere. I had studied animals' messages years ago, realizing now, from the inner eye, and elsewhere. Gratefully I again expressed my love and honor to them and elsewhere that they were still speaking to me.

A very precious and ongoing reminder came often, especially from horses and trees to me:

"Always be aware of your dignity!"

This process is my ongoing, high heel moment unfolding in my life, leaving me often speechless with a deep feeling of being blessed and elsewhere that they were still speaking to me.

—*Birgit Bonin, ND*

The pinnacle of my professional journey came on the day I was honored with the Global Vision Award by Johnny Regan at the Broward County Convention Center. This moment marked my profound realization that an award symbolizes the recognition of a vision realized. Before meeting Johnny, the true essence and manifestation of a vision eluded me.

My path to this achievement was not straightforward. After falling victim to a financial crime, I faced a three-year suspension from practicing law. This challenging period forced me to reinvent myself and embark on a new career. I envisioned creating a television channel, which I named "Laws of Life." My aim was to produce webcasts and podcasts to empower entrepreneurs, sharing their stories and messages. I hosted a weekly networking group on Zoom, uniting entrepreneurs from around the globe.

Through this platform, I had the privilege of interviewing over 4,000 individuals, including notable figures such as Dr. Khalilah Camacho Ali, Dr. Jo Dee Baer, PhD, Forbes Riley, Nancy Grace, and, of course, Johnny Regan. It was only upon receiving the award that I truly understood I had journeyed from darkness into light. This recognition reaffirmed my purpose: to connect with the world and help entrepreneurs attract abundance.

—Blanca Perper Greenstein, Esq.
www.lawoflife.com

When I was honored and selected to sing the leading role in Puccini's Iconic Opera *Tosca* I was an accomplished and gifted classically trained vocal musician, having sung multiple roles in Europe and North America at my young age of 24. Although winning the audition and lead role was exhilarating, I felt insecure. This demanding role really was more suited for a soprano, twenty years older, but I exhaled my insecurities and just went for it: thinking that I may never have another opportunity to do this again! Prior to singing the grand finale aria, "Vissi d'Arte," the role demanded that I run around the stage like an Olympic Athlete running a 100 meter dash. My gift of being able to multitask in life kicked in. My Grand Finale, although in my mind, wasn't my best, thought it was a **true** Finale fitting the role of Floria Tosca. Fifty plus years later, I still get exhilarated by my musical Olympic Feat of singing 'over' a full Orchestra! A true high heeled moment nailed like a Soprano high "C"!

—Kathleen Heler
Opera Singer/Fashionista Retired

To create a better world is my ultimate goal. Yes—from what I can remember things about my life, I was always curious—some say—nosey, but I say curious and adventurous.

So just to open up a little about what I am curious about. Born into a business family I enjoyed the discussions and debate and the deliberations among adults. I can still close my eyes and replay events and complete scenarios as I was really into it all. I found it fascinating that with sustained thinking and planning people hadd the capacity to idenitfy a problem and/or take action and fix or improve that which was seen to need improvement. And sometimes—the solution arrived at eliminated the issue completely.

Now imagine living among dynamic positive adults who loved me and encouraged me to think out my own solutions!!!

In a sense—I was given my own runway to find and use my superpower—I discovered how to make myself happy by stripping down anything and conquering it. I learned to read at a young age and read everything and anything I wanted. That is Power and a High Heel Moment.

—Dr. Margaret M. Noguera, MD
Bossladynogs@outlook.com

I stepped up to the podium in the tranquil sanctuary to deliver my mother's eulogy. This was my high heel moment—an experience of being a fully integrated and expressed woman. Looking over the sea of faces, my heart swelled with sorrow and pride. I was honoring the remarkable woman who had given me life, and now, in her final moments, I had the privilege of giving back to her.

Before moving my mother from Philadelphia to Boston, a meditation group clarified my soul's mission: to provide a haven where she felt loved and appreciated. From 92 to 96, she lived with my husband and me. She thrived, laughing more, her eyes sparkling with youthful joy. With support, she knitted scarves for her family. This role reversal was challenging and deeply rewarding, embodying my mission to reciprocate her love and care.

Her funeral was a celebration of our shared journey—a testament to the transformative power of love and care. In that moment, I stood tall, not just in my high heels, but in the essence of who I am: a daughter, a lifegiver, and a fully expressed woman.

—*Anne Borow-Lawrence, MEd*

I always felt a deep desire to help others by sharing my life experiences. Growing up amid struggles and personal losses, I found solace in writing, filling journals with my thoughts and dreams. After years of personal development, I began writing in public spaces, becoming a beacon of hope for many. Now, I travel the world, encouraging others to align to their highest outcome, find their inner strength, and persevere despite life's difficulties. My journey from personal struggle to transformational coach and published author has transformed my life and touched countless others, proving the incredible impact of sharing one's experiences.

—*Anna M. McKee*

They say that women have superpowers because we can multitask. We can work and still take care of our children and home. I still brag about the time in my life when I felt like I was a real-life SuperWoman. I set out with a goal and did not allow anything or anyone to deter me from it. I desperately wanted to obtain an undergraduate degree. During this time in my life, I held several titles. I was a wife, a mom of two young children, and a full-time employee. I enrolled in college and took as many night and weekend classes per semester as possible. I graduated three years later. Not only did I crush this goal, but I also decided to continue my education and immediately began an accelerated graduate program. I graduated one year later.

—*Dr. Annette Watson-Johnson*

There was a high heel moment when we all shared how much being in this book meant to each of us and having the ability to bring in top notch women from around the world to share their inspiring stories.

—*Barbie Layton*

Driving into the CNN Center in Atlanta at midnight for the Medical Miracles Conference amid COVID and the riots made me realize and celebrate what saying "YES" to opportunities meant!

I met and spoke to Dr. Joselyn Elders, Former Surgeon General for the United States, who told me that listening was one of the most essential skills. I also met Dr. Marc Siegel, who reinforced that people should think for themselves and trust the process they uncover to find answers. When I spoke to Dr. Drew, he shared that it was necessary to (1) Be Clear on What You Do, (2) Follow Your Instincts, and (3) Do the Right Thing. I also met Dr. Oz on Zoom and later in real life.

Saying "YES" to life and opportunities like this have helped me step into more than one High Heel Moment…and I am grateful.

—*Betty (Elizabeth) A. Norlin*

Needing to sell my house fast in a challenging market, I had ambitious goals! I wanted an offer within three days of the listing and a bidding war to get a great price. I was determined to make my property stand out and attract eager buyers. My realtor said, "It would be a long shot."

My strategy was driven by urgency and a desire to maximize the value of my home. I went unconventional and contacted my friend Charlotte Spicer for energy work. Charlotte cleared out my family and pets' energies and made the home feel open and inviting. I made a detailed vision board showing my house surrounded by loving light and peace. My vision board had my dream price and goal for the date sold.

The end result was an accepted offer that Monday, with a bidding war that got me the desired price.

—*Cathy Vergara, APRN*

My most recent high heel moment began when I had the honor of being invited to a knighting investiture. This honor is something most people will never have the opportunity to see. It led me to be invited to three more after that, in which I began noticing things I could do to make it an even more epic occasion. I had the goal to plan one in the future.

That day arrived when my dear friend asked me to plan the first ever in Florida. It was in six weeks. A large order, especially for an event of such proportion. I have to say I delivered epically. It was everything a royal knighting investiture should be—opulent, ornate, and elegant. When I received the large applause from all the celebrated guests and royalty in the room, I thought, "I have accomplished my vision."

—*Cristina Candullo-Dody*

My first recording contract offer came when I worked at a popular nightclub in a very lovely hotel. An artist development agent for Atlantic Records in New York heard me singing with the band and gave me a song to learn.

I met him in the lobby the next night before work and sang it for him. He said he would bring me a contract when he returned to town, which he did. I took it to my lawyer, and it was approved.

Unfortunately, he expected me to do more than sing. I ripped up the contract, returned it, and kept my self-respect.

—*Cynthia Hammel-Knipe CPE*

In 1997, I found myself in the middle of the biggest financial crisis in the history of Asia. Businesses were shutting down; fortunes were lost; people were even jumping off buildings! I couldn't leave our eight employees in the lurch, so I went through my nest egg to support them for nine months. It was my time to put Bucky's wealth 'win-win' wisdom to practice amid the devastation. Though financially, that seemed like a big mistake, it was one of the biggest blessings. I came back wealthier, more robust, wiser, and with the certainty that I could always trust myself and my decisions.

—*Dame Doria Cordova*
www.moneyandyoudistinctions.com

My marital adventure began in 1974 with a U-Haul truck and destination: Jacksonville, Florida. I quickly had to adjust to deployments, getting an ID for access to the base, and finding a pay telephone down the road at the 7-11 Convenience Store. Survival skills and finding a "tribe" with other wives in the 'same boat' was key! Six moves to four states in seven years—home became where I dropped my bags. I learned patience waiting on movers, lost boxes, broken furniture, extended deployments, and Snail Mail—but Joy comes when the ships return safely. The ship's crew sacrifice much, as do the amazing families that are also on this journey as a Navy wife and children. That's why my email has been my 50-year nickname: mermaid_central@yahoo.com

—*Debby Armentrout*

Negotiating contracts to recruit for large successful companies such as Microsoft and Texas Instruments happened because of taking risks at the right time and place. The fantastic lady in charge of HR for software hires did not like public speaking even though she had a PhD in harpsichord; yes, she did, and she had an MBA. She asked me to do it. I was 24. I was the main speaker at the welcome breakfasts for interviewees flown in for the events. It was because I wore cowboy boots to a meeting with my suit in front of her and other VPs. They complimented me. I said the oil companies, the tech companies, and even EDS are finally letting go of high heels and pantyhose as absolute non-negotiables for women. This funny episode got me to a whole new level in my career!

—*Deborah Dennis*

As I entered prison, I was given a number to replace my identity. I died that day! I had to dig out of a dark, wet, and lonely grave of my soul. Trapped in lies that consumed me with the humiliation of what I had become grabbed me like a vice gripping me so tight I had to surrender.

As I started climbing the mountains' highs and lows, it was exhausting, making every muscle ache, especially my heart. This journey has kept me moving forward, giving me this high heel moment and a new identity in Christ!

—*Desiree Peacock*

There came a moment when destiny took shape at the click of my high heels on a polished stage floor. I entered a pitch competition that would change my life. I had never done anything like this, but I knew: "You have to do this."

Winning that pitch competition was more than a triumph—it was a crescendo of courage, a testament to resilience forged in the fires of doubt. As I flew to Detroit, anticipation hummed in the air, mingling with the whispers of my disbelief turned determination. Standing there, under the spotlight's embrace, I was so nervous and excited! I felt the power of words cascading like a waterfall of possibility. I stumbled but came out of it with fierce strength and determined drive. At that moment, every syllable spoken carried the weight of dreams realized, igniting a flame within each listener's soul. It was not just a speech; it was a symphony of strength, each word a note resonating with the melody of empowerment and change.

And I haven't stopped. I was just accepted into another accelerator with more pitch competitions, and I help organize events for other Founders— My heels haven't stopped clicking since.

—*Dominique Brun*

March 1984. I was involved in a new venture/start-up company, scheduled to meet with the founder and private investors. Shortly before the meeting, I was diagnosed with a potentially life-threatening parotid tumor, had surgery, and ended up with some facial paralysis. Wearing suede boots and a high-necked designer dress to cover the bandage on my neck, I attended the meeting. We received funding, and I eventually recovered my facial expression!

—*Gloria Kurz, JD, SRS*

I could have danced all night! My beautiful eldest daughter found her prince charming. At her wedding I felt illuminated in my high heels and danced all night, just three years after splitting my knee cap, and two surgeries. I could feel no pain! I just kept dancing until 4am. Filled with joy and gratitude for those sacred moments of bliss and transcendence.

Much love and light to all courageous souls. Please keep dancing and remember *"it's never too late to regenerate."* —Metta Bhavana

—*Dr. Golda Joseph, PhD*

I have had several. My biggest high heel moment came about five months after I started treating my daughter for retinal detachment in both eyes with bioidentical hormones. The retinal specialists who had been following my daughter's case showed me her OCT scan, which had appeared markedly abnormal at first, but by the end of the 5 months in which I had been treating her with quantum biofeedback and bioidentical hormones, both her vision and her OCT scans were absolutely normal, which made it unnecessary for her to take a course of high-dose prednisone.

—*Dr. Hepsharat Amadi, MD, LAc*

In the face of adversity, the true test of strength often lies in our ability to rise above challenges with unwavering determination. It's in these high heel moments, when the weight of the world feels overwhelming, that we must summon our inner resilience. Imagine the scene: facing trials and tribulations, you dig deep within yourself, reaching beyond your comfort zone, and unleashing the power that resides in every one of us. This is where we find our inner lioness, fierce and unyielding, ready to confront whatever stands in our way. The roar of this lioness symbolizes our refusal to be defeated, our commitment to fight for our dreams, and our relentless drive to overcome obstacles.

As we embrace this inner strength, we not only conquer the immediate challenges but also soar to new heights of personal growth and achievement. Each struggle becomes an opportunity to tap into a deeper level of courage and resilience. By channeling this powerful force, we transform our adversities into triumphs, proving to ourselves and the world that we are capable of greatness. It is through these moments of profound struggle that we discover our true potential, allowing us to rise, roar, and conquer, emerging stronger and more victorious than before.

—*Dr. Jacqueline Mohair, PhD*

My "High Heel Moment" isn't about wearing heels—it's about stepping into a role with confidence, capability, and integrity. It's about those pivotal instances when you realize that trust is the foundation of leadership, a lesson I learned early and to this day from my dad.

Years ago, I was driving a large tractor, and inside were my dad, my husband, and my newborn daughter. On one side of the tractor was the road, and on the other side, a cliff. My dad quietly gestured for me to move an inch to the right. Then another inch, then another. No words were spoken, yet I trusted his directions implicitly. That 'inch by inch' story became a defining moment in my life and career.

Growing up, I watched my father lead with quiet strength and unwavering principles. True leadership isn't about being the loudest in the room, but about being useful (the other options are dead and useful dead when you grow up on a farm. His lessons were simple yet profound, and I apply those lessons every day—with my teams and me.

My own leadership journey is based on the values my father exemplifies and building confidence and trust with my own teams to push them beyond their limitations to accomplish great things. In the end, it's not about the shoes you wear, but the steps you take that define your leadership journey.

—Tricia Benn
Partner & Chief Executive Officer
C-Suite Network™
Podcast & TV Host, Business Disruptor

My high heel moment began during a pivotal time in my life, filled with challenges and self-discovery. While navigating the end of a complicated relationship, I found the strength to rediscover my worth and potential. This experience was a turning point, pushing me to embrace my true self and pursue my passions with renewed vigor.

Through this journey, I realized the importance of self-love and resilience. I took bold steps to build a life that reflected my values and aspirations. This transformation was not just about leaving behind what no longer served me, but rather, about stepping into a future filled with possibilities.

Each stride I took in those high heels symbolized my commitment to myself, my dreams, and the empowering belief that I could overcome any obstacle. In this moment I have marked the beginning of a new chapter, one where I stood tall, confident, and ready to embrace the world on my terms.

—*Karen Rudolf*

Steadfast, clear thinking, and heart-centered—each describes my journey as a caregiver to my late husband. I smile with a glint in my eye as I describe how "I'm an artist, not a medical professional" and share some of the nightmarish stories of caring for him as his health deteriorated. His health adventures started like a shot out of a cannon. It was a hospital misdiagnosis that turned into a plethora of diagnoses, two surgeries, three hospitals, and four months of hell for both of us. But, during these four months, I dug deep, found my voice, and reestablished the creative seed within my soul. Each time a new curve ball came at me, I learned to pivot and think outside the box with a solution. I often say that creativity saved me and helped me establish it as my superpower.

Because of my creative attitude and calm thinking during stressful times, I am asked to teach others how to do the same thing. Because of how I handled myself during my husband's illness, I was appointed to the Sentara Northern Virginia Medical Center's family patient advisory board. As a result, I made a difference in his life and other patients. I firmly believe that every action we take affects all living things. Now, several years after his passing, I find I'm still being called on for my thoughts on how to care for a loved one—but in a creative, more holistic way. In recent times, I find myself being called on to help my aging parents. When they didn't know what to do, I could see, connect, and put things in place to help them age gracefully at home. I'm a creative connector. Through all these and other life experiences, I grabbed the paintbrush of life and created a colorful canvas called my life.

—*Kathy Strauss, CCFC*

I worked in the pharmaceutical industry, and we were honored to have Dr. Les Brown come to our national convention to speak! At that moment, I knew my life would never be the same again. I am usually cautious when encountering strangers inviting me to go anywhere with them. My high heel moment was when I decided to spend the entire day with Les Brown and his team! From that time spent, I partnered with Les Brown and began traveling with him nationwide to train people how to start a seminar business and earn money by sharing their stories. That tour ultimately led to me having a talk show on PBS and The Word Network. I also became the Balance expert on an NBC affiliate station. I am glad I put my stilettos on and stepped out of my comfort zone to yield a result I would have never experienced if I stayed in flats!

—*Kim Jacobs, MBA, BD*

A huge dream came true in 2023—a long five-year immigration journey, holding a dependent visa, I became a permanent resident. I moved forward with my vision of creating my first company in the United States, '*3 Wins International LLC*—a second company I founded, all by myself, and my third including partnerships. I worked for different local agencies when I graduated as a Graphic Designer. Although I enjoyed the design work, I never liked having a boss. That was the main reason why, in 2005, at 22, I started my own company: '*más-in*,' where we specialized in wedding stationery design and printing. As my slogan says: "Here is where the magic happens." We have had a blast during the last 19 years, still thriving, even though I chose to scale back during the pandemic. My second company was a collaboration with my brother Gerardo Ibarra and Rodrigo Trujillo. We became partners in '*Astillero 88*' back in 2015. We were dedicated to designing and creating custom furniture from reused materials, solving space issues, and meeting customer needs with eco-friendly products. Keep going, keep moving… dreams come true if you hold space for your vision and take action.

—*Laura Ibarra, AbD*

I had an unprecedented winning streak of my first 13 motions. A senior partner directed that I review and revise another's brief because "we have to win this one." I performed exceptionally well in my first job as an attorney. So, with permission neither requested nor granted, I ordered a round of Champagne for all partners, associates, and staff after our Christmas Party, then winked my eye at the senior partners. They just raised their eyebrows and chuckled.

—Leilani Alesh, Esq.
Reiki Practitioner

Feeling comfortable in my life, I was still intrigued that even in retirement, there may be more to living an abundant life. Kicking and screaming, I reluctantly attended a Women's Retreat Weekend based solely on relationships. What I discovered during that weekend was the first relationship began with me. When I understood that living in self-acceptance and high self-esteem was my choice, my life has never been the same. I am the only person that has the power to choose for me. I am the author of my life.

—Linda Huff

I remember being a Certified Nursing Assistant (CNA) and watching some of my favorite nurses care for residents at a local assisted living facility. I admired their compassion and knowledge. As I watched them work each shift, I thought to myself, one day, I would be just like them. Recently, I was named Best Nurse of Otero County (2024) in Alamogordo, New Mexico. Not only is it an honor, but a dream come true. Being put into the same category as so many amazing nurses is something I never imagined but I will never forget!

—Lorina K. Sanchez, MSN, RN

My high heel moment was realizing how amazing, inspired, and dedicated Dr. Jo Dee Baer and her team are to creating a book of excellence with impact for thousands of women. *The Essence of a Woman* is head and shoulders above other collaboration books I've participated in, where my chapter was edited only once. These dedicated women edited my chapter three times! They have added so much to the experience of this book.

—*MarBeth Dunn, M.Ed.,* Somatic Healing Expert
Energy Healer, Empath, and Intuitive

When I was initially asked to be a speaker at the Woman of Achievement National Pageant, a woman's entrepreneurial pageant competition for female leaders, I could never imagine that this opportunity would then lead me to me being asked to represent the state of Pennsylvania as a contestant the following year. This experience was completely out of my comfort zone. I never imagined or even saw myself being in a pageant. As a speaker the year prior, I chose to speak on *Looking at the Woman in the Mirror*. Little did I know that speech would ring true in my own life when I had to look in my own mirror to uncover a new found confidence and appreciation of my value and contribution to the competition. I went on to be awarded the Ambassador Crown that year, and the following year was selected to be Legacy Crown Holder, as the first African American woman to hold the title in pageant history.

—*Ambassador, Dr. Nephetina L. Serrano*

I was at the Warrior Camp in 2017, where we had to wake up super early. I was in a hurry and accidentally mistook my purple eyeliner for my brow pencil and applied it to my eyebrow instead.

I had no idea until the afternoon when we were dancing around the room, and my roommate saw my face and cried out, astonishingly startled that my brows were PURPLE!! I was dancing around the room and facing so many people. Oh my!! Hey, perhaps some may have thought it was a new fashion trend! Amen.

—*Dr. Nitikul Solomon, MD, MSHA, ABIHM*

I believe one of my greatest moments occurred during the Health-a-Pedia symposium in Florida. I was surrounded by knowledgeable, talented, renowned, and famous individuals for several days. Prior to going, I was nervous because I was an amateur compared to them when it came to public speaking, writing, promoting, etc. However, I realized I could and DID rise up to the level to provide my expertise along with the other authors. My professional life has been evolving for the past two years, and the symposium has thrust my desire to "move outside my box" from being a provider to greater things! Thank you to all my H.A.P. family!

—*Shannon L. Roper, FNP-BC*

I never imagined myself entrenched in the finance industry, let alone being regarded as a subject matter expert. It all started with a realization after facing financial hardships and navigating through uncertainty. At first, I felt out of my depth—what did I know about money management? Yet, with determination fueled by those experiences, I immersed myself in studying the intricacies of the industry and its profound impacts on communities and individuals, particularly women. From those early tribulations emerged a newfound passion and understanding. Today, I find myself humbled yet proud to be recognized as a leading authority in finance, sought after for insights that influence policies and empower others to navigate their financial landscapes confidently.

From the throes of financial challenges to being ranked among the top in the country, my journey has been nothing short of transformative. It underscores the importance of turning adversity into opportunity. Standing at the pinnacle of my profession, I am reminded that every setback was a stepping stone towards achieving expertise that allows me to make meaningful contributions and inspire others in finance and beyond.

—*Dr. Shirley Luu*

I never wanted to have children because of a debilitating fear of pain.

As giving birth without pain is 'impossible' without pharmaceutical drugs—which I am opposed to taking under any circumstances—it became something I wrote off as a teenager in science class—re: graphic birthing videos!

But something changed when I learned how to clear my subconscious and societal limiting beliefs, which were holding me back in life.

Beliefs like 'birthing equals pain' and 'you cannot squeeze something the size of a melon out of a hole the size of a grape!' I methodically cleared these beliefs and wrote a book as I went.

The day came when I thought: *"Wow, this had all better be true, or I will have to throw my published book. 'Natural Pain-Free Birth,' in the bin."*

Of course, I had the most beautiful experience with the birth of my son, Oliver, and published my book with the birth story as the final chapter. My daughter, Millie, came in the same magical way four years later.

People still find it hard to believe that it is possible to have a natural and utterly pain-free birth. Women, I admonish you: "Dare to do the impossible and do the work to make it happen."

We are all capable of absolutely magical accomplishments, and we deserve to have these experiences!

—*Sonja Rechnitzer*

One of my most embarrassing moments was also a high heel moment… literally! Sixteen years ago, I was at the Marriott Marquis in NYC, to speak to approximately 1,000 computer science engineers about the newest releases in technology.

I was separated from my infant at home and was on the phone multitasking that morning in the hotel room. My other children had needs that I quelled on the phone. I rushed to the lobby to check out with my bags in hand. I was in a hurry to make sure that I had enough time to set up in the large auditorium.

Using my hands expressively at the counter, I noticed that I still had a grip on my breast pump at the end of the conversation!! Thank goodness the young man who checked me out that morning was clueless!

—*Renée Brown, CEO*
Next Level Recovery

After months of planning with my team, it was showtime! My office was co-hosting a regional campus event with over three hundred educators, parents, and community members to share progress on a particular academic endeavor.

I have convened several significant professional events, but this one was different. Why? It was the first public event that I had after my health challenges, which took away my mobility, stability, and ability to walk securely in balance. I worked hard for two years to regain full strength in my knees and legs. I was finally ready to be glammed up in a wardrobe that did not have to be accessorized with flat cushioned shoes.

As I mounted the stage to serve as mistress of ceremonies, my flowing green floral dress was styled with signature green pumps. I love green because it signifies growth, blessings, restoration, and transformational health progress. I literally and boldly stepped into my high heel moment while harmonizing in my head, "I'm coming out, I want the world to know, got to let it show, " by Diana Ross. It was a #GOOD Day!

—*Dr. Tyra Good*

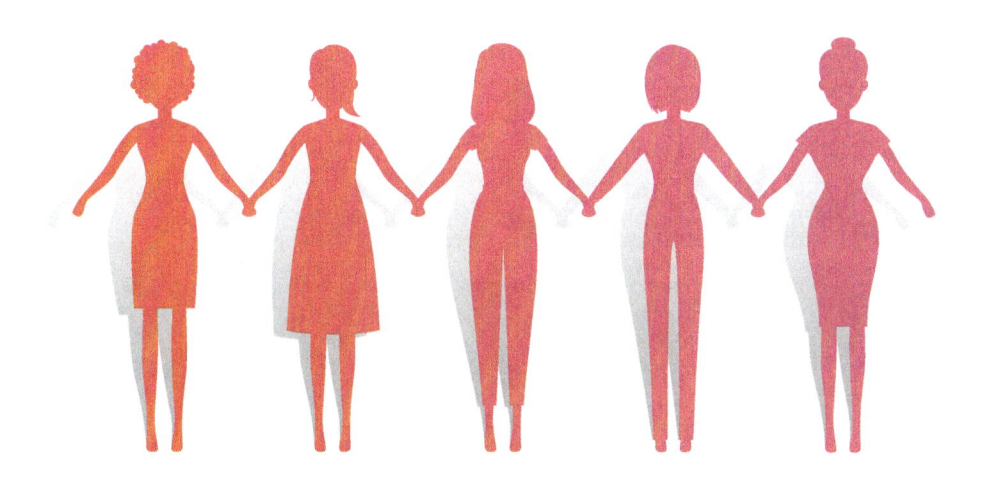

High Heel Moment | 433

434 | The Essence of a Woman — Legacy Lady

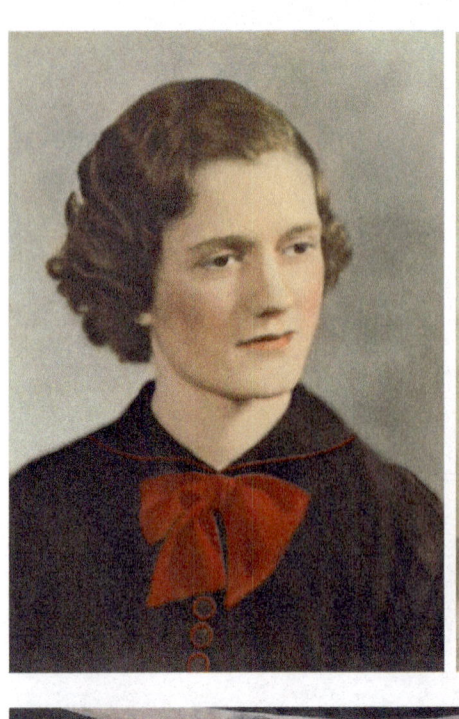

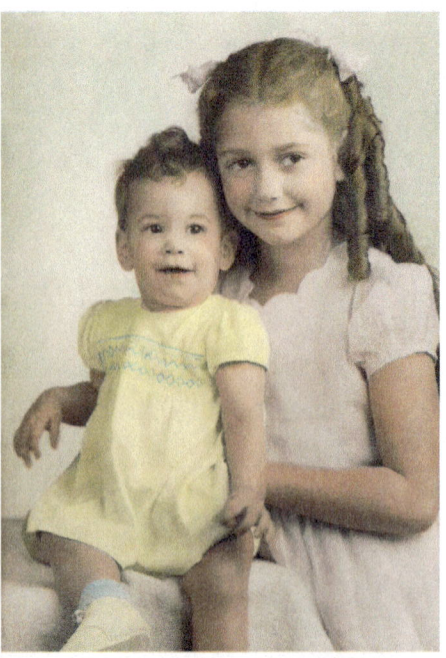

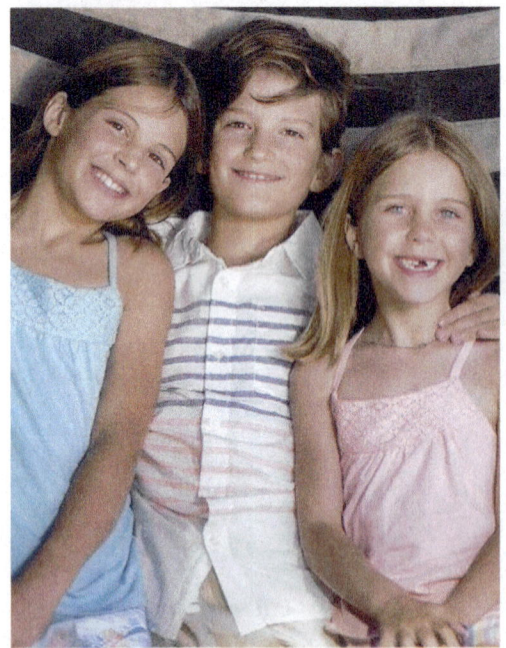

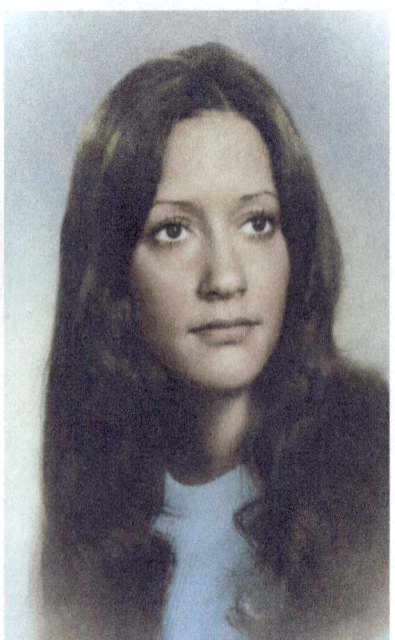

Legacy Lady

Women living with high self-esteem seek out other women, both personally and professionally. Empowered women are in tune with their inherent essence that lay their egos aside. They attract and seek out women who have the life that they want—like the inner connectivity of these paper dolls pictured below. Any woman fully expressed and fulfilled does not go it alone. She has unearthed the core significance that she simply cannot.

We honor the women who have blazed the trail for each of us, paving the road for a smoother ride on the highway of an empowered life—Women Supporting Other Women: The Power of the Universe.

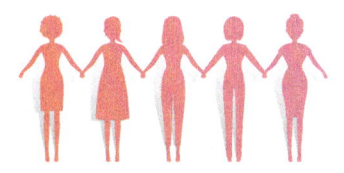

My first coach and mentor in Business, Corporate Health Coaching, and in life was the iconic Mary Kay Ashe, Founder of Mary Kay Inc. Professionally, leading the billion dollar empire on the premise of a true P & L: Not Profit and Loss but rather "People and Love." Personally, marrying Mel Ashe on a Thursday, she was such an irresistible woman to her husband that he bought/brought her a gift every week on Thursday for their entire 35 years of marriage.

—*Dr. Jo Dee Baer, PhD*

My legacy lady in life is my mother; Antoinette D. Martin who is the woman who gave me life—both to myself and my twin brother, Sean. Even during his untimely death with his tragic murder last year, she displayed the ultimate love in sacrifice in celebrating his death as a celebration of life. My other legacy lady, Dr. Jo Dee Baer, while working together for the last five years, showed me this same support and love through my grief and family healing with my brother. I honor them both.

—*Allison Anne Martin*
Virtual Assistant

In the tapestry of my life, one figure stands out as a beacon of resilience and love—my paternal grandmother, Grandma Rosie. Her journey began in turmoil, escaping a Russian pogrom and sailing to America at six years old. Upon arriving in Philadelphia, her parents fell ill and passed away, leaving her an orphan. Her older brother and sister took her in, forming a new family unit. She contributed by taking on sewing projects for her sister, honing skills that served her throughout her life.

Never having had a formal education, Grandma Rosie was incredibly smart and feisty. At 85, she decided to learn to read and write English, sitting with me to read children's books, showcasing her lifelong commitment to learning and self-improvement.

Grandma Rosie showered me with love and unwavering belief in my potential. She raised four sons, all of whom became successful men. Her legacy of resilience and familial love continues to shape my life, a true legacy lady whose influence endures.

—*Anne Borow-Lawrence, MEd*

In my lifetime, I have had amazing experiences, met extraordinary people, and received priceless guidance along the way. No one was as impactful in course-correcting my trajectory as Kerry Kronenberg (Kerry K). I was on a decade-long journey of self-discovery when I started working with Kerry and her like-minded tribe of seekers. We focused on new levels of personal responsibility and learned, as Kerry demonstrated what leadership represents. She offered me the opportunity to continually meet myself where I was, with no judgment, and a willingness to hold space in love and compassion. She exemplified kindness and empathy in a raw, real, and unapologetically authentic manner. Her example allows me to continue stepping further into my truth, exploring, expanding, and growing in a supportive environment. Kerry not only stood as an example of a beautiful healing light, but she also led me to recognize much of my potential as I lead and support others through my experiences. I use many frameworks and processes in coaching from Kerry's teachings. She is an extraordinary teacher and mentor, and she exemplifies—in every way—the true essence of a woman.

—*Anna M. McKee*

My legacy lady is First Lady Michelle Obama. Michelle used her platform to fight childhood obesity via The Healthy, Hunger-Free Kids Act. She changed nutrition standards for the National School Lunch Program by requiring that schools serve more fruits, vegetables, whole grains, and fat-free and/or low-fat milk more frequently and less starchy vegetables or foods high in sodium and trans-fat. By having more food options, the recipients utilizing this food program can live healthier lives into their adulthood. These food options may also break some of the diseases that plague underrepresented communities with health disparities. We can thank her for this.

—*Dr. Annette Watson-Johnson*

I want to acknowledge my Oma, Sigrid, who had to flee Latvia in 1939. She spoke multiple languages and landed in Germany, where my wonderful mother was born, and immigrated to Canada. They rebuilt their wealth with hard work and perseverance. She called me "Oma's Sunshine" and believed in me in a way I had never experienced before. She taught me about unconditional love and took me on a special trip when I was 12 to the historic Miramar bungalows in Montecito, California to bond with me. She worked for the government of Ontario, Canada and had multiple retirements because she was so beloved. Her smile was megawatt. She always had gifts and was generous to a fault. Her attitude and example inspired me to be generous as well.

—*Barbie Layton*

Grandmother Norlin—my legacy lady. I was the first born of her first-born son and named after her. Her attitude was "I was perfect in every way." (It took me a long time to unlearn that or live up to it—probably a little bit of both! LOL!) When I would write her letters, she would circle my errors and send them back to me. That began my foundation of being an author and helping others. She loved me unconditionally, believed in me when I did not believe in myself, and guided me through life with her strong, powerful personality.

—*Betty (Elizabeth) A. Norlin*

My mother, Brenda Cagle, is a pillar of strength and has an unwavering faith in God. Her journey has been difficult and has been filled with continuous learning and personal growth, embodying resilience and integrity. She has always fought for what is right, inspiring me to do the same. Her dedication to self-improvement and her relentless pursuit of knowledge have left an indelible mark on my life. Her example of living with purpose and faith has shaped my values and driven me to strive for excellence in everything I do.

—*Cathy Vergara, APRN*

The woman who has had the greatest influence on my life is my mother. I watched as she raised 7 kids while still helping my father manage multiple businesses, and take care of my grandparents. My mother was always incredibly active in our schooling and never missed any event. When my youngest brother was a toddler she survived a brain aneurysm. As the oldest, I have always been a help to her. It was my responsibility to "be in charge" when she needed me and I continued to be responsible well into adulthood. During this time, she owned a gym, continued to help run my father's businesses, was taking care of one of my grandmothers who was ill, and had a toddler. While she was in the hospital I took on her routine and was amazed at how much she did in a day. She is our family's support system and because of her, I am the woman I am today.

—*Cristina Candullo-Dody*

My legacy lady would be my Aunt Ruth. She always encouraged me to believe in myself and my abilities. She was one of the first women to break through the corporate ceiling. She became the first woman Vice President of Mountain Bell in 1969. The original phone company in Colorado. She instilled confidence and bravery in every female she met.

—*Cynthia Hammel-Knipe, CPE*

My 99-year-old mother, who now has "good dementia," was a fabulous example of living a life of "sufficiency"—meaning that she had access to enough resources for us to have a good, prosperous, comfortable life in the 1950s in Santiago, Chile.

She was a hair stylist who owned a beauty salon in her early '30s, where she rented stations to other stylists. She had products for sale and hired resource-poor workers to provide supplies for her. She was a humanitarian and constantly prospered for others in her successful life. I was even encouraged to be a "little cashier" in her salon, as young as six years old. My first training on handling money!

Can you imagine? I don't know if you realize how different the world was then, especially in a Catholic country in Latin America! No matter what came her way, she surpassed it. She inspired me to go for my entrepreneurial dreams. She has been an example for me to commit to a purpose-filled life where I create wealth as I add value to others. Now, she continues to teach me as she expresses gratitude daily through the "fog" of dementia. Mamacita, my best teacher by example—for nearly a century!

—*Dame Doria Cordova*
www.moneyandyoudistinctions.com

Hermine Tobolosky, mother of the Texas Equal Rights Amendment, took several young career women into her home so we could roll up our sleeves and work with her. We learned what it takes to make things happen over time; we saw the importance of being able to care for ourselves.

—*Deborah Dennis*

Linda Huff is a mentor, friend, and the most substantial person to me. She has touched my soul with her kindness, wisdom, and love. She has touched many lives through the Women's Refuge where I had the pleasure of meeting her. I have seen her be selfless, understanding, and compassionate like no one else, she is truly remarkable. The Christ-like character she has shown has not only changed my life but many others as well. Thank you!

—*Desiree Peacock*

Legacy Lady | 439

Dr. Jo Dee, you're my legacy lady for pushing me to pursue and embark on this journey. For believing in me and giving me space to share my passion with the world.

—*Dominique Brun*

Female role models weren't well-publicized in the pre-internet era of my youth. I was later inspired by talented trailblazers Anne Morrow Lindbergh, a 1928 Smith College graduate, pioneer aviatrix, writer, wife, mother, and the first woman to receive the Hubbard Medal of the National Geographic Society (1934), and jurist Ruth Bader Ginsburg, a woman of many "firsts." She was a wife, and mother, balanced a baby, and caregiving for her husband (also a law student) while at Harvard Law School (1956–1958), and then spearheaded gender equality, battled sexism, and co-founded the ACLU Women's Rights project.

—*Gloria Kurz, JD, SRS*

My legacy lady is the Venerable Dr. Rina Sircar. She was my Theravada Buddhist studies professor, incredible healer, nun, and meditation teacher for several years. Rina was my Divine Mother incarnate. Her unconditional love and warmth were incredible. She was my mentor, best friend, healer, and sister, all-in-one. I was honored to be her scribe and translator to help her bring her ancient healing practices and knowledge from her teacher, the Very Venerable Taungpulu Tawya Kaba-Aye Saydaw, to America. Together they carried the ancient forest traditions of Theravada Buddhism from Burma to Boulder Creek, California from my invitation in 1977. She is the first female teacher in the U.S. to bring ancient wisdom teachings, meditation, and chanting practices from the oldest forest monk Buddhism tradition. They are both fully realized saints. I am grateful and awed that I could be of service to World Peace in this lifetime by their side.

May All Beings Be Healthy, Happy, and Holy! Much loving kindness always.

—*Dr. Golda Joseph, PhD*

The legacy lady that I would like to mention is named Gage Tarrant. I met her more than 20 years ago when I first got my first quantum biofeedback device, the QXCI. She was one of my first teachers on how to use the device and later on I took training from her as well when I upgraded to a new model of the quantum biofeedback device, called the SCIO. Gage runs the Institute of Stress Sciences MND NRG, which puts on weekly webinars about quantum biofeedback for practitioners and has put together many online courses for training people in quantum biofeedback. Gage is incredibly bright and energetic as well as being very compassionate. She is a great teacher and I am so glad to have been taught by her.

—Dr. Hepsharat Amadi, MD, LAc

My granny the great, as I always called her, Iris Rose Bailey, was born in Poplar Workhouse in London, United Kingdom, to an "insane mother." When she was old enough, her father took her in, but she was passed from one violent auntie to the next, each time staying only until they grew tired of her.

Despite her harsh upbringing, two husbands who treated her horribly, and a life of poverty, she embodied resilience and grace. She made strength look invincible and brokenness look beautiful. She carried the weight of the world on her shoulders, yet it seemed like a pair of wings.

This year, Granny the Great began her spiritual journey in heaven. Rest easy, Queen Iris. Your spirit inspires me every day to be the best wife and mother I can be, regardless of life's challenges. I adore you and miss you deeply.

—Jennifer Louise Kerr

Reverend Alma Stevens, known to me as "my legacy lady," has been a pivotal figure in my Spiritual journey since 2010. Her unwavering support and wisdom have profoundly influenced my growth, development, and understanding of myself, the world, and human nature. Under her guidance, I have learned to navigate life without personalizing or judging others, allowing me to stand firmly within my true nature. She has taught me to live from the heart, embrace the love of all things, and find beauty in everything around me.

Throughout the years, our relationship has evolved from that of a student and mentor to one of deep friendship and mutual respect. I am incredibly grateful for the experiences we have shared and the bond we have formed, which I now cherish as a family. Together, we continue to contribute to each other's expansion, enriching our lives and the lives of those we touch. Forever grateful for the connection.

—Karen Rudolf

Best friend, wife, mother, aunt, Nana, confidant, teacher, cheerleader—not to mention—gourmet cook, avid knitter, art lover, opera lover, animal lover, sailor, world traveler, and a power kibitzer. Each of these describes my mom, Lois Strauss. I learned from her and have some favorite stories of my mom. Whether it involved a dog, fish, gerbil, frog, or even a cow, I think the gerbil was my favorite.

Growing up, we had a menagerie of critters—it always seemed that each of our dogs became "her dog" and the frog and gerbils became "ours"! Our gerbil lived in an old fish tank that sat proudly on one of the counters in our kitchen. My brother and I took turns taking care of them, as my mom refused to—she was deathly afraid of rodents. One morning she came down to prepare breakfast for us and it wasn't just any morning. We heard a scream, "the gerbil got out!!! COME DOWN STAIRS NOW!" Running down, we saw the mesh top was laying on the kitchen floor and one gerbil remained in the tank, the other got out! To no avail, we couldn't find it before everyone had to leave for work and school. As my Dad left, he told her, "If you see the gerbil, catch it!" With all of us gone, my Mom spots the gerbil behind the dryer. She called my Dad to come home immediately and he did. The capture scene that plays in my head still makes me giggle. Our laundry room was very tiny and was also the back entrance to the house. In a space approximately 7' wide by 10' long, you had the washing machine and set tub on one side with a 2' walkway and opposite was the refrigerator, freezer, dryer, and broom closet. As my Dad looked for the gerbil, the milkman made a delivery. In the 1960's it was common for women to wear pencil skirts and tight girdles to do chores. Asking the milkman to help catch the gerbil, the plan was to push the dryer out and then poke the back of it with a yardstick to coax it out. My Dad then said to my mom, "When the gerbil runs from behind, you grab him!" He poked, the gerbil ran and all they heard was a loud thud. But, it wasn't any thud—my Mom, wearing her tight pencil straight skirt and girdle, jumped on top of the washing machine!!

Besides making us laugh at her antics, she was a gracious hostess and an amazing cook. Mom was a lot of things to me, but the warmth of her heart always showed brightly. She could walk into a room of strangers and within a short time, know everyone in there—including their entire life story. We called her a power kibitzer. I only share a bit, as her light shines brightly in my heart and memories. Mom was my everything, my cheerleader, my confidant, and when dementia took her mind from us, I realized how powerful stories were to me. For my mom, *I love you.*

Remembering Her

Smile because she has lived.
Open your eyes and see all she's left.
Be full of the love you shared.
Be happy for tomorrow because of yesterday.
Cherish her memory and let it live on.
Do what she'd want: smile, open your eyes, love and go on.

—*Kathy Strauss, CCFC*

I owe all that I am and hope to become to my Mommy! My Mom raised me as a single parent in a low-income housing project. She worked every day, came home, and did things for me and my siblings like she wasn't tired. My Mom instilled in me that regardless of our physical environmental limitations, I could be anything I decided to become! She enrolled me in Young Author conferences, pageants, cheerleading, Student government, and debutante balls. I was groomed to be a leader because of my Mom.

I can never write about Legacy Ladies without acknowledging the contributions of my Great Grandmother—Vater Perkins, who I had the privilege of caring for until she passed at 96 years old. My Dad and Mom divorced when I was very young. However, my Dad's sisters (Aunt Erma and Aunt Sadie) have both been my earth angels, showing up for every important event in my life since childhood. They are both tremendous leaders, and I would not be who I am today without their support! Their Mom, my Grandmother Tomcena Clark, was always present in every aspect of my life! She taught me leadership and how to be a public speaker. She was a charter graduate and basketball player at Bethune-Cookman College. Grandma Clark passed at 96 years old.

My maternal Grandmother, Mary Kee, taught me the importance of owning real estate. With no higher education, she became the owner of 6 homes that she was able to rent out in her community prior to her transition from this earth at the age of 78. She was very strict, but loved very hard! My mother's two friends (Ms. Margaret and Ms. Wilhemina) gave me hand-me-down brand-name clothing during childhood. This gesture made me feel trendy, and I always felt like I had everything growing up. A childhood teacher, Ms. Cynthia King, referred to me as a debutante, teaching me elegance and poise. Growing up in the projects, this opportunity changed my life.

I am blessed with a community of *Legacy Ladies* who have left an indelible mark on my life. As I continue to build my personal legacy, there will be a piece of each of these women imparted as I salt the earth!

—Kim Jacobs, MBA, BD

Laura Elena Parra López took on the massive endeavor to preserve the memories of Anastacia Monsiváis Navarro, her grandmother, by keeping a journal during each visit to her place. This continued for many years with the loving intention of capturing the 107 years of Anastacia's life and preserving it for the next generations in the family. Now, that journal has turned into one of the many books published by Laura Elena Parra, my mother. Mamá Tacha, as we used to call Anastacia, is my great-grandmother. She lived as a strong, passionate, sensitive, solitary, and straightforward woman whose inheritance will flow through my veins and the generations to come. I can proudly say that I am a true testimony and fruit of many Legacy Ladies.

—*Laura Ibarra, AbD*

Forthright, brave, honest, of high character, principled, extraordinarily accomplished, deeply caring, elegant, refined, cosmopolitan. I'm still searching for a set of words to encompass the appreciation, admiration, and respect I have for Madeleine Albright. From a child refugee, fleeing persecution from fascist anti-semites bent on murdering the rest of her family, to going tête-a-tête and toe to toe on the world stage with the toughest of men, dominating the narrative and leading the way. As a world leader, she pulled no punches in acknowledgment of harsh truths. After serving as US Secretary of State and US Ambassador to the UN, she continued her commitment to improving the human condition through advisory services to heads of state, and academic prowess in the field of foreign relations, with comprehensive and complex understanding. I only wish I could have been in one of her classrooms. I wish I'd have had a chance to work with her. I will forever hold Dr. Albright in the highest esteem. By her yardstick, I know I've miles to go.

—*Leilani Alesh, Esq.*

She is strong. She is beautiful. She is gentle. How could she not be? She came from a family of five sisters, all of whom share those same traits, having to learn how to do life together from a very young age. She taught me the importance of a soft heart, even when the world around you can be so cruel. I've never seen her wear a cape, but I know she has one, somewhere. When asking me to describe a lady of legacy, she is her… She is my world. She is my namesake. She is my grandma.

—*Lorina K. Sanchez, MSN, RN*

I want to acknowledge my Mom, Shirley, who attended law school as a single mom and was one of only three women in her class. She became a US attorney back in the 1950s and went on to become a Circuit Court judge in New Jersey. After moving to Florida, she continued her practice well into her 80's. She set a powerful example for me of what a woman can do, pushing the boundaries of society, and being a wonderful mother.

—MarBeth Dunn, M.Ed. Somatic Healing Expert
Energy Healer, Empath, and Intuitive

My mother is such a woman who paved the way and passed the baton of greatness to me to further that legacy. She has consistently been the rock of our family. She was a caretaker for my brother for thirty-six years before his passing, sacrificing her life in many ways to care for him, all those years from birth. She is an excellent role model who exemplifies how to press through adversity and challenges. She went to school later in life and received first her Associate, then her Bachelor, and then her Masters. She is determined and was the first of her siblings to graduate from college.

Beautiful in and out, she exemplifies Christ in thought, word, and deed. No matter what she endured, she never gave up. A prayer warrior, she taught me how to pray and travail in the Spirit. She loves God above all else. She is one of the reasons why my Christian walk is so dedicated, why I serve in the manner that I do; I realize that no matter my title, servant is the greatest of all.

My spiritual mother, Winifred Morris, also has a significant impact on my life. She has always been the epitome of brilliance, class, and elegance. She is an excellent first lady and church mother and indeed is a leader in her own right, a formidable example to women in ministry. I gleaned from her masterful public speaking skills.

These women of legacy exemplified greatness for me to emulate in my unique way when pursuing God's destiny for my life. It is the legacy of a woman's distinction, a social mandate embedded in all women, that allows her to confidently pursue her authentic eminence, her distinct essence, knowing as Psalm 46:5, NIV affirms, "God is within her, she will not fall." She, indeed, is a phenomenal woman, like that of Maya Angelou's poem. Honor her for all that her hands have done, and let her works bring her praise (Proverbs 31:31).

—Ambassador, Dr. Nephetina L. Serrano

My inspirations stem from several female mentors, including the Divine of compassion: Kwan Yin, Goddess Isis, Mother Mary, Outstanding Oprah, Legendary Louise Hay, and Amazing Esther Hicks (Abraham)—*Law of Attraction.*

—*Dr. Nitikul Solomon, MD, MSHA, ABIHM*

I am so grateful to have had a Grandmother who was first and foremost loving and nurturing! If I stayed a week with her and my Grandfather, she always hugged me as if she hadn't seen me in a month…every morning!

Her name was Rhoda-Marie, and she knew how to confidently self-advocate, her example of that would stay with me for the rest of my life. Grandma enjoyed fashion modeling when she was young. Later, she became a hairdresser.

Her real interest was always in the wellbeing of each and every family member. She was quite detail-oriented and memorized our plate to mouth patterns. Any deviation always begged questions! It was really important to her that we all enjoyed our meals together. I thought she was pretty cool, she was married in an elegant suit in the 1930s.

—*Renée Brown, CEO*
Next Level Recovery

Billie Lynn was a strong, independent woman whose wisdom and character demanded respect. She took me under her wing during those pivotal teenage years, and I will forever be grateful for the time she spent nurturing me. She taught me to stand in my beliefs, to believe in myself, and not to conform to society. She saw something in me that others did not, and I attribute part of the success I have achieved in life to her. Thank you Mrs. Lynn for going above and beyond your responsibility as a teacher to be a role model to so many others like me!

—*Shannon L. Roper, FNP-BC*

To me, my grandmother epitomizes what it means to be a legacy lady. Widowed at a young age, she courageously took on the responsibility of managing our family's farmland, showcasing remarkable resilience and business acumen. She didn't shy away from hard work, often in the fields herself, yet her legacy extends far beyond mere labor. What truly set her apart was her compassionate approach to business. Despite the challenges she faced, she conducted herself with integrity and kindness, always putting the well-being of others before profit.

Her generosity was legendary. I recall how she would often give to those in need. She instilled in me a profound lesson about the importance of giving back and showing gratitude to the less fortunate in our community. This act of selflessness left an indelible mark on me, teaching me the value of empathy and the significance of supporting others.

My grandmother's legacy is not just about her achievements as a businesswoman or her resilience in adversity—it's about her unwavering commitment to kindness and compassion. She exemplified how success is measured not only by financial gains but also by the positive impact we have on those around us. She remains my ultimate role model—a true legacy lady whose lessons continue to guide and inspire me every day.

—*Dr. Shirley Luu*

Sue Baldwin was an influential businesswoman in an era when no women were in the boardroom is my legacy lady. Sue was always the only one, and I was lucky enough to be there alongside her on several projects—in an era where women were cutting each other down rather than supporting one another. I will always remember Sue for her support and encouragement in my first years in business.

I started working with Sue during my Work Experience placement in High School in 1989, and went on to work under her when she was Director of Marketing at SCA Packaging in Belgium in 1995.

She showed me that being a woman was an asset—not a liability—in our ability to envision, multitask, and persist toward a common goal.

But most importantly, she gave me my first positive belief in the form of a small poster she had made and pinned on her office door:

'The Impossible Just Takes A Little Longer.'

A sentence that has shaped my career and my life.

The strength I have drawn from this above phrase has helped me achieve what some have called 'miracles'—for me, it is just 'normal,' 'purposeful,' and 'life.'

—*Sonja Rechnitzer*

Alleda Travillion Good: The original #GOODGirl. Period! Your infectious smile, laughter, and heart built communal bridges of unity, hope, and joy like no other. The world was your dance floor and you would spontaneously do a one-two step, shake, or roll bounce as the sound of drum beats, horns, or marching bands alike unleashed your soul. You will forever be my big cousin. A Legend. A legacy lady. Live, Love, Laugh like Leda!

—*Dr. Tyra Good*

Old Women in the Locker Room

Old women in the locker room
undress for the water aerobics class
at the local community center,
push their fleshy breasts into too-small cups
of faded swimsuits, and swollen feet
into bright colored sandals.
Eager as girls, they head for the pool
chatting in several languages, holding off
the ravages of time one more day.

Husbands long gone,
sustained by their children,
skin deeply wrinkled and bodies sagging
from years of toil and stress,
their unfailing courage astounds me.

No reporters come to interview them,
no medals are awarded to them,
no platform is theirs on which to speak.
Unnoticed and invisible they survive
to return day after day,
the brave old women in the locker.

—June Mandelkern (age 100)
Award winning poet
Author page: https://shorturl.at/BXKsS

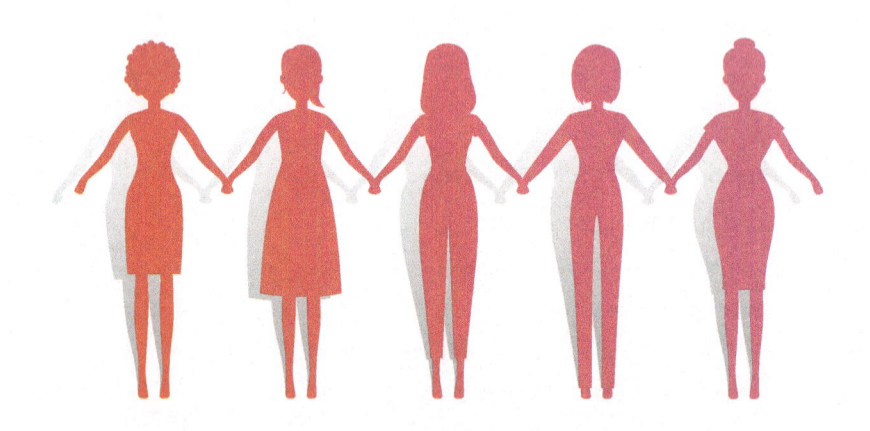

The Young Women

The young women, I love to see them
clutching books tightly in their arms
or pushing strollers to the library
and the shops on Main Street,

Legs sturdy or slim
brightly encased in patterned tights,
long sweaters hanging loosely
according to the fashion of the day,
with sneakers or practical shoes
and jackets snugly fastened
against the winter chill.

American to the core,
they know the world awaits
the sound of their voices
and the firm tread of their heels
in the corridors of power.

We, my friends and I,
their mothers, aunts and grandmothers
who have walked the paths they walk today,
we spread our canopy of love
beneath their wings
and, awestruck, watch them as they fly.

—June Mandelkern (age 100)
Award winning poet
Author page: https://shorturl.at/BXKsS

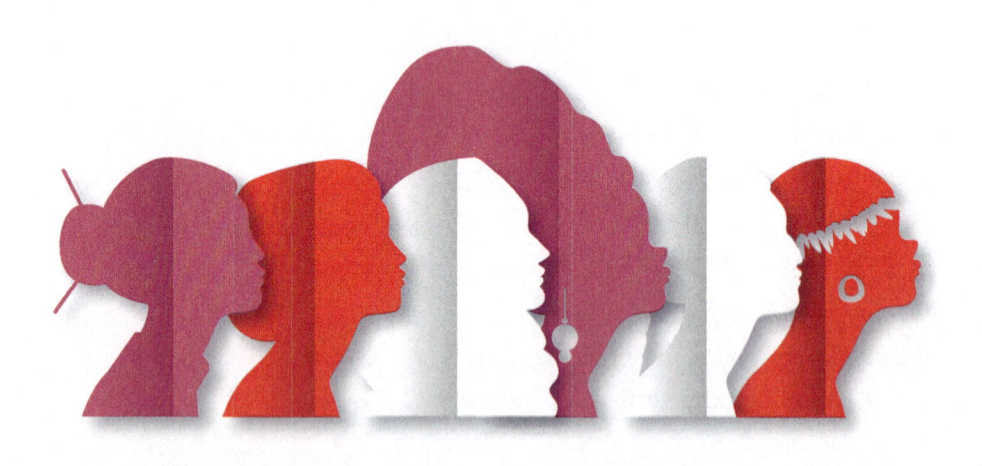

Author Resources

SPIRITUAL PILLAR

Dr. Khalilah Camacho-Ali
Author, Actress, Filmmaker, Motivational Speaker, Philanthropist
United States
E-mail: TKO2020@yahoo.com
www.MamaAliToday.com

Dr. James Marinakis, ND, HmD, Acu.Phys.
Boca Raton, Florida, United States
E-mail: dr.marinakis@gmail.com
www.vitalessence.com
www.ppi-international.com

Shannon L. Roper, FNP-BC
Family Nurse Practitioner
Roper's Health Oasis
Carlsbad, New Mexico, United States
www.ropershealthoasis.com
E-mail: shannon_roper@ropershealthoasis.com
Facebook: www.facebook.com/ropershealthoasis
IG: @shannonroper11
LinkedIn: www.linkedin.com/in/shannon-roper-a030a8289

Resources
The New Catholic Answer Bible, "A Virtuous Woman Speaks with Wisdom and Kindness" Proverbs 31:26

Dr. Nephetina L. Serrano
U.N. Global Ambassador for Peace, Relationship Expert, Co-founder
Covenant Rescue 911 501c3
Philadelphia, Pennsylvania, United States
E-mail: drserranoministries@gmail.com
www.marriageCEOs360.com
www.covenantmarriagesinc.com
Facebook: www.facebook.com/drnephetinaserrano
IG: @drnephetinaserrano

www.linkedin.com/in/dr-nephetina-l-serrano-977a633/ ("A journey of a thousand miles begins with a single step," 2024)

www.threads.net/@drnephetinaserrano?xmt= AQGzIdZmkq2svXX63rwOo5fEpE7cLApdjjLeCRixsyObk0M

Resources

Scriptures marked NIV are taken from the New International Version (NIV): Scripture taken from *The Holy Bible, New International Version®*. Copyright 1973, 1978, 1984, 2011 by Biblica, Inc.™. Used by permission of Zondervan.

Debbie Morales
Executive Director
Women's Refuge of St. Johns County
St. Augustine, Florida, United States
E-mail: debbiemorales77@yahoo.com
www.womensrefugeofstjo.com
Facebook: www.facebook.com/thewomensrefugeofstjo

Resources

Holding On When You Want to Let Go: Clinging to Hope When Life Is Falling Apart by Sheila Walsh

How to Forgive Ourselves Totally: Begin Again by Breaking Free from Past Mistakes by R.T. Kendall

TOTAL Forgiveness Experience: A Study Guide to Repairing Relationships by R.T. Kendall

Desiree Peacock
Christian Counseling
Liberty University
United States
E-mail: peacockdesiree4@gmail.com

Dr. Nitikul Solomon, MD, MSHA, ABIHM
Holistic Physician
Doctor Niti
United States
E-mail: Nitikuls@hotmail.com
www.DoctorNiti.com
Facebook: www.facebook.com/DoctorNitikul
IG: @doctornitiheals/
X (Twitter): @DoctorNitiheals
LinkedIn: www.linkedin.com/in/dr-niti-solomon-732490a

Resources

https://navuturesorts.com/blog/chakras-explained-the-7-chakras-you-need-to-know-about

MENTAL PILLAR

Jennifer Louise Kerr

Co-founder at MindKite Wellbeing | Mental Health First Aid Trainer | Expert in Mindset & Performance Coaching

United Kingdom

E-mail: Jenniferlouisekerr@gmail.com

www.MindKitementalhealth.com

Facebook: www.facebook.com/profile.php?id=100009653316775

IG: @ jennifer.louise.kerr

TikTok: www.tiktok.com/@jenniferlouisekerr

Kathy Strauss, CCFC

Creationeer | Creative Connector

ImageWerks LC | photography & art

Myrtle Beach, South Carolina, United States

E-mail: kathy@imagewerks.net

www.imagewerks.net

Facebook business: www.facebook.com/imagewrks

Facebook personal: www.facebook.com/kathy.strauss1

Facebook: www.facebook.com/wine.nibbles.scribbles

IG: @imagewerks

LinkedIn: www.linkedin.com/in/imagewerks

X (twitter): @imagewrk

Resources

Rhonda Byrne. *The Magic.* www.thesecret.tv/products/the-magic-book/

Jill Bolte Taylor, Ph, D. *My Stroke of Insight: A Brain Scientist's Personal Journey.* www.drjilltaylor.com

Ted Talk: Jill Bolte Taylor's "Stroke of Insight."
https://www.ted.com/talks/jill_bolte_taylor_my_stroke_of_insight

Ted Talk: Tina Seelig. *InGenius: A Crash Course in Creativity.*
https://youtu.be/gyM6rx69iqg

Mel Robbins. *The High Five Habit.* 2021.

Whitney Freya. www.whitneyfreya.com

Published books:

Ignite Your Faith. (compilation book). My chapter, "Making an Impression." 2023

Health-a-Pedia: Putting the Pieces Together in Foundational Health. (compilation book). My chapter, "Creating the Art of Your Strength." 2024

Kathy Strauss. *Kaleidoscope: Redesigning Your Life. Tapping into your inner artist for healing and inspiration.* Forthcoming.

Coloring Your Spirit: designs & meditations to spark the creative in all of us. 2017

52 Weeks of Gratitude: 52 positive words that can change your life & the way you think. 2019.

Positive Spirit: an intentional & mindful journey through coloring & journaling. 2023.

Lorina K. Sanchez, MSN, RN

Forensic Nurse

Alamogordo, New Mexico, United States

E-mail: lorinasanchez@gmail.com

www.thesanenurse.com

Facebook: www.facebook.com/lorina.sanchez.75

IG: @lorina.sanchez

LinkedIn: www.linkedin.com/in/lorina-sanchez-5b28852b0

Resources

National Sexual Assault Hotline: 1(800)656-HOPE (4673) or online chat available at www.online.rainn.org

Victim Support Systems: 1(425)252-6081 or www.victimsupportservices.org

World Health Organization (WHO). (2024). Violence Against Women. www.who.int/news-room/fact-sheets/detail/violence-against-women#:~:text=A%20 2018%20analysis%20of%20prevalence%20data%20from%20 2000%E2%80%932018,partner%20or%20non-partner%20sexual%20violence%20 or%20both%20%282%29.

Anne Borow-Lawrence, MEd

The Science of Well-being

EnVisionCCS

Boston, Massachusetts, United States

E-mail: anneblawrence@gmail.com

www.envisionccs.com

Facebook: www.facebook.com/anne.borowlawrence

IG: @artof_aliveness

LinkedIn: www.linkedin.com/in/anne-borow-lawrence-3b18b933

The Art of Aliveness, Let Your Spirit Soar

YouTube: Art of Aliveness Chronicles with Annie B.
www.youtube.com/watch?v=1CWqfZPxIXY

Resources

Dr. Ruth Richards: "Everyday Creativity and the Healthy Mind"
Yale University: Coursera: The Science of Well-Being
www.MarthaGraham.org
VIA Strength Finders
The Art of Aliveness, Let Your Spirit Soar

Betty (Elizabeth) A. Norlin
President and CEO
What Is Holistic Health, LLC
Tampa, Florida, United States
E-mail: whatisholistichealth@gmail.com
E-mail: transform@bettynorlin.com
www.bettynorlin.com
Facebook: www.facebook.com/whatisholistichealth
LinkedIn: www.linkedin.com/in/bettynorlin
IG: @WhatIsHolisticHealth
Speaker Hub: bit.ly/BettyNorlin
X (Twitter): @WhatIsHolisticH
YouTube: www.youtube.com/@whatisholistichealth3474 (Check out Playlist Vagus)
Podcast: www.behealthyinahurry.com

Renée Brown
President and CEO
Next Level Recovery, Sober Living Properties, and Medical Mindshare
Salt Lake City, Utah, United States
E-mail: improvefostercare@gmail.com
E-mail: reneeb@nextlevelrecovery.com
www.nextlevelrecovery.com
www.soberlivingproperties.com
www.medicalmindshare.com
Facebook: www.facebook.com/profile.php?id=61560982367321
Facebook: www.facebook.com/NextLevelRecovery
Facebook: www.facebook.com/SoberLivingProperties
LinkedIn: www.linkedin.com/in/reneebrown360

Resources

www.ImproveFosterCare.org—
   Platform to improve foster care through legislative change.

www.ForeverHomesforFosterKids.org—A nonprofit that reunites children with family internationally You can also support child reunification efforts when you purchase the international award-winning book, Do No Harm
www.amazon.com/Do-No-Harm-Tragedy-Continues/dp/0981919952

The world's first free gamified school for business—www.mannyfestation.com Manny Lopez assists entrepreneurs to market and the proceeds educate thousands of foster children in business nationwide.

Fostering Great Ideas: www.fgi4kids.org. Resources for everyone.

EMOTIONAL PILLAR

Dr. Jacqueline Mohair, PhD
President; Trinity School of Business
United States
www.trinityschoolofbusiness.org
themohairs@gmail.com

Sonja Rechnitzer
CEO, Global Trainer
Intuition Wisdom Institute
Brisbane, Australia
E-mail: 1@intuitionwisdom.com
www.IntuitionWisdom.com
Facebook: www.facebook.com/SonjaRechnitzer
Facebook: www.facebook.com/IntuitionWisdomInstitute
YouTube: www.youtube.com/@IntuitionWisdom

Karen Rudolf
Creator | Empowerment Coach, Catalyst for Change
Tranquil SOULutions, LLC
United States
E-mail: Karen@TranquilSOULutions.com
www.TranquilSOULutions.com
Facebook: www.facebook.com/karen.rudolf.14
IG: @tranquilsoulutions/
LinkedIn: www.linkedin.com/in/tranquilsoulutions
Linktr.ee: https://linktr.ee/tranquilsoulutions

Resources

A SOUL-opreneur's Stress Relief Checklist at: www.karenrudolf.com/freegiftfromkaren.com

Calendly: www.calendly.com/tranquilsoulutions/30-minutes-meet-greet

Check out our Podcast: *Awakening Potential*:
https://open.spotify.com/show/4YWLGUPg3rWtumXl084oEJ

Grab yours complimentary: *A SOUL-opreneur's Stress Relief Checklist* at: www.freegiftfromkaren.com

Cynthia Hammel-Knipe, CPE

Certified Professional Electrologist | Previous Director of Continuing Education, American Electrology Association, AEA | President, Colorado Association of Electrology, 20 years | Currently: Vice President, CAE | Esthetician, Permanent Make-Up Artist | Certified Iridologist, Applied Kinesiologist | Master Herbalist

Integrated Wellness Services, Inc.

United States

E-mail: crhkiws@gmail.com

www.electrology.com

#hammelknipe

IG: @cindyrhk

LinkedIn: www.linkedin.com/in/cindy-hammel-knipe-5a113034/

Resources

Electrolysis, Thermolysis and the Blend. A.R. Hinkle

Milady—Guide to Esthetics. Bickmoore

Spontaneous Healing. Dr. Andrew Weil

International Board of Electrolysis Certification Study Guide. Patsy Kirby CPE and various experts in the field of Electrology, Dermatology, Endocrinology and Health

CPE is the International Board of Electrology Certification Credential

American Electrology Association, IBEC Study Guide. Patsy Kirby CPE and various experts in the fields of Electrology, Dermatology, Endocrinology and Infection Control.

MarBeth Dunn

M.Ed., Kundalini Yoga Instructor, Reiki Master, Matrix Energetics Practitioner, Empath and Intuitive

Destination Empowerment, Inc.

Florida, United States

E-mail: marbeth@marbethdunn.com

www.marbethdunn.com

Facebook: www.facebook.com/marbethdunn1

Facebook: www.facebook.com/MiracleMindsetwithMarBeth

IG: @marbethdunn
LinkedIn: www.linkedin.com/in/marbethdunn

Barbie Layton
CEO
Barbie Layton Quantum Enterprises, LLC
United States
E-mail: intuitivebarbie1@gmail.com
www.barbielayton.com
www.theinfinitylifeusa.com
Facebook: www.facebook.com/barbie.layton.5
IG @barbielaytonofficial
LinkedIn: www.linkedin.com/in/barbielayton
Threads @barbielaytonofficial

Leilani Alesh, Esq.
Creative
A Sante LLC
United Kingdom
E-mail: LeilaniAlesh@icloud.com
www.privatelyplaced.com
www.bloomingzenies.com

Resources
[i] Bessie Smith was a famous blues singer who tragically died after a car accident. She was allegedly denied a blood transfusion by a hospital designated "No Colored People."
www.grunge.com/942393/the-truth-and-myth-behind-the-1937-death-of-bessie-smith/

Anna M. McKee
Personal Development Consultant, Embodiment Coach
AM Developments
United States
E-mail: anna@iamdevelopments.com
www.iamdevelopments.com
Facebook: www.facebook.com/anna.mckee.330
IG: @iamdevelopments
LinkedIn: Anna McKee

PHYSICAL PILLAR

Dr. Glen Depke, ND
E-mail: glen@depkewellness.com
www.depkewellness.com
Dr. Glen Depke is a Traditional Naturopath since 1985

Cathy Vergara, APRN
APRN
United States
E-mail: cathyarnp@gmail.com
www.newhoperegeneration.com
www.thelifelinecenter.com
Facebook: www.facebook.com/cathy.c.vergara
https://www.spiritualinsightsradio.com/#

Dr. Annette Watson-Johnson
Author, CEO, President, Wellness Ambassador
Dynamic AWJ Products LLC
United States
E-mail: justgetwellseamoss@gmail.com
www.dynamicawjproducts.com
Facebook: www.facebook.com/dynamicawjproductsllc
Facebook: www.facebook.com/JustGetWellSeaMossProducts
IG: @Justgetwellseamoss
LinkedIn: www.linkedin.com/in/annette-watson-johnson-0b3b94245/
YouTube: www.youtube.com/@justgetwellseamoss5625
Tik Tok: www.tiktok.com/@justgetwellseamoss

Dr. Hepsharat Amadi, MD, LAc
Medical Doctor, Licensed Acupuncturist
Dr. Amadi's Holistic Health Center
United States
E-mail: dramadi@dramadi.com
www.greatnaturaldoctor.com
www.dramadi.com
Facebook: www.facebook.com/DrHepsharatAmadi

IG: @greatnaturaldoctor
LinkedIn: www.linkedin.com/in/hepsharat-amadi-01159125
YouTube: www.youtube.com/@dramadi
TikTok: www.tiktok.com/@realdramadi

Resources

Book about Natural Hormone Balance by Hepsharat Amadi, MD, LAc (available later this year)

What Your Doctor May Not Tell You About Menopause by John R. Lee, MD

What Your Doctor May Not Tell You About Perimenopause by John R. Lee, MD

The Wisdom of Menopause by Christiane Northrup, MD

Overcoming Thyroid Disorders by David Brownstein, MD

Safe Uses of Cortisol by William McK. Jeffries

Why Do I Still Have Thyroid Symptoms by Datis Kharrazian

Normal Blood Tests Aren't Good Enough by Ellie Cullen

From Hormone Hell to Hormone Wellby C.W. Randolph, Jr., MD and Genie James, M.M.Sc.

Dr. Tyra Good

Associate Professor of Education

GOOD Knowledge Connections, LLC / Elms College

United States

E-mail: tyragood@gmail.com

Business Facebook: www.facebook.com/drtyragood

Personal Facebook: www.facebook.com/tyrathegooddr/

Instagram: @tyrathegooddr

X (Twitter): www.twitter.com/tyrathegooddr

LinkedIn: www.linkedin.com/in/drtyragood

Resources

Addressing Implicit Bias in Women's Health. 2021. Nursing@Georgetown.

Logan, S., & Good, T. (Eds.). (2022). *Black Women Navigating Historically White Higher Education Institutions and the Journey Toward Liberation*. IGI Global.

Science, Innovation and Technology Summit: Chronic Pain in Women—Focus on Treatment, Management and Barriers. 2020. Healthy Women.

Sustainable Development Goals: 17 Goals to Transform our World

Dr. Golda Joseph, PhD

M.A. East West Psychology and Integral Counseling | PhD in the Philosophy of Nutrition

Regeneration Health, Inc.

United States and Panama

E-mail: drgolda@gmail.com
www.regeneration.com
Facebook: www.facebook.com/drgoldajoseph
IG: @drgolda/
LinkedIn: www.linkedin.com/in/drgolda/

Resources

Human Life—New Organic Thinking to Practice Spiritual Science Study: by George and Gisela O'Neil

Man on the Threshold: The Challenge of Inner Developments by Bernard Lievegoed

Citizens of the Cosmos: Life's Unfolding from Conception through Death to Rebirth by Beredene Jocelyn

Rudolf Steiner Archive: rsarchive.org—*Study of Man—Lectures on Human Development*

FINANCIAL PILLAR

Dr. Shirley Luu
Financial Planner and Insurance Broker
Shirley Luu & Associates (SLA): Financial Services and Insurance
McLean, Virginia, United States
E-mail: luushirley@gmail.com
www.shirleyluuassociates.com
Facebook: www.facebook.com/shirleyluuassociates
IG: @shirleyluuassociates
LinkedIn: www.linkedin.com/company/shirley-luu-associates
YouTube: www.youtube.com/results?search_query=Shirley+Luu

Resources

IUL ASAP by Shirley Luu
https://www.amazon.com/IUL-ASAP-Financial-Generate-Tax-Free/dp/0578907054
https://worldreporter.com/shirley-luu-empowering-financial-literacy-and-security/
The Power of Zero by David McKnight
The Retirement Miracle by Patrick Kelley

Donna Dawson, FCCA
Certified Accountant
Australia
www.proverbsforthesoul.com
E-mail: donna@proverbsforthesoul.com

Dominique Brun

CEO, Founder, Coach
DominoFX Group
United States
E-mail: dominique@dominofxgroup.com
www.dominofxgroup.com
linktr.ee/dominofxgroup.com
Facebook: www.facebook.com/dominofxgroup
IG: www.instagram.com/thedomino_effect_/?hl=en
X (Twitter): www.twitter.com/dominofxgroup
LinkedIn: www.linkedin.com/in/dominofxgroup
YouTube: www.youtube.com/channel/UCViXjE4nsxoWYdV304DJ8uA

Resources

Claim Your FREE Business Credit Building Guide:
https://financeguide.dominofxgroup.com/

Want more tips and info about this resource, let's connect! Book a call, email or schedule your Funding Planning Session today. https://plan.dominofxgroup.com/

Workshop: How to Get $50k+ in 0% Interest Funding:
https://api.profitlifter.com/widget/form/10otYhXUTXYgwZ68oV98

Newsletter: Subscribe on LinkedIn to stay connected with the best resources to grow your business:
www.linkedin.com/build-relation/newsletter-follow?entityUrn=7187592978859773952

Laura Ibarra, AbD

Founder and CEO of más-in (Torreón, Coah. México) and 3 Wins International LLC (Greenville, S.C., USA).
Mexico and United States
PhD Student in Social Research; MBA and Master of Arts in Strategic Design and Innovation.
Master Interpreter of the DISC Model (English and Spanish).
E-mail: laura@3winsinternational.com
www.3winsinternational.com
Facebook: www.facebook.com/Laura.Ibarra.Creative
IG: @laura.ibarra.creative
LinkedIn: www.linkedin.com/in/lauraibarracreative

Resources

Hill, N. (1937). *Think and Grow Rich*. The Napoleon Hill Foundation.
www.3winsinternational.com
www.mas-in.com
ww.thebriefjoy.com

www.ahamsc.org
www.naphill.org
www.luisjimenezcoaching.com

Gloria Kurz, JD, SRS
Principle
Mansions & Manors®
United States
gloria@mansionsandmanors.com
www.mansionsandmanors.com
Facebook corporate: mansions_manors
Facebook personal: www.facebook.com/gloria.kurz1
IG: @gloriajkurz
LinkedIn: www.linkedin.com/in/gloriakurz/
X (Twitter): @mansionsmanors
X (Twitter): @kurzgloria

SOCIAL PILLAR

Tiffany Haddish
Comedian, Actress, New York Times Best-Selling Author: "The Black Unicorn" and "I Curse You with Joy"
United States
https://shop.tiffanyhaddish.com/collections/shop-all
IG:@tiffanyhaddish
YouTube: @thaddish
#icurseyouwithjoy

Dr. Jo Dee Baer, PhD
Certified Health Coach; Holistic Nutritionist; Board Certified NLP Trainer
Foundational Health; *Health-a-Pedia*
United States
E-mail: jodee@healthcoachjodee.com
www.drjodee.com
www.healthapedia365.com
Facebook: www.facebook.com/healthapedia365
Facebook Public Figure: Dr. Jo Dee | www.facebook.com/profile.php?id=61558578356855

IG: @HealthCoachJoDee; @HealthaPedia365
LinkedIn: www.linkedin.com/in/drjodeebaer/
LinkedIn: www.linkedin.com/company/health-a-pedia/
YouTube: www.youtube.com/@HealthaPedia365

Resources

Holy Bible: NIV Version

Life on Your Terms. Rex Sikes

Coco: Will You Be my Friend. Dr. Seuss

"I am Woman" song by Helen Reddy: All rights reserved

United Nations symbol all rights reserved

Publications

Ignite the Hunger in You anthology book with Dr. Les Brown chapter: "From Tummy Ache to Transcendent Health." 2020.

Ignite your Wisdom. anthology book: Chapter: "Feel Your Real." 2021.

Ignite your Faith: anthology book: Chapter: "Messengers on the Shoulder." 2023.

21 Days to Your Best You: Keys to a Life of Excellence. Dr. Jo Dee Baer, PhD 2023.

Health-a-Pedia" Putting the Puzzle Pieces Together in Foundational Health. Dr. Jo Dee Baer, PhD and Dr. James Marinakis, ND, HmD, Acu.Phys. 2023.

Kim Jacobs, MBA, BD (Balance Doctor)

Host of The Kim Jacobs Show | Founder, Gabe's Heart Foundation

eWomenNetwork.com—Charlotte Managing Director

United States

E-mail: kimjacobs@ewomennetwork.com

E-mail: kim@thebalancedoctor.tv

E-mail: kimjacobs@ewomennetwork.com

www.kimjacobsconsulting.com

www.gabesheartfoundation.org

Facebook: www.facebook.com/Thekimjacobsshow

Facebook: www.facebook.com/thebalancedoctor

IG: @Thekimjacobsshow

IG: @Kimjacobsthebalancedoctor

x (Twitter): @Kimthebalancedr

LinkedIn: www.linkedin.com/in/thekimjacobsshow/

YouTube: www.youtube.com/@KimJacobsShow

Deborah Dennis:
XtraGrow, LLC
Dallas, Texas, United States
E-mail: Deborah@XtraGrow.com
www.XtraGrow.com
www.XtraGrowFoundation.org
Facebook: www.facebook.com/XtragrowNutrition
Facebook: www.facebook.com/XtraGrowFoundation
IG: @XtraGrow

Resources
Deborah@XtraGrowFoundation.org
Deborah@XtraGrow.com
David@XtraGrow.com

Cristina Candullo-Dody
Owner—Co-founder
Cristina Candullo Events; Zeta Mu Phi; Illuminate
United States
E-mail: cristina.candullo@gmail.com
www.cristinacandulloevents.com
www.zetamuphi.com
www.illuminatezeta.org
Facebook: Zeta Mu Phi: www.facebook.com/profile.php?id=100064659915085
IG: @CristinaCandulloEvents
IG: @zetamuphi
IG: @illuminateltw

HRH Princess Dr. Moradeun Ogunlana
UN Ambassador, Nigeria
Founder and CEO African Women's Health Project Interntional
AWHPI GLOBAL
Nigeria and United States
Nigeria E-mail: deunogunlana@gmail.com
www.awhpi.org
www.princessmoradeun.com

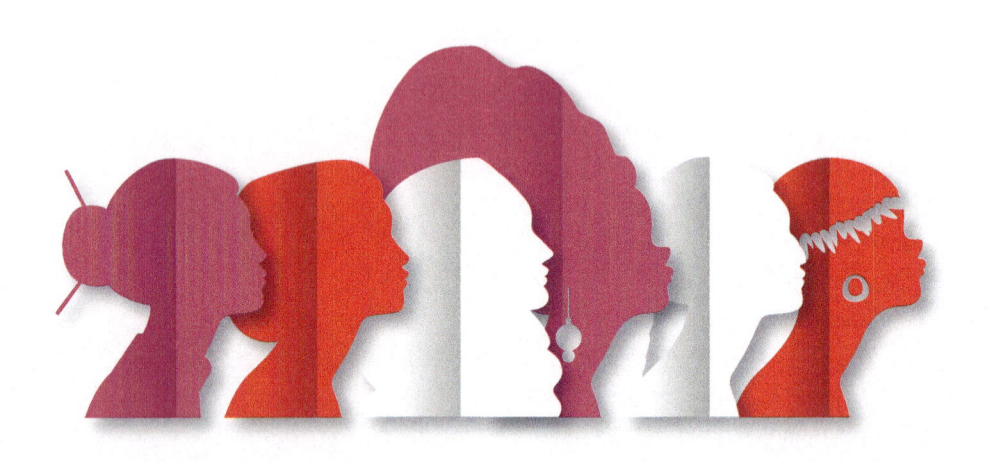

Author Acknowledgements

SPIRITUAL PILLAR

Dr. Khalilah Camacho-Ali

Thanks to my five amazing children for their love and support, and to Allah for my eternal hope, passion, and vision.

Dr. James Marinakis, ND, HmD, Acu.Phys.

My Family, the Marinakis Clan (Heracleidae) Greece

Photography: Meg Pukel Photography

I'm dedicating my efforts regarding this book, *The Essence of A Woman*, to the most significant female of my life, Ahisha Marinakis. I may have fathered her, what a privilege, but she has taught me more about the importance of the female essence in all things, than any one in this life. She did this with her generosity, kindness, perseverance, tenacity, and endurance. Ahisha is an emanation of the divine female essence. Her namesake is of what may be the first name and acknowledgment of a goddess, recognized by people prehistoric. This entity Aisha was called on by people during the formation of civilization whenever there was a problem so dire that it threatened their existence and the organization of life. The entity Aisha is called on when mankind cannot go on without that spirit to solve a problem. I received her name inside myself before she was born. But I had never heard the name before. It had not become popular until quite a while after her birth. I saw the spelling of the name on a business card of a doctor who worked for me in California, whose father was the physician to the last emperor of China. Although Ahisha would never say these things about herself, like her brother, Ulysses, they were more than their mother and I could have ever hoped for to share this human experience. Had I done one thing to leave this world a better place than when I got here, I have succeeded in them.

Shannon L. Roper, FNP-BC

Photographer: Ashley T. Kajiki

I would like to thank Robert for his guidance, support, and, most of all, unconditional love along my journey.

I also want to thank my parents, sisters, and my children for their never-ending support through all my life journeys.

Dr. Nephetina L. Serrano

I give God all the Glory for the things he has done and is still doing in my life. For in Christ there is no failure.

To my amazng husband, Dr. Richard Serrano for 35 years in covenant: thank you for your friendship, love, support, and most of all, your prayers.

Thank you to my beautiful Mom, Elder Emma Jean Brant, for being the true essence of a woman for without you there is no me.

Claudia S. Crammer you are a gift and I am blessed to have you on my team.

And lastly, to any and every woman that has made an impact in my life, you all matter and I thank you from my heart.

Debbie Morales

Thank you to the late Ed and Joan Clements, Linda Huff, Mama Myrtle Hollingsworth, Mr. Dennis Hollingsworth, and The Women's Refuge of St. Johns County.

Also, thank you to Mr. Herbert Beck, GospelBlue Productions: Photography/Videography: https://www.gospelblue.org/ or facebook.com/GospelBlue/.

Desiree Peacock

Thank you to my family, Linda Huff, the late Joan Clements, and the Seminole Community Church family.

Dr. Nitikul Solomon, MD, MSHA, ABIHM

My daughter, Natalie Solomon, is my rock.

My beautiful friend, Renée Brown, inspires and supports me.

Dr. Jo Dee Baer: an empathetic, understanding, and patient super mentor.

MENTAL PILLAR

Jennifer Louise Kerr

To my husband, words cannot fully capture the depth of my gratitude for your unwavering love and support. Thank you for seeing the real me beneath the armour and for standing by my side with steadfast patience and strength. Your belief in my potential and your relentless encouragement have been my guiding light on this journey. Even on the days when I resist and push back, your love remains unshakeable.

—All my love, Little Jen

Kathy Strauss, CCFC

Photography and hair/makeup: Gillian Claire—Gillian Claire Photography and Trei Helms/Myrtle Beach Hair & Makeup

Thank you to my late husband—GC Schow, who, no matter what health challenges he faced, always encouraged me to reach for my dreams. If it wasn't for him, I would not have learned to dig deep into my creativity and faith. A heartfelt thank you to my mom and dad for smiling with a push to follow my artistic vision. My Dad is and has been my source of inspiration for resilience and creativity. He's shown me that even late in life and after a long, loving marriage to my mom for 63 years—you can move on and find love, and encouragement, and live creatively! And finally, to my old college friend Pete Denio. He's taught and is continuing to teach me that the trait of patience is truly a virtue. Encouraging me to embrace the natural world and to truly see everything with my eyes and my soul.

Lorina K. Sanchez, MSN, RN

Thank you, first and foremost, to my mom for your unconditional, and unwavering love. You're my hero!

Thank you to all of the women who have impacted my life through your support, strength, and courage to help create the woman that I have become today!

A special thank you to my photographer: Trish Flores Photography.

Anne Borow-Lawrence, MEd

I could never have participated in this amazing collaboration without the endless love, patience, encouragement, and support of my dear husband Jim Lawrence. My parents, Willard and Florence Borow, without whom I would not be here…their love, support, guidance, and inspiration are with me every day and with every breath I take. Dr. Jo Dee Baer for seeing the bright light in me and trusting who she has always known me to be—a leader and guide of women on behalf of them living their most extraordinary and fulfilled lives. To my brothers and sisters-in-law for their love, insights, and undying support. I am grateful to all of my dear friends and mentors along my journey. Thank you Lynne Damianos for the beautiful photos.

Betty (Elizabeth) A. Norlin

Thank you to my family, friends, colleagues, and students who have taught me the gift of love, tenacity, perseverance, and grit. Thank you to my Chi Omega chapter at Troy State that taught me the true essence of being a woman.

Thank you to my mentors: Lethia Owens, Women of Audacious Faith; Clint Arthur and Ali Savitch, Celebrity Entrepreneurs; Dr. Wayne "The MangoMan" Pickering and Buddy Lee who have grown and challenged me along the way; G. Randall James who believed in me and our ideas as we started our initial business venture together, and to the many others who have influenced me, and now you. Also, to my National Speakers Association Central Florida Chapter for their grace and guidance.

Special mention to my family, who have walked through the challenging path of the "health hiccups" I have had along the way, and blessed and guided me with their love and support: Luci Norlin, Judy Norlin, Lori and Mike Mondor, Andre and Robby Mondor and the multitude of friends I call family.

Most of all, thank you to my Creator for blessing me with life and the mission to share my lessons with others.

Renée Brown

To Kevin and Eddie and in memory of Danny, Anna, and all of the foster care children.

In memory of my Grandparents who gave me enough love to last a lifetime.

To my loving husband and beautiful daughters, as well as to my extended family.

To my work associates/board members who continuously have love for our clients and journey with them in wellness.

To Dr. Jo Dee Baer: Thanks for all of your love and encouragement!!

To supportive friends in my life: Julia, Yolanda, Chrissie, Tina, Michelle, Gina, Beatrice, Tina, Silvia, Eldi-Mira, Debbie, Tess, Laura, Denise, Katrina, Antonella, Carmen, Hallie, Niti, Jim, Lina, Amy, Wendy, and anyone I may have left out!

To the friends who have supported me through this chapter: Niti, Richard, Kathy, Denise, Katrina, Tselane, and Evie

And to my parents, everything happens for a reason and I'm glad to have you back in my life as well as my children's.

EMOTIONAL PILLAR

Dr. Jacqueline Mohair, PhD

I extend my deepest gratitude to Dr. Nephetina Serrano and Dr. Jo Dee for their invaluable support and wisdom in the creation of this book. Your dedication to the mission of healing and empowerment has been a guiding light throughout this journey. To all the incredible women who participated in this mission, thank you for your courage, your stories, and your unwavering commitment to transformation. This book, *Emotional Intelligence: A Journey of Healing, Trust, and Transformation*, is a testament to the power of collective strength and the enduring spirit of women everywhere.

Sonja Rechnitzer

Daniel, Oliver, and Millie Rechnitzer—my husband and children who have taught me everything I know about intuition, purposeful living, and unconditional love.

Ernst, Roswitha, and Ines Gegenhuber—my parents and sister, who have shaped me into the strong woman I have become.

My dear friends, who stand by and support me every step of the way on this crazy journey.

Karen Rudolf

To my children, Dana, Amy, and Erica thank you for your love, patience, and unwavering support. You are my inspiration and my greatest joy. Your belief in me gives me the strength to pursue my dreams and the courage to overcome challenges. I am eternally grateful and still learning from each of you and the light you bring into my life.

My deepest gratitude to Reverend Alma Stevens. Your unwavering faith and belief in me have been a guiding light on my journey. Thank you for your constant encouragement and for inspiring me to keep moving forward, even when the path seems uncertain. Your support has been invaluable, and I am profoundly grateful for your presence in my life.

To Dr. Jo Dee Baer, thank you for taking me under your wing and seeing me in a way I hadn't seen myself, especially in the realm of health and well-being. Your guidance and belief in me have been transformative, and I am deeply grateful for the community you've welcomed me into and the opportunity to be a part of, and the friendship forged.

Cynthia Hammel-Knipe, CPE

Susan Melching—CIDESCO Friend and Mentor

Helen Kunze—Owner/Instructor Rocky Mountain College of Electrology

Alex Schlough—Photography and Technical Support

BSMM—University of Colorado—Denver and Boulder

Ultima College of Beauty

Don Edwards—School of Holistic Healing and Iridology

Nature's Sunshine—herbal Specialist Course and various certifications

Steven Horne—Tree of Life Institute—Various courses on Flower Remedies and Herbal Remedies

MarBeth Dunn

A special thank you to Harrison, Shanna, Chelsea, Dr. Jo Dee, and my sister authors.

Barbie Layton

Dr. Jo Dee Baer for putting this book together.

My Oma, God rest her soul, and her unconditional love.

Leilani Alesh, Esq.

Thank you, Wilson Vasconcelos, for your eye, and the beautiful photo.

Thanks, AFF, for always being there, always being fair, for your insights and genius talent.

Thank you Audrey Fitzhugh Barr for your resolute bearing and virtue as you raised me. The best mother award is yours.

And thank you to my sisters in Brazilian Voices. You bring me joy!

Anna M. McKee

Thank you to all those who believed in me until I believed in myself. And to my children Jamael, Malik, and Ari thank you for choosing me; I am eternally grateful.

PHYSICAL PILLAR

Dr. Glen Depke, ND

I would first like to thank Dr. Jo Dee Baer, PhD for her passion, compassion, and dedication to releasing *The Essence of a Woman*. The countless hours that go into writing a book is difficult enough, and putting together such a compilation of expertise that has been accomplished by Dr. Jo Dee, takes a whole other level. She has what it takes to reach the finish line. And Dr. Jo Dee reached this finish line to help you find your "Essence of a Woman." I would also like to thank the more than 7,627 women I have personally worked with over the last 24-plus years for helping push me to always learn more to continually help every woman find the optimal version of themselves. Lastly, thank you to all the other authors for sharing their levels of expertise in this amazing work of art, *The Essence of a Woman*!

Cathy Vergara, APRN

I would like to extend my deepest gratitude to my love, James. His unwavering support and love have allowed me to flourish and continue my never-ending journey of growth. To my mom—your strength and conviction are inspiring, without it I would not be here today—literally! To my children, family, and friends your encouragement and understanding have been invaluable. Thank you for believing in me and standing by my side.

Dr. Annette Watson-Johnson

I want to thank God for entrusting me with this beautiful gift of herbalism, entrepreneurship, and the vision to build wellness platforms to help people get mentally, physically, and spiritually well as he has instructed me to do so. I want to praise God for my late parents Elder John and Addie Watson. They both helped me to comprehend that God doesn't make mistakes and that my gifts are granted to me, and I am blessed for it. I thank my children Provine M. Cosby Jr. and Octavia M. Cosby for all they do to support me. Thanks to my husband Reginald E. Johnson for being my rock when I needed him. Hats off to my best friend Tammy Watkins and Goddaughter Tamala Watkins, and a huge shout out to my cousin Lizette, you are always willing, and ready to assist and support me when I need you. I cannot forget my countless customers who use their testimonials to encourage others to use my products to get the results they received. I love you all. Thank you to the team members of *The Essence of a Women*, who have made it possible for me to spread my message throughout the world.

Dr. Hepsharat Amadi, MD, LAc

Thank you, Desiree Dubounet, for inventing Quantum Biofeedback, one of my daughters for showing me how hormones can be crucial to overall health, Kevin Clark for making it easier to attend acupuncture school, and Kamau Kokayi, MD, for being a great role model of holistic medicine in Family Practice.

Dr. Tyra Good

I would like to acknowledge my mother, Joan Faith Pollard-Raiford, whose unwavering and sacrificial love supported me through this healing process. Mom, your own life is a testament to God's miraculous healing power. Thank you to all the prayer warriors—Minister Kay Brown and Warriors of Holiness in Power Ministries—and to my family, friends, and colleagues who sent care packages and cards of encouragement. Finally, I would like to acknowledge the life and legacy of my late friend and colleague, Dr. Antoinette "Bonnie" Candia-Bailey. Her life has left a lasting impact and elevated a national discussion on women's health and the treatment of black women in higher education.

Dr. Golda Joseph, PhD

I am grateful to my family and the many global communities that I have served.

I am in deep devotion and reverence to all the spiritual hierarchies that guide every thought, feeling, and action I perform and respectfully offer back with every breath I take.

FINANCIAL PILLAR

Dr. Shirley Luu

Thank you to my partner Hoang Vu and my kids, to my Mom, and to all my friends, business associates, and of course, all of the clients who have shown me the trust and given me the privilege of structuring and managing their life and retirement accounts.

Donna Dawson, FCCA

To my girls—life is for the living, live it to the fullest and don't settle. Love always and forever. Love, Mom.

Dominique Brun

To God, whose unconditional love and grace saved me and uplifted my spirit.

To my mother, whose unwavering support has been my foundation, and my fathers, who never ceased believing in me.

My family, who always stood by my side, and my handsome fiancé Felix, whose love transformed my world.

To my children, my guiding light and constant inspiration.

To Annabella Gutman for inspiring me and for her mentorship. And to Shawn Fair and Dr. Jo Dee for pushing me to put myself out there, and be vulnerable and confident in my craft.

Laura Ibarra, AbD

I deeply appreciate my family, friends, and mentors. Thanks to those who have been by my side: Your love and support have been instrumental in making this possible. Special thanks to my Mom, Laura Elena Parra López, my Dad, Gerardo Ibarra Solis, my brother Héctor Gerardo Ibarra Parra, and my brother, sons and daughters in heaven; you are my core team!

Gloria Kurz, JD, SRS

Thank you to Rick, my family, friends, clients, and my amazing team at M&M—Maureen, Mark, and Maria. This wouldn't have been possible without your support and understanding.

SOCIAL PILLAR

Dr. Jo Dee Baer, PhD

The Late Dr. Hulda Clark, ND—Extra-Ordinary Mentor

Dr. Jim Marinakis ND, HmD, Acu.Phys.—Mentor, Teacher, Coach, and Partner

A. Justin Sterling Co-founder of the Sterling Institute

Meg Pukel Photographer: www.megpukel.com

Tomosaski Photography https://family.tpphoto.com

My "Big Sister" Kathleen Heller and her husband of 54 years, Wayne (family nickname: Homer Dingus) who've been my shining lights to displaying the social pillar of love—with their marriage moniker: humor in all things. My sons Carl and Evan whose wisdom and strength have made me a better woman since birth.

My husband, Bob, an accomplished author of 14 internationally acclaimed books, who's mentored, loved, elevated, and encouraged me through this process once again.

Kim Jacobs, MBA, BD

Thank you Dr. Jo Dee Baer for choosing me to go on this wonderful adventure with you and these distinguished collaborating authors. I want to thank God for allowing me to be an ambassador of Christ on this earth. I am extremely thankful for the parents He gave me. My Dad, Bishop Elijah Jackson (Mrs. Ann) and my Mom Ella Mae Spratley. Thank you to Jerome Mitchell and Claude Spratley for being in my life. Thank you to my two earth angels I call Aunts, Elder Erma Mason (Arthur), and Sadie Jones (Deacon William). Thank you to my five children (Frank Jr., Ivan, Gabriel, Jeremiah, and Jayla) and my niece Sharday who supports and loves me unconditionally. Thank you to my siblings Javon, Ron (Jacci), and Felicia (Breehon), and to my brother, Jerome. My cousin Vee, who is like a sister to me. Thank you Uncle James (Talma) for being a wonderful uncle and Father figure to me. Thank you to all of my grandparents, because each of you imparted some wisdom that I carry with me daily. Thank you to all of my aunts and uncles. Thank you to my nieces and nephews and their beautiful mothers Dez, Jacci, and Katrina. Thank you to my cousins Ebony, Sherronda, and Alacia for our cousins' lunches. Thank you Nikki, for being a great cousin. Thank you to all of my family—I love you all, and I am grateful God made us family. Thank you Mrs. Jacobs for you and my mom helping me with my children over the years. Thank you to Les Brown for believing in me and serving as my mentor. Thank you to my best friend Shawn Hall for being my support system. Thank you to my friends Tonyia, Davida, Tyra, Elisa, Carrianne, Clarissa, Ernetta, Vickie, Pam, and Lawanné. Thank you to my church mothers and church family for praying for me. Thank you Bishop Stenneth and Lady Beverly Powell for being my spiritual leaders for over 20 years. Thank you, Mother Patricia D. Lofton, Mother Barbara Lockett, Mother Barbara Anderson, Mother Julia Harper, Dr. Marcia Alston, Mother Marie Talbert, and Evangelist Clara Walton. Thank you, Bishop Anthony L. and Pastor Harriet Jinwright for believing in me. Thank you Pastor Selwyn and Cassandra Davis for being so supportive. Thank you, Dr. Lotus Riché and Angie Elting. Thank you Mrs. Margaret Blackwell, Ms. Wilhemina, and Ms. Cynthia King (Childhood Teacher). Thank you to the Board members of Gabe's Heart Foundation. Thank you to Sandra Yancey for allowing me to serve as The Managing Director for eWomen Network in Charlotte, NC. Thank you to all the Mother Dreamer members. Thank you to all of my students who have taken my course "How to Start Your Show from Scratch." Thank you to Dr. Tina J. Ramsay for including The Kim Jacobs Show in the CTR Media Network family. Thank you, Mackenzie Rhoades, for being a part of The Kim Jacobs Show team. Thank you to everyone I have connected paths with on this journey called life.

Deborah Dennis

Texas Business and Professional Women.

Texas Business and Professional Women's Foundation (Hermine Tobolowsky Scholarship).

BPW International (International Federation of Business and Professional Women).

Cristina Candullo-Dody

I want to thank my husband Tony "DreamMaker" Dody for always encouraging me to make my dreams a reality.

I want to thank my parents for instilling good values in me and raising me to be the person I am today.

I want to thank Jona Hall for her hard work in creating Zeta Mu Phi and Illuminate. I'm so proud to be a co-founder and contributor to such a great cause.

Lastly, I want to thank my family, both biological and in-laws, and my closest friends for always being supportive.

HRH Princess Dr. Moradeun Ogunlana

I am deeply humbled to be a part of *The Essence of a Woman* by Dr. Jo Dee Bear, a motivational and empowering book that features an incredible lineup of global leaders, including award-winning actress Tiffany Haddish, Khalilah Ali (wife of Muhammed Ali), and other remarkable individuals. A woman's essence can be seen by more than just the eye. Each woman is intricately wrapped by layers and layers of qualities, which make up her very fundamental nature and her essence.

As I reflect on this journey, it becomes difficult to describe the essence of a woman by mere words alone. The actual meaning of being a woman can only be sensed by the heart. I am reminded of the love and support that has fueled my passion to write from the heart. As a Royal, family is everything! To my family, who are the essence of my existence, I extend my heartfelt gratitude. My three beautiful Princesses: Lola, Bolade, and Shola—my LOBOSH Legacy, and my heartbeats, Glamma's babies, Prince Richard and Prince Remi—you are my rock, my everything. I love you all to the moon and back!

I also want to express my deepest appreciation to everyone who has supported us on this incredible journey. To the women who have inspired me with their strength, resilience, and determination, I am forever grateful. Your stories have ignited a fire within me to write this piece in this amazing book, and I hope that it will do the same for our readers.

I would like to extend my gratitude to my AWHPI Global Foundation global families, who have been a constant source of support and inspiration. Your dedication to empowering women and girls around the world is truly remarkable, and I am honored to be a part of this community.

I also want to acknowledge my circle of amazing ladies with the First Ladies Forum and Economic Development Global Summits platforms in Dubai, UAE, and Doha, Qatar. Your leadership and commitment to creating positive change in the world are truly inspiring, and I am grateful for the opportunities we've had to connect and collaborate.

Thank you to my loved ones, who have endured my absence, distraction, and creative chaos. Your unwavering encouragement and patience mean the world to me. I also extend my gratitude to my editors, designers, and publishers, who have worked tirelessly to shape this book into its final form.

To our readers, I am honored that you have joined us on this journey. May the stories of the empowered women who have inspired me resonate with you, ignite a fire within you, and inspire you to embrace your strength, beauty, and potential. Thank you again for being part of this journey. May we all continue to rise together, empowered and unstoppable.

Author Acknowledgements | 479

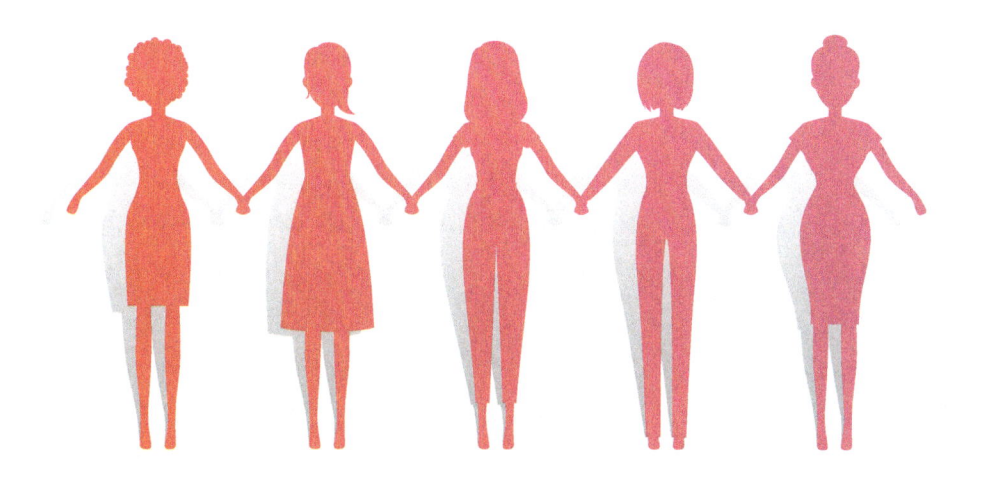

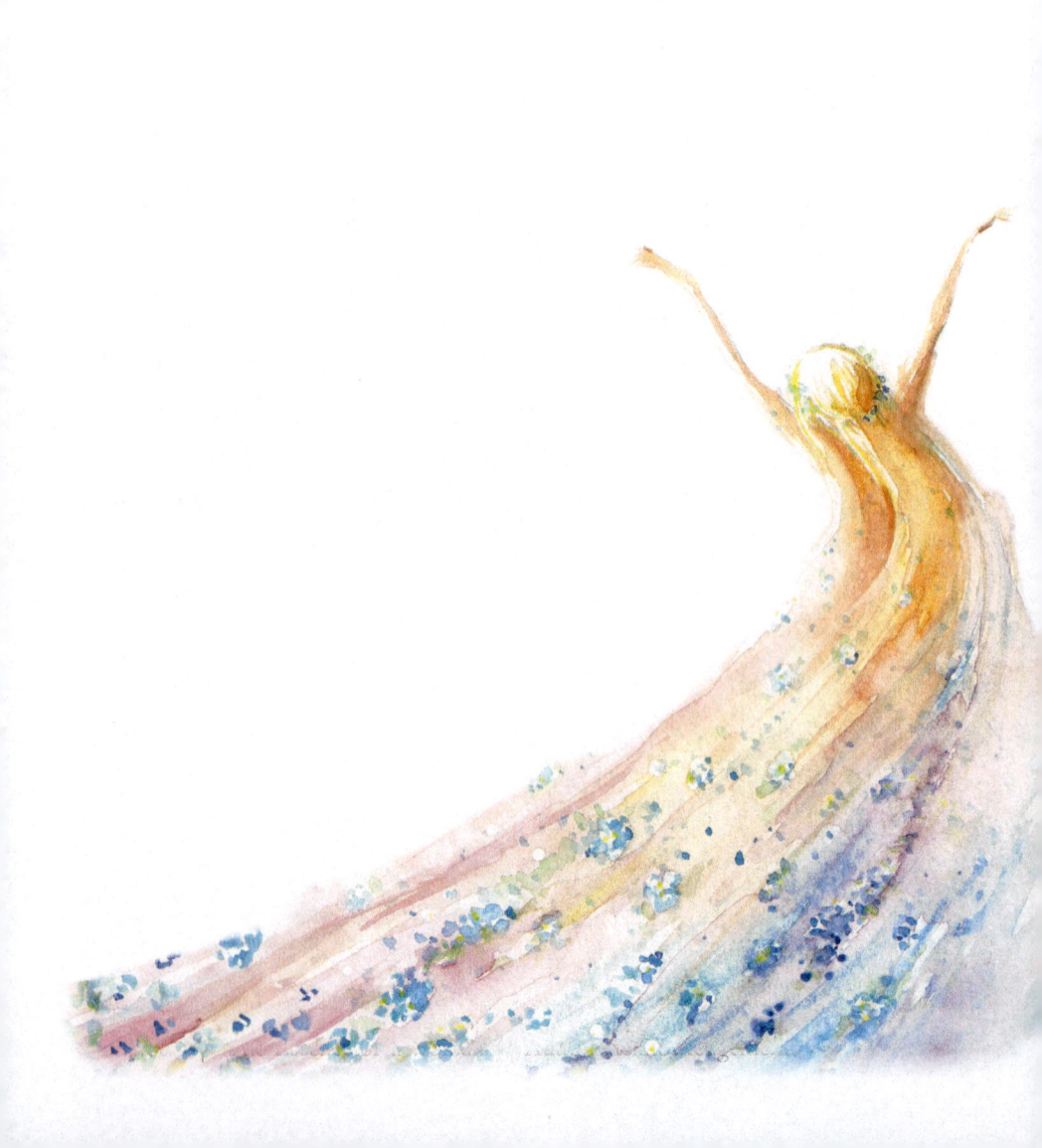

Conclusion

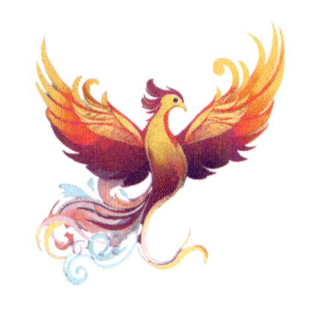

The Beatles sang about it with the words:

*"All you need is love,
Love is all you need.."*

The Scriptures elevated it in Corinthians 13:13: ESV

*"So now faith, hope, and love abide, these three;
But the greatest of these is love"*

Every woman embraces this unique 'love':

*L - Leading with
O - Optimism
V - Valuing
E - Everything*

We Women's Essence invoke our love to you…..

Love Freely

Life's most persistent and urgent question is, "What are you doing for others?"

—Martin Luther King, Jr.

Love Freely

The only way for us to love freely is to let the love that already exists in our hearts flow effortlessly. You can do this by practicing good communication, expressing your feelings honestly, and giving unconditional love, which requires not placing any conditions on how you accept another person. It requires the strength to set personal boundaries, but the ability to still fully accept everyone with an open heart. This is a pure example of God's love. Our natural state is to be in a state of unconditional love, but we have moved away from our true nature. We spend too much time and energy protecting our hearts. Despite the illusions of suffering that we have attached to our experience of love, we need to relinquish the negative perceptions we have about giving and receiving it.

By putting protection around your heart, you prevent love from flowing freely. Love is always ready and wants to flow effortlessly between people, but we have to choose to let go of the fear so this energy can flow in and out of our hearts. We are meant to embody love. When we do not give and receive unconditional love, we can feel that something important to our survival is missing. We operate defensively, all the while longing for love.

When we step into the place of being willing to love unconditionally, the love flows freely and we embody unity. When we allow energy to flow in and out of our hearts, we realize it is not love that hurts. Unconditional love for ourselves and others is our natural state when we vibrate higher throughout our bodies and our souls, and we can project other loving situations to us. We can project love onto all aspects of the world, and in this state, the entire world can be raised as we picture the planet Earth in complete peace and harmony. To maintain high consciousness and remain connected to the healing energy of the Holy Spirit, letting down barriers to love is essential.

Discovering Self-Acceptance

If you're on a serious mission for spiritual and personal growth, there is no self-judgment to be made. To be awakened in this human form, you cannot judge yourself or others, because we are all at the right space and time. We are not here to make enemies and pass judgments, and there are no mistakes. Because we are human, we are here to learn about ourselves.

We all have gifts that are specific to our earthly life experience. It's self-judgment that prevents us from moving into our gifts, purpose, and commitment to the **Holy Spirit**. You are here to awaken through your human form. One part of the Awakening is the acceptance of who you are in this human form because there is something you came here to do. A good example of this is my life and the difficulty I had in letting go of the life I wanted to live to accept the life I was meant to live.

As a healer, I have not always wanted to accept who I am. Some time ago, I spoke with a close friend who said to me, "I don't know who you are anymore. You talk, walk, and look differently than you used to. You're doing things you never used to do. You cry sometimes because you don't like all the ways your life has changed. I wonder, who are you? And even though I don't fully know who you are, I do know that you have to accept who and what you are. You should be used to all of this change by now."

Once I got to the point in my life when I could look in the mirror and truthfully say, "I accept you. I accept you. I accept who I am now," I would blink to confirm. From that point on, every time I thought of myself and the newness of my healing gifts and life as I had come to know them, and said, "I accept you," I began to feel better and more gifts began to open up for me. In addition to self-acceptance, I also had to undergo a period of balancing the feminine and masculine energies within me that had worked against each other.

The left side of your body relates to the feminine aspect of your consciousness; the right side of your body relates to the masculine aspect. We need the feminine energy to be present and strong in ourselves and across the planet right now. For so long, the dominance of male energy and consciousness has remained in the forefront of our personal lives, and this imbalance of the feminine and masculine energy has caused internal and external conflict on many levels, affecting each and every one of us, including me.

For years, a part of me did accept who I am now and what I'm doing, but it wasn't full acceptance. These parts of ourselves must be in balance because they represent both aspects of the Holy Spirit, which is one and all, encompassing both energies. As I said "I accept you," I felt as if I was being healed through balancing the feminine and masculine aspects of my consciousness. Self-acceptance is a vital tool that continues to help me fully tap into higher consciousness. When we accept both the feminine and the masculine, this begins to calm the overbearing aspect of the masculine energy and creates an opening for balance to be felt, accepted, and integrated on a personal and internal level, so it can then manifest on the external, global level.

Women have been encouraged to act more male oriented and to develop the masculine aspect of themselves to survive in this culture. Women have used this energy to get the right to vote, to fight back after being beaten down mentally or physically, to find productive and meaningful work, to raise strong children, and ultimately, to survive. However, we don't have to continue using forceful energy in the same way that we did in the past to be strong in this world, even if this has previously been the way of the world.

We are no longer of the time when the male perspective has to determine what feminism, womanhood, personal strength, leadership, and power will encompass. We can be strong, loving, and empowered peacemakers. We don't have to be strong with dominance and force.

My life is proof that you can indeed be a powerful, strong, and effective leader who stands in love of the Divine feminine and makes decisions from a place of love. Despite the challenges many of us face, including my own, we can still go and do the work of God as our calling from a strong and powerful place within ourselves. Whether you are a man or a woman, there is a place for both masculine and feminine energy to work together in Christ Consciousness. The voice of the peacemaker who walks this new energy into existence to heal our planet, our bodies, and our souls can do this in a loving way and still be heard.

—Kimberly Meredith
Celebrity Medical Intuitive Medium; Holistic Practitioner
Author: *"'Awakening to the Fifth Dimension:*
Discovering the Soul's Path to Healing"
www.thehealingtrilogy.com

Be Bright
Bold
Happy
You

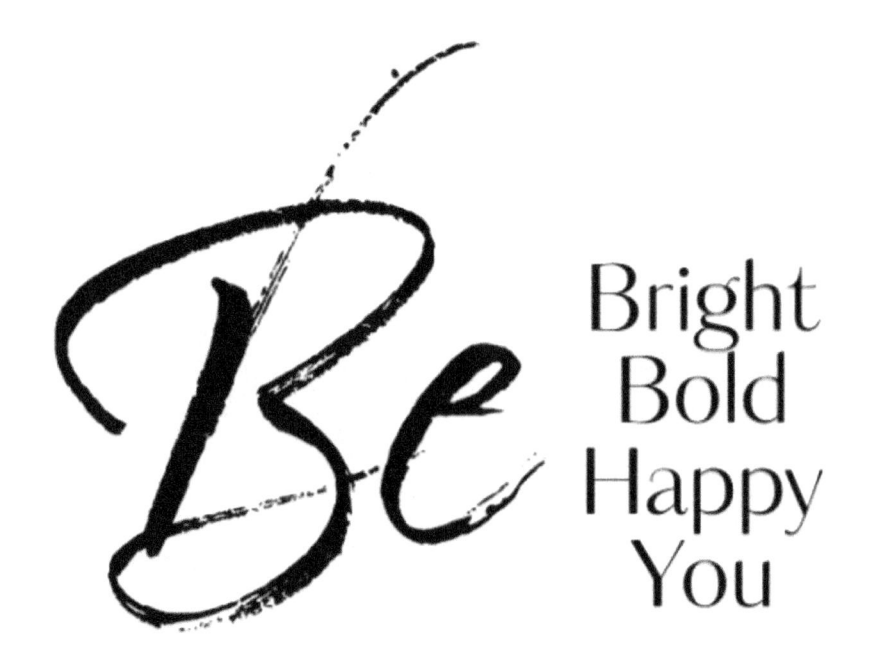

My heart torn and misused.

I arose from my dark night,

My SOUL again took flight!

Attuned and unleashed in this hour,

In my Universe?

I AM Power!

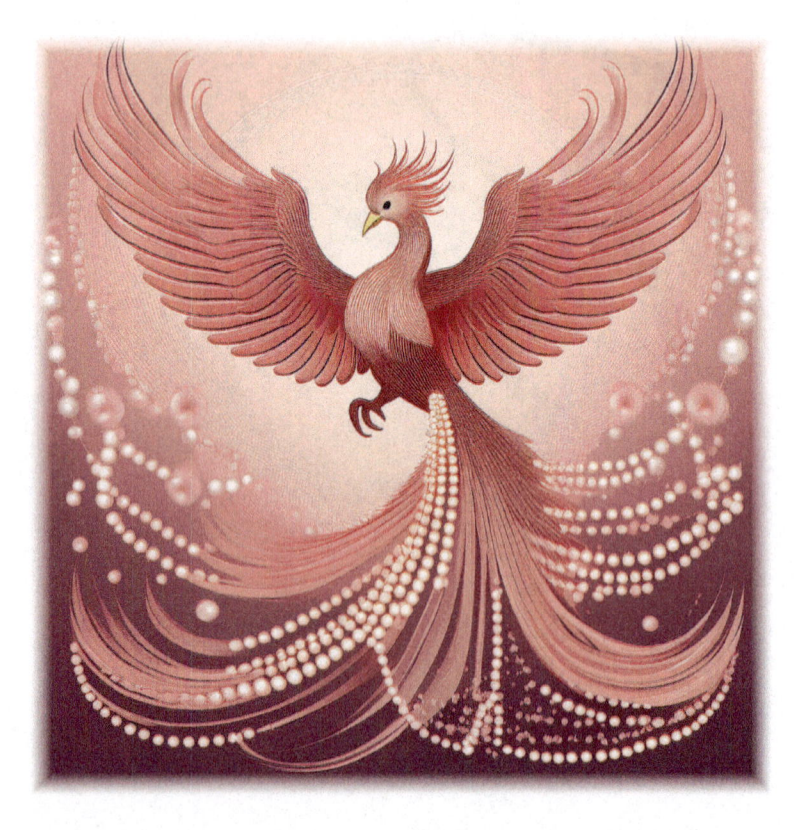

We Women of Essence Write

For the exhausted woman who showers a few minutes longer to cry with the cascading water.

For the woman hidden in the bathroom, because she needs a few minutes of tranquility.

For the woman who is so tired that she struggles to continue.

For the woman who would give anything to feel like herself again.

For the woman who gives a sigh of relief when everyone leaves the house.

For the woman who just can't let the past go.

For the woman who desperately battles with self-confidence when wearing denim pants.

For the woman who just wants to look pretty again.

For the woman who just wants to get through these hot flashes.

For the woman who can only find self-worth in achievement.

For the woman who begs for identity beyond her children.

For the woman who is only empowered by perfectionism.

For the woman who orders pizza for her family because there was no time to make dinner.

For the woman who feels alone, even when she's accompanied by those she loves.

We "Women of Essence," all say to You:

You're worth it all.
You are important.
You deserve it.
You are enough.
You are unique.
You are wonderful…
WE ALL LOVE YOU!. 💯

Universal QR Code

The Essence of a Woman Collaborative

Dr. Jo Dee Baer website

"The Essence of a Woman"
Unleash the Feminine Soul

*Eleven countries sharing the global sisterhood with our
tapestry in health, healing, and hope for humanity:
the United States, United Kingdom, Panama, Mexico, Colombia, Belize,
Croatia, Germany, Australia, Nigeria, and the Philippines.*

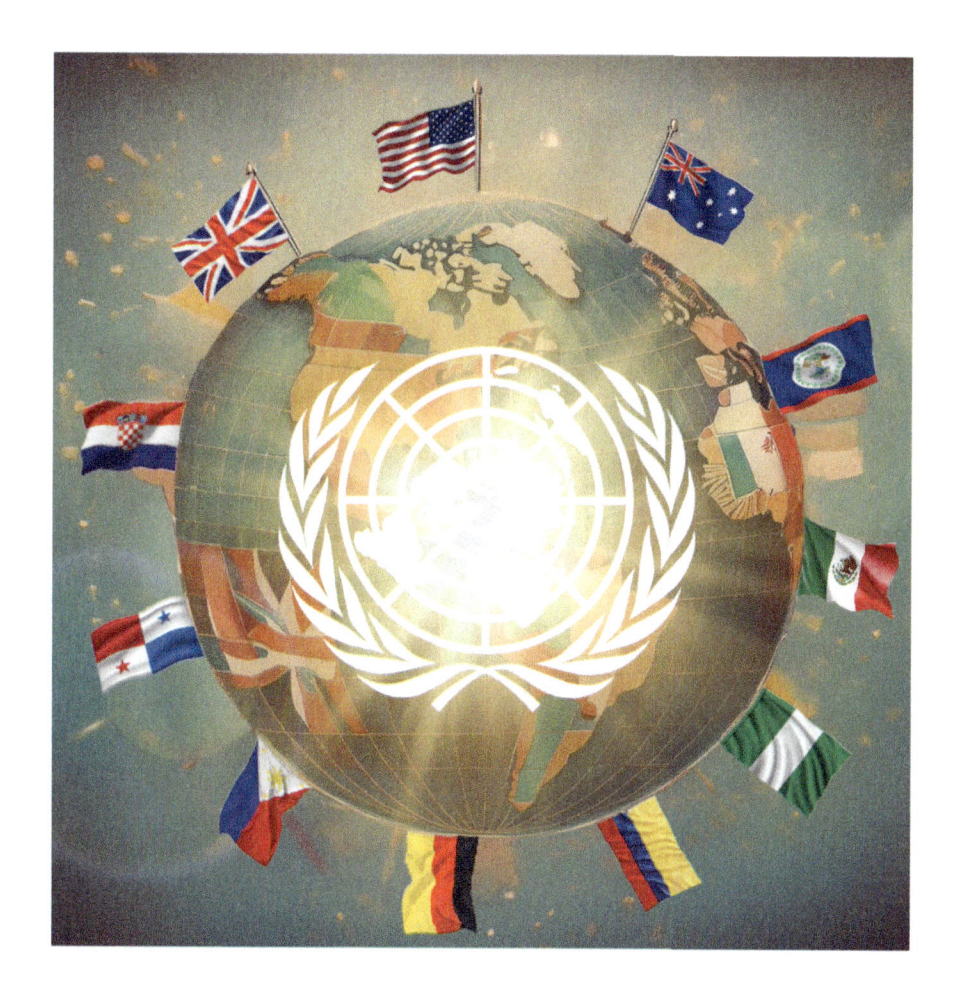

The POWER of the UNIVERSE!

Printed in Great Britain
by Amazon

49196904R00294